psychopharmacology
in the
practice of
medicine

psychopharmacology in the practice of medicine

Edited by
Murray E. Jarvik, M.D., Ph.D.
Professor of Psychiatry and Pharmacology
University of California, Los Angeles
School of Medicine; Chief, Psychopharmacology Unit
Brentwood Veterans Administration Hospital
Los Angeles, California

Foreword by
Louis Jolyon West, M.D.
Professor and Chairman, Department of Psychiatry
and Biobehavioral Sciences;
Director, Neuropsychiatric Institute
University of California, Los Angeles
School of Medicine
Los Angeles, California

APPLETON-CENTURY-CROFTS /New York

Library of Congress Cataloging in Publication Data

Main entry under title:

Psychopharmacology in the practice of medicine.

    Bibliography: p.
    Includes index.
    1.   Psychopharmacology.   I.   Jarvik, Murray E.
RC483.P778   615'.78   76-45749
ISBN 0–8385–7950-7

Prentice-Hall International, Inc., London
Prentice-Hall of Australia, Pty. Ltd., Sydney
Prentice-Hall of India Private Limited, New Delhi
Prentice-Hall of Japan, Inc., Tokyo
Prentice-Hall of Southeast Asia (Pte.) Ltd., Singapore
Whitehall Books Ltd., Wellington, New Zealand

PRINTED IN THE UNITED STATES OF AMERICA

Cover design: Judy Forster

contributors

Robert D. Ansel, M.D.
Clinical Instructor of Neurology, Department of Neurology, University of California, Los Angeles, School of Medicine, Los Angeles, California

Erin Charles Bick
Senior Information Specialist, General Foods Corporation, Technical Center, White Plains, New York

Dennis P. Cantwell, M.D.
Assistant Professor, Department of Psychiatry and Biobehavioral Sciences, University of California, Los Angeles, School of Medicine; Neuropsychiatric Institute, Los Angeles, California

Jonathan O. Cole, M.D.
Director of Clinical Research, Institute of Research and Rehabilitation, Boston State Hospital; Psychiatrist, McLean Hospital, Boston, Massachusetts

Michael H. Ebert, M.D.
Acting Chief, Section on Experimental Therapeutics, Laboratory of Clinical Science, National Institute of Mental Health, Bethesda, Maryland

Carl Eisdorfer, M.D., Ph.D.
Professor and Chairman, Department of Psychiatry and Behavioral Sciences, University of Washington, School of Medicine, Seattle, Washington

Everett H. Ellinwood, Jr., M.D.
Professor of Psychiatry and Director, Behavior Neuropharmacology Section, Department of Psychiatry, Duke University Medical Center, Durham, North Carolina

Robert O. Friedel, M.D.
Associate Professor and Vice Chairman, Department of Psychiatry and Behavioral Sciences, University of Washington, Seattle, Washington

Ronald Gallimore, Ph.D.
Associate Professor of Psychology, Department of Psychiatry and Biobehavioral Sciences, University of California, Los Angeles, School of Medicine, Los Angeles, California

John P. Geyman, M.D.
Professor and Vice Chairman; Director, Residency Network Program, Department of Family Practice, University of California, Davis, School of Medicine, Davis, California

Stanley Glick, M.D., Ph.D.
Professor of Pharmacology, Mount Sinai School of Medicine of the City University of New York, New York, New York

Donald W. Goodwin, M.D.
Professor and Chairman, Department of Psychiatry, University of Kansas Medical School, Kansas City, Kansas

v

Frederick K. Goodwin, M.D.
Chief, Section on Psychiatry, Laboratory of Clinical Science, National Institute of Mental Health, Bethesda, Maryland

David J. Greenblatt, M.D.
Acting Chief, Clinical Pharmacology Unit, Massachusetts General Hospital; Assistant Professor of Medicine, Harvard Medical School, Boston, Massachusetts

Ellen R. Gritz, Ph.D.
Research Psychologist, Brentwood Veterans Administration Hospital; Assistant Research Psychiatry and Biobehavioral Sciences, University of California, Los Angeles, School of Medicine, Los Angeles, California

Jerome H. Jaffe, M.D.
Chief, Psychiatric Research, Department of Biological Psychiatry, New York State Psychiatric Institute; Professor of Psychiatry, College of Physicians and Surgeons, Columbia University, New York, New York

Murray E. Jarvik, M.D., Ph.D.
Professor of Psychiatry and Pharmacology, University of California, Los Angeles, School of Medicine; Chief, Psychopharmacology Unit, Brentwood Veterans Administration Hospital, Los Angeles, California

Donald J. Jenden, M.D.
Chairman and Professor, Department of Pharmacology, University of California, Los Angeles, School of Medicine, Los Angeles, California

Reese T. Jones, M.D.
Associate Professor of Psychiatry in Residence, Langley Porter Neuropsychiatric Institute, University of California, San Francisco, San Francisco, California

Keith F. Killam, Ph.D.
Chairman and Professor, Department of Pharmacology, University of California, Davis, School of Medicine, Davis, California

Harold S. Levenson, Ph.D.
Director, Coffee Research, General Foods Corporation, White Plains, New York

John C. Liebeskind, Ph.D.
Professor of Psychology, University of California, Los Angeles, Los Angeles, California

Horace W. Magoun, Ph.D.
Professor Emeritus, Department of Psychiatry and Biobehavioral Sciences, Neuropsychiatric Institute, University of California, Los Angeles, School of Medicine, Los Angeles, California

Charles Markham, M.D.
Professor, Department of Neurology, University of California, Los Angeles, School of Medicine, Los Angeles, California

William H. Oldendorf, M.D.
Professor of Neurology, Reed Neurological Research Center,

University of California, Los
Angeles, Los Angeles, California

Donald A. Overton, Ph.D.
Associate Professor, Department
of Psychiatry, Temple Medical
School, Eastern Pennsylvania
Psychiatric Institute, Philadel-
phia, Pennsylvania

Dell L. Rhodes, Ph.D.
Department of Psychology, As-
sistant Professor, Reed College,
Portland, Oregon

Karl Rickels, M.D.
Professor of Psychiatry and
Pharmacology, Psychophar-
macology Research Unit, University of Pennsylvania, Philadelphia, Pennsylvania

Robert T. Rubin, M.D.
Adjunct Professor of Psychiatry,
Department of Psychiatry and
Biobehavioral Sciences, Univer-
sity of California, Los Angeles,
School of Medicine, Harbor Gen-
eral Hospital, Torrance, Califor-
nia

Edward J. Sachar, M.D.
Director, New York State
Psychiatric Institute; Chairman,
Department of Psychiatry, Col-
umbia University College of
Physicians and Surgeons, New
York, New York

Jon F. Sassin, M.D.
Associate Professor of Neurology
and Psychobiology, University of
California, Irvine, Orange,
California

Richard I. Shader, M.D.
Associate Professor of Psychiatry; Director, Psychopharmacology Research Laboratory, Harvard Medical School,
Massachusetts Mental Health
Center; Director of Training and
Education, Massachusetts Mental Health Center, Boston, Massachusetts

Ronald K. Siegel, Ph.D.
Associate Research Psychologist,
Department of Psychiatry and
Biobehavioral Sciences; Adjunct
Associate Professor, Department
of Psychology, University of
California, Los Angeles, School
of Medicine, Los Angeles,
California

Shepard Siegel, Ph.D.
Associate Professor of Psychol-
ogy, McMaster University,
Hamilton, Ontario

Jim L. Turner, Ph.D.
Assistant Research Psychologist,
Department of Psychiatry and
Biobehavioral Sciences, Socio-
Behavioral Group, University of
California, Los Angeles, School
of Medicine, Los Angeles,
California

Abraham Wikler, M.D.
Professor of Psychiatry and
Pharmacology, Department of
Psychiatry, University of Ken-
tucky Medical Center, Lexington,
Kentucky

preface

The primary care clinician is the health professional to whom an individual turns when he first feels he has medical or psychological problems, or when he thinks he needs a checkup. The first professional contact may be a physician, psychologist, social worker, counselor, nurse, minister, attorney, resident, intern, or medical student. On the other hand, a nonprofessional—friend, relative, or merchant—may advocate self-medication and the sufferer may turn to over-the-counter drugs, official "nondrugs" such as tobacco, alcoholic or caffeinated beverages, or even illegal "street drugs." However, a great number of symptomatic individuals will visit a physician, who is likely to prescribe a psychotherapeutic agent.

The purpose of this book is to help practitioners understand such drugs and how to use them. Each chapter was written specifically for this book by an authority in his field, and each author has presented his own point of view in his own style. I have tried to organize and also to digest these chapters. The book is divided into five parts, to each of which I have written an introduction. Also, to help integrate the book, and to present my own point of view, I have provided a commentary for every chapter, which I hope may furnish the basis for instruction or review.

The proliferation of psychopharmacologic literature today has become virtually unmanageable, and one of the aims of this book is to pinpoint the most important facts. References following each chapter will guide readers who wish to expand their knowledge of a particular topic. While sources of information about drugs are plentiful, they must be approached judiciously. Drug advertisements are usually the most flamboyant and the least objective. Package inserts and the information contained in the *Physicians Desk Reference* are more sedate and represent the results of an interaction between the Food and Drug Administration and the pharmaceutical manufacturer. However, these sources are largely enumerative and fail to consider the relative importance of each point discussed; the information, therefore, is of limited value. The voluminous restrictions and indications in the package insert, while not binding on the physician, may nevertheless be used as evidence in a malpractice suit, as may any other published information about drugs.

In the final analysis, the physician must use his best clinical judgment in advocating the use of any medication. He must be certain that every patient has adequate informed consent. Hopefully, the information in this book will serve not only to give the reader a better perspective on the indications and contraindications of a drug, but will also help the therapist to discuss drug actions with his patients.

In addition to practical points of clinical usefulness, we have included descriptions of basic findings where applications have not yet been worked out. This is to emphasize the point that basic research and advances in medical practice are inextricably intertwined and neither should be sacrified at the expense of the other. We have also attempted to bring together current concepts of mechanisms of action of different psychoactive drugs.

I would like to express my appreciation to a very large number of individuals who contributed to the conception of this book. I owe special gratitude to Mrs. Evelyn Stone, whose persuasion, inspiration, and advice provided the motivation for launching this project. Obviously, I am most deeply indebted to all the scientific and clinical authorities who contributed their skill and knowledge and time in writing the chapters that constitute this book. Special thanks are due to Mrs. Rivia Gately and Miss Irene Watanabe, who assisted in the difficult task of preparing the manuscript. I was encouraged and advised by many of my colleagues too numerous to mention, but those I consulted most often were Dr. L. J. West, Chairman of the Department of Psychiatry, University of California at Los Angeles (who has written the foreword); Dr. Donald J. Jenden, Chairman of the Department of Pharmacology, University of California, Los Angeles; Dr. Manuel Straker, Chief of Psychiatry Services, Brentwood Veterans Administration Hospital; the residents and house staff in psychiatry at the Brentwood Veterans Administration Hospital and at the Neuropsychiatric Institute, University of California at Los Angeles, as well as the students in my class at the School of Medicine, University of California at Los Angeles, Psychopharmacology M239. Of course I want to thank my wife, Dr. Lissy Jarvik, for both her professional and nonprofessional encouragement, benevolence, and advice in my pursuit of this venture. Finally, I want to express my obligation to Ms. Hilary Evans and Mr. Steven Abramson of Appleton-Century-Crofts for their help at every stage of the production of this book.

M.E.J.

contents

foreword

Drugs possessing psychotropic qualities have been employed in the healing arts from the beginning of recorded human history, and undoubtedly long before that. In fact it is probable that substances like alcohol, opium, cannabis, Indian snake-root (*Rauwolfia serpentina*, containing reserpine), and henbane (*Hyoscyamus niger*, containing scopolamine and atropine) were prominent among the earliest medicaments ever administered by one person to another to produce a specific desired effect in the context of a therapeutic relationship.

Today, sales of such medications represent a substantial portion of the profits of the pharmaceutical industry. The total annual volume of pharmaceutical business is now over $6 billion (wholesale, all drugs, 1975). Drugs acting primarily upon the nervous system are estimated to account for nearly a third of the total. Of these, almost half the expenditures go for tranquilizers, followed—in descending order—by analgesics, psychostimulants, appetite suppressants (other than amphetamines), barbiturates, other sedatives, amphetamines, and anticonvulsants.

More than 200 million prescriptions a year are written by physicians for psychotherapeutic adjuvants (tranquilizers, anodynes, sedatives, hypnotics, antidepressants, and stimulants) in the practice of medicine. Nearly a billion dollars was spent by the American pharmaceutical industry in 1975 for advertising directed at the country's 322,836 physicians. That is more than $3000 per doctor per year—and not all of the doctors are in practice by any means. More of this advertising concerns psychopharmaceuticals than any other single type of medication.

There is every reason to believe that the proportion of medication prescribed for psychotherapeutic effect will continue to increase. Furthermore, it seems very likely that in the future an increasing proportion of nonpsychiatrists will be responsible for decisions to administer drugs for psychotherapeutic purposes. These nonpsychiatrists will also be following the patients who require such medications, many of them for protracted periods of time. There are several trends that justify such a projection.

For one thing, in recent years there has been a decline in the percentage of medical graduates who choose psychiatry as a specialty. At the same time, we have seen a sharp increase in the number of young physicians committed to primary care. The designation, primary care physician, applies not only to those who become family physicians, but also to a new generation of pediatricians, internists, and obstetricians who take a more holistic approach to their patients, and who are psychotherapeutically oriented. Furthermore, the increased emphasis upon psychiatry in medical education has led many of the recently graduated physicians toward a greater understanding of the ubiquity of psychotherapeutic opportunities in medical practice, together with a greater general sense of competence in office psychiatry. Such competence includes knowledge of the ways in which psychotropic medications can be integrated with other aspects of the doctor–patient relationship to yield the greatest possible therapeutic benefit in each case.

There is no doubt in my mind that the future of psychiatry as a specialty lies to a considerable degree in improved working relationships between psychiatrists and other specialists, including primary care physicians. To fulfill this role it seems clear that the psychiatrist of the future will necessarily be an expert, not only in medical psychology, psychophysiology, and psychotherapy, but in psychopharmacology as well. Much of his work in liaison with colleagues will involve discussions and decisions about the psychotherapeutic employment of medications old and new.

As these various trends become manifest, an increasingly obvious need emerges for a good new reference work on psychopharmacology for the practicing physician. For some time, various colleagues have been urging Dr. Murray E. Jarvik to organize such a book. Certainly Dr. Jarvik is uniquely well qualified to provide leadership for this venture. He completed his Ph.D. in psychology at the University of California, Berkeley, and earned his M.D. at the University of California, San Francisco. He then spent two years at the Yerkes Laboratory of Primate Biology at Orange Park, Florida, followed by two years as a neuroscientist at Mt. Sinai Hospital and Columbia University in New York City. His subsequent distinguished career as a researcher at the interface of behavioral science, pharmacology, clinical medicine, and psychiatry then unfolded at Albert Einstein School of Medicine, until he came to UCLA in 1972.

For years Dr. Jarvik held a coveted career research award from the National Institute of Mental Health. Presently Professor of both Psychiatry and Pharmacology at UCLA and Chief of the Psychopharmacology Unit at the Brentwood Veterans Administration Hospital, Dr. Jarvik has been a highly influential figure in the rapid development of psychopharmacology as a field of study over the past 20 years. In organizing, editing, and contributing to this book, he continues his own fine tradition of scholarship that is both basic and, at the same time, practical. In this he has been joined by an outstanding group of colleagues, each of whom I congratulate for contributing to this important new addition to the literature on psychopharmacology.

While this book is basically intended to meet the needs of medical practitioners, I believe it will also prove useful to medical students, to residents in various specialties, and to many of the nonphysicians in mental health-related fields who wish to expand their understanding of the growing role of psychotropic substances in the practice of medicine.

Louis Jolyon West

psychopharmacology
in the
practice of
medicine

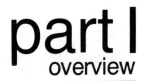

part I
overview
psychopharmacology
in medical practice

Introduction

Psychopharmacology as a recognizable separate discipline first came of age in the mid-1950s, when reserpine and chlorpromazine were introduced for the treatment of psychoses. The discovery of this demonstrably effective and easily available treatment for a serious psychiatric condition and its rapid and wide acceptance had a profound effect upon our understanding of brain functions and ultimately revolutionized the practice of psychiatry. Electroconvulsive shock therapy and psychosurgery, used since the 1930s, required elaborate instrumentation and elicited much opposition, not always rational. Moreover, a happy concatenation of political events and changing social mores helped launch psychopharmacology on its productive path. Those were the days of a bountiful Congress, of Senator Lister Hill and Representative John E. Fogarty, who were shepherding larger and larger appropriations bills through the United States Congress to encourage progress in medical research and to develop medical institutions, such as the National Institutes of Health.

The thalidomide disaster had not yet occurred and the Kefauver amendments to the Food and Drug laws restricting the pharmaceutical industry were yet to come. Every major drug firm had a psychopharmacology department and drugs were created and sold to treat every conceivable form of psychologic or psychiatric problem. The years 1955 to 1960 were expansive and optimistic for psychopharmacology.

1

The almost simultaneous appearance of drugs that could produce and alleviate psychotic states further stimulated the development of psychopharmacology. Drugs have been used for "recreational" or self-medicational purposes since the dawn of history, but the discovery of the potent psychotogenic and hallucinogenic action of lysergic acid diethylamide (LSD), by Hofmann in 1943, was the forerunner of scientific and lay interest in hallucinogens during the 1950s. Possible military usefulness of these drugs for incapacitating purposes was an early goal of the United States government agencies, but some psychiatrists and other scientists were interested in the clues that drug-induced model psychoses could furnish for the understanding of naturally occurring psychoses (Jarvik 1967). Later hallucinogenic drugs and social change became interwoven. Alienated members of society have always used drugs (eg, Moreau de Tours 1845), but mass communication in modern times publicized drug taking as never before. It started with the beatniks (1940s to 1950s) and continued with the hippies (1960s to 1970s). Writings of Aldous Huxley, Timothy Leary, Ken Kesey, and others had a profound influence on drug use. The onset of the escalation of the Vietnam war in the early 1960s led to the greater alienation of young people in society, and "drug" experimentation as a protest and for escape was one consequent spinoff. Even in the "straightest," "squarest," most conservative segments of society, curiosity about drugs grew, and ministers and maiden aunts spoke freely of pot and acid (marijuana and LSD). Rock music groups, such as the Beatles and the Rolling Stones, popularized drug use but so did *Life, Time,* and *Playboy.* As Frank Barron (1967) put it, the chemical with the greatest influence on the drug-seeking behavior of the public was printer's ink.

Meanwhile the mechanisms of action of psychotropic drugs were investigated and led to greater understanding of the workings of the brain. For example, it soon became evident that biogenic amines (5-hydroxytryptamine, norepinephrine, dopamine) were intimately involved in the action of drugs such as reserpine and chlorpromazine. Work on the synthesis and metabolism of these amines won Julius Axelrod the Nobel Prize. Many other brilliant scientists applied their talents to the study of psychotropic drug actions and some of their work will be described in this book. During the 1950s it became clear that the brain was more than just a complicated electrical switchboard; it was a chemical factory where drugs could have fairly specific actions if they could penetrate the blood–brain barrier.

Many of the substantive advances in psychopharmacology during the last decade have come from contributions from the basic biologic sciences, molecular biology, chemistry, histology, and neurophysiology. Our greatest need in this area is to understand the etiology of various forms of mental disease and the mechanism of action of drugs that influence mental disease. This means localizing, if possible, parts of the brain disrupted by disease and analyzing the biochemical changes associated with emotional and cognitive disorders. It means discovering where drugs go in the body; especially in the brain; determining whether specific receptors are involved; and finding out how behavioral changes induced by drugs are produced in the brain (Iversen 1975, Snyder 1974).

To be sure, the functioning human brain does not yield its secrets easily, while encased in its bony chamber. Complex information is coded in electrical and chemical forms and intricate instruments are needed to retrieve that information. Models of human psychiatric disorder can be produced in animals only with the greatest difficulty; fear and anxiety somewhat easily, depression and mania perhaps, psychosis perhaps not at all. In fact psychiatric illness characterized by disorders of thinking, perception, and mood manifests itself in those very functions that distinguish humans from even their nearest primate relatives (language and emotion). Thus, it is controversial whether such diseases as schizophrenia, depression, or neurosis can be found or reproduced in animals even in a minimally analogous form. Aberrant behavior can be induced by administration of drugs such as reserpine, LSD, and amphetamine. But how closely the resulting behavior resembles human psychopathology is still a matter of debate. If animals could be bred with the same type of genetic defect as human schizophrenics or manic depressives, research in psychopharmacology would proceed with much greater speed (see pp 205, 219).

By contrast the chemistry of psychopharmaceuticals is very amenable to study. The exact three-dimensional structure of most psychopharmaceuticals now in use is well known. The physicochemical properties of drugs have been investigated intensively. The nature of the chemical bonds, which hold atoms and molecules together in aqueous and lipid media, have been characterized. Drug solubility and ionization are of particular importance and there is a respectably large amount of literature on the subject. Whether drugs will dissolve in fat or water, or whether they are acidic or basic, makes a big difference in determining, for example, whether they will be absorbed in the stomach and intestines and whether they will get into the brain (see p 35).

Slight changes in structure can radically modify the actions of a compound (see p 35). The structure of a compound determines its weight, whether it is liquid, solid, or gas or whether it is lipid or water soluble; most important, it determines how that compound fits into the molecular structures of other classes of compounds, such as enzymes or postsynaptic receptors, manufactured by the body. The drug-receptor interaction is of great concern to the pharmaceutical chemist who is seeking to improve the specificity or the potency of a particular compound. It also interests the biologist who wants to understand the nature of the receptor and the function that it might play in the life of the organism. Generally speaking, highly potent drugs are thought to influence specific receptors, whereas relatively weak drugs are likely to be much less selective in their sites of action. Thus, potent drugs like botulinus toxin and LSD undoubtedly fit only into certain tightly prescribed receptors and easily pass barriers, whereas drugs like ethyl alcohol or chloroform possibly combine with a large variety of structures, or have difficulty passing barriers (see p 167).

Of greatest importance in understanding the mechanisms of action of a drug is the identification of receptors. If a drug can be considered a key, then its structure implies a great deal about the structure of the lock or bodily receptor, since they must fit one another. Much of the early work in pharmacology centered on the identification of the receptor upon which the neurotransmitter, acetylcholine, worked. A vast amount of work on structure–activity relationships of analogs and antagonists of acetylcholine has resulted in reasonable inferences about the nature of the cholinergic receptor (see p 35). Another family of drugs in which agonist–antagonist relationships have been studied in great detail is the narcotic analgesics, relatives of morphine. Unfortunately, specific antagonists have not been found for most drugs. Where there are pure antagonists, ie, drugs that only oppose and have no other action of their own, the drug they oppose can be controlled very well, its action terminated at any time. A good example of a relatively pure antagonist is naloxone, which stops most actions of morphine and related narcotics but has virtually no action of its own (see pp 145 and 437). It would be very useful if antagonists could be found for all drugs, particularly to stop toxic actions but also to control desired actions. We now have agonists and antagonists for histamine, acetylcholine, 5-hydroxytryptamine, norepinephrine, dopamine, gamma aminobutyric acid, and many other substances, with more on the way.

Molecular biology has produced a revolution in science during the past quarter century. Small wonder that so many Nobel prizes have been awarded in this area. Indeed, the study of macromolecules has yielded the secret of life in DNA. Now we have a good idea of how genetic information is carried and how it is translated into the formation of an organism. Unfortunately, we know considerably less about how information is acquired during life, how it is learned, and how it is remembered. The secret of the nature of the memory trace in the brain is perhaps the last frontier of biologic science. It appears that the nature of changes at the synapse, resulting from experience, is the key to the problem and some progress has been made in this area. Evidence is quite strong that synapses located in certain areas of the brain have been specialized for learning, whereas other synapses, such as those in the spinal cord, are practically immutable. Thus, it is necessary to interrelate localization of function with localization of drug action.

Within the body, chemical compounds are distributed unevenly and segregation usually has some functional significance. Thus, iron is found mostly in blood, iodine mostly in the thyroid, and calcium in bones. These examples with simple inorganic elements may also be illustrated with more complex organic compounds such as hemoglobin in blood and melanin in skin. Ever since the days of Thudicum (1962) the localization of compounds in the brain has been of special interest. In recent years the perfection of specialized histochemical techniques has allowed us to map the location of different chemicals, particularly neurotransmitters, in the brain. It has long been recognized, particularly by freshmen medical students, that the brain is the most complex organ in the body. One hundred years ago a great many names were given to various parts of the brain, the function of which is still not clear. Some functions that have been more or less localized and which are important to psychopharmacologists are various types of sensations and perceptions, motor activities, reward and punishment, and activation (see p 61). There is still a great deal of speculation about the locus of higher mental functions, such as thinking, learning, and memory. The more we learn about the neurophysiologic substrate of these functions, the more rationally we will be able to determine whether and how drugs can influence them.

Sensory and motor functions can be more or less directly observed and measured. A great deal more inference is required for psychologic functions. Methods of objectifying subjective events are discussed in several chapters (see pp 47, 61, 219, 309). In recent years the development of electronic technology has enabled engineers to design instruments that measure both behavior and electrical activity in the brain. Furthermore, computer technology now enables the investigator to analyze complex relationships between electrical activity of the nervous system and behavior and the influence of drugs on both of these functions.

There is fairly wide agreement that the simplest prototype of human behavior is the simple spinal reflex arc. Here a sensory stimulus gives rise to a highly predictable motor response of fairly constant intensity and duration. In a two-unit reflex arc (for example, the knee jerk or patellar reflex) there are only two types of nerve endings and, therefore, possibly no more than two neurotransmitters. But drugs may act not only at synaptic transmitter sites but anywhere on the surface of the two nerve cells as well as inside axons and cell bodies to affect a multiplicity of organelles and subcellular structures. Furthermore, the nutrition and external milieu of these cells might be influenced by drugs. Other extraneuronal actions of drugs might be on receptor structures or on effectors (eg, muscles or glands). So, even in a simple reflex arc there are a great many drug-sensitive processes.

More complex behavior could be considered an elaboration of the reflex arc with the intercalation of intervening variables (Tolman 1959; Hebb 1949). A complex network of neurons between stimulus and response allows for infinitely greater variability in responsiveness to stimuli and for vast modulation, which would be characterized by such variables as activation, motivation, and mood. The ability of the organism to introduce long delays between stimulus and response is possible only with the development of mechanisms subsuming learning and memory; we are just beginning to discover how some of these might be drug sensitive or resistant.

Of course the clinician is most concerned with people who come to him with complaints or illness. Every illness, no matter how physically based it might seem, has a psychologic component, whether it is pain, or fear, or insomnia. It is important to decide whether psychopharmacologic treatment is appropriate, and if it is, to select the appropriate drugs to treat these symptoms. Disorders whose manifestations are obviously psychologic, such as obsessions or compulsions, also may be amenable to drug treatment. Discussion of the effectiveness as well as the dangers of such drug treatment should be of interest to most medical practitioners, even though it will become apparent in the following pages that panaceas are not yet available for the treatment of psychologic and psychiatric disorders.

References

Barron F: Motivational patterns in LSD usage. In DeBold RC, Leaf RC (eds): LSD, Man and Society. Middletown, Conn, Wesleyan University Press, 1967, pp 3–19

Hebb DO: The Organization of Behavior. New York, John Wiley, 1949

Iversen SD, Iversen LL: Behavioral Pharmacology. New York, Oxford University Press, 1975

Jarvik ME: The psychopharmacological revolution. Psychol Today 1:51–59, 1967

Moreau de Tours JJ (1845): Hashish and mental illness. In Peters H and Nahas GG (eds), translated by Barnet GJ. New York, Raven Press, 1973

Snyder SH: Madness and the Brain. New York, McGraw-Hill, 1974

Thudicum JLW (1884): A Treatise on the Chemical Constitution of the Brain, with a New Historical Introduction by Drabkin DL. Hamden, Conn, Archon Books, 1962

Tolman EC: Principles of purposive behavior. In Koch S (ed): Psychology: A Study of a Science, Vol 2. New York, McGraw-Hill, 1959, pp 92–157

psychopharmacology: past, present, and future

commentary

Even though there has been a quantum increase in the study and use of drugs for behavioral purposes, the roots of psychopharmacology are ancient and date from prehistoric times. The science of chemistry really developed in the nineteenth century, providing the basis for modern pharmacology, which developed in the latter part of that century. One man stands out during this era and could be called the father, or perhaps the grandfather, of psychopharmacology, Emil Kraepelin. He was also one of the founders of modern psychiatry, but was strongly influenced by Wundt's development of experimental psychology. The amalgamated methodology of these two men has had a profound influence to this very day upon scientific psychopharmacology.

Dr. Siegel emphasizes the literary and romantic element in the history of drug use. There is also the parallel development of physiologic and chemical knowledge, and of classic pharmacology (Heymans 1967). Clearly, psychopharmacology is only in its infancy, but progress during the past 25 years gives us room for optimism for its future growth.

References

Heymans C: Pharmacology in old and modern medicine. Ann Rev Pharmacol 7:1–14, 1967

psychopharmacology: past, present, and future

Ronald K. Siegel, Ph.D.

Most historians date the start of psychopharmacology to 1952 with the introduction of chlorpromazine to psychiatric therapy, but the term was originally coined in 1920 by Macht. The linguistic roots are far older than that. The term *psychopharmakon* was first used by Reinhardus Lorichius of Hadamar in 1548 to refer to prayers of comfort for death. The *pharmakos* in ancient Greece was the sacrifice in primitive ceremonies. Later, when human sacrifice was abandoned in Greece, the term *pharmakoi* came to mean "human medicine" and was applied to poisons and drugs. The word *drug* is of Teutonic origin and simply means a "dry herb." The origins of all those herbs, drugs, poisons, and medicines go back still further in time. They go back millions of years before the dawn of man.

Prehistory

Plant Evolution

In the beginning of the Mesozoic Era, some 225 million years ago, the coal-swamp flora and fauna were disappearing while angiosperms and reptiles were beginning their evolutionary advance. The angiosperms rapidly became dominant and the evolution of their plant chemistry eventually led to the science of psychopharmacology.

First, angiosperms started to produce hydrolyzable tannins. There is little knowledge concerning the role of tannins in plants, but these substances do act as antifungal agents for plants and, for animals, they are bitter tasting, inhibit protein digestion and enzyme activity, and cause liver lesions if taken in excess. Second, angiosperms started to produce aromatic amino-acid-based alkaloids, substances that constitute major groups of psychopharmacologic agents. As a general rule, alkaloids have no known function in plants and no one really knows why plants produce them. However, alkaloids taste bitter, like the tannins, but have a wider range of physiologic activity, including psychologic, teratogenic, and toxic effects. They act as extremely effective feeding deterents, and it has been argued that many of the naturally occurring plant drugs are evolutionarily justified in terms of the maladaptive effects they could have on herbivores (Bever 1970, Eisner and Halpern 1971). Indeed, Swain (1974) has noted that these major changes in plant chemistry coincided with the sudden extinction of the dominant life in the animal kingdom, the dinosaurs. These giant reptiles, unlike the birds and mammals that followed them, failed to evolve effective mechanisms with which to detect and /or detoxify the alkaloids. Subsequently, changes occurred in the thickness of dinosaurs' egg shells, there was an increase in the size of their hypothalamus (indicative of stress), and their fossils have been found in contorted positions suggestive of alkaloid poisoning.

Animal–Plant Interactions

Today, some 65 million years later, veterinarians are well-acquainted with the contorted bodies of grazing horses, cattle, and other animals that have accidentally ingested lethal amounts of highly toxic alkaloidal plants such as species of Senecio, Datura, and Nicotiana. Similar accidents have occurred in man. For example, a group of soldiers, sent to Jamestown in 1676 to put down Bacon's Rebellion, ate the young shoots of Datura as a pot green and became severely intoxicated for several days. Datura (containing scopolamine, atropine, and hyoscyamine) has since been known as "Jamestown" or jimson weed. Anthony's legion had a similar Datura experience during a retreat in 38–37 B.C. Periodic outbreaks of ergotism, resulting from accidental ingestion of a rye fungus, Claviceps purpurea, were common in the Middle Ages and even in this century. Epidemics occurred in France as far back as 857 A.D. and as recently as 1951. In 944 A.D., 40,000 people died of the disorder.

Not all of man's encounters with naturally occurring durgs were accidental. Early man learned much of his basic psychopharmacology from observations on animal-plant interactions.

Folklore and mythology are replete with examples of man's discovery of psychopharmacologic agents through observations and modeling of animal behavior (cf. Siegel 1973). The legendary discovery of coffee, purportedly around 900 AD, was made by an Abyssinian tending his herd of goats. The herder noticed that his animals became abnormally "frisky" after eating the bright red fruit of a tree that was later isolated and identified as coffee (Taylor 1965). In Yemen, another herder discovered that his goats exhibited signs of extraordinary stimulation after eating some leaves. The shepherd himself found the leaves quite stimulating after a day's work. Since that time, the use of the leaves (qat leaves containing the alkaloids cathine, cathedine, and cathenine) spread throughout the entire country (Abdo Abbasy 1957). Similar stories are told about the discovery of 22 other psychoactive drugs including alcohol and Cannabis.

The names of many plants reveal something about their observed effects on animals (cf. Folkard 1884). Some were named for their apparent aversive or attractive properties. Henbane (Hyoscyamus niger containing atropine and scopolamine) seems to have derived its name from its effect upon poultry. Similarly, Leopard's Bane (Doronicum pardalianches) caused the death of leopards who ate it; Sheep's Bane (Hydrocotyle vulgaris) poisoned sheep; Swine Bane (Chenopodium rubrum) killed swine; fly-agaric (Amanita muscaria) killed flies that landed on it; wormwood (Absinthium spp. or absinthe) drove away insects and insect larvae; Flea Bane (marigolds) repulsed fleas and other insects; and Cow Bane (Cicuta virosa or hemlock) killed cattle and other grazing animals. Indeed the Iroquois Indians employed hemlock roots for suicide, and the classic suicide of Socrates was performed with hemlock.

Other plants were identified by the attraction that animals displayed toward them. Catnip (Nepeta cataria containing hallucinogenic nepetalactone oils) attracted cats who eagerly ingested it; Hare's lettuce (Lactuca spp.) was allegedly used by rabbits for stimulant and medicinal effects and later by man as an opium substitute for narcotic and stimulant properties; Dog Grass (Triticum caninum), Swine Grass (Polygonum aviculare), Pigeon Grass (Vervain), and Goose Grass (Galium aparine) all attracted their respective namesakes. Pigeon Candy was an early vernacular name for hempseeds (Cannabis spp.) derived from stimulating effects on pigeons (Levi 1957, p 499). Such effects were also observed by the ancient Greeks who adopted the habit of eating hempseeds after watching finches do so (Schultes 1970).

Early Experimentation by Man

Despite the benefit of animal observations, early man developed psychopharmacologic experience for beyond that obtained by animals. On the basis of archaeologic findings, the use of alcohol, opium, and *Cannabis* developed early in man's prehistory. Indeed, man's exploitation of plant drug resources has been claimed to date from 40,000 BC to 10,000 BC (Flannery 1965). Hunting and gathering societies of man were in excellent positions for such experimentation. The relative ease of fermentation in stored foods accounts for the early use of alcohol. According to Blum (1969), the use of hackleberry wine and beer date to 6400 BC in Anatolia, while predynastic Egyptian farmers, c. 4500 BC, learned to maximize fermentation and alcoholic content by malting their grain or sprouting it before grinding.

Archaeologic evidence from Greece and Cyprus show ritual opium use as early as 2000 BC. Hempseeds, together with a cauldron and stones used in their smoking, have been found in excavations in Central Europe and dated c. 430 BC. Hempseeds were also used by Pythia, the priestess of the Delphian oracle (cf. Caldwell 1970a). However, the use of *Cannabis* is far older; a Chinese treatise on pharmacology (2737 BC) refers to medicinal uses of *Cannabis*. Other archaeologic evidence indicates tobacco smoking among American Indians in 200 AD. Some scholars have argued that the chewing of Kava, betel nut, and coca leaves were practices dating from Paleolithic times.

Perhaps the most intriguing development in applications of drugs was self-administration through smoking. Probably no animal models existed for this behavior. Accidental encounters and sniffing of vapors or burning plants may have occurred. Morphine or nicotine, since they penetrate the blood-brain barrier, may have reinforced such accidental behavior. It has been speculated (cf. Siegel et al 1976) that the smoke itself is inherently evocative of visions and mystery—a natural medium for shamanistic practices. Other virtues of magic may have included tobacco smoke's use as a "smoke screen" to conceal the movements of shamans or to blow onto affected parts of people undergoing curing. The white clouds of smoke are also suggestive of and associated with rain clouds and play an important part in many primitive ceremonies for securing rainfall.

History

Ancient, Classical, and Medieval

The written record of psychopharmacology is almost as old as writing itself. The earliest prescription involving psychoactive drugs appeared in an Egyptian papyrus dated 3700 BC. The Ebers Papyrus, c. 1550 BC, contains remedies including wine, beer, wormwood, henbane, and mandragor among others. Rig-Veda medicinal uses of plants in India are claimed before 1600 BC and drug therapies described about 1000 BC.

Undoubtedly, there were many "psychopharmacologists" who contributed to such early knowledge, but we have scant information on them. According to Homer, the mythologic Circe was polypharmakos, or "one who knows how to use drugs" (cf. Caldwell 1970a), but he also referred to some real physicians and surgeons of the time in the same way. Indeed, psychopharmacotherapy also arose in ancient Greece; it was studied by Helen of Troy and popularized by Homer in what Caldwell (1970b) terms "the golden age of psychopharmacology." A popular drug of the time, still unidentified but suggested to be Cannabis or opium, was used with great knowledge "against sorrow and anger" and "to survive despair." Aristotle, Pliny, and Dioscorides, as well as lesser known herbalists and botanical writers, wrote extensively of the medicinal or curative properties of psychoactive plants (cf. Folkard 1884).

Perhaps the best example of early experimentation in psychopharmacology derives from pre-Columbian Aztec pharmacology. A series of impressive sixteenth-century documents have detailed the achievements of Aztec medicine and these include Father Sahagun's General History of Things of New Spain and other books by Francisco Hernandez, physician to Phillip II (cf. Del Pozo 1967). Interestingly, the medicinal and pharmaceutical mixtures described in these texts did not employ sorcery or magic, but "could be used by anybody without devices or spells for supernatural powers" (Del Pozo 1967, p 66). The Aztecs developed applied uses for over 461 plant drugs, many of which they discovered among the psychoactive-rich flora in the New World and some of which have still not been identified. The Aztecs had chocolatl, ololiuqui (Rivea corymbosa containing D-lysergic acid amide), peyotl, picietl (tobacco), pulque (a beer made from mescal), toloatzin (Datura inoxia), marihuana, and Psilocybe mushrooms among others. Such drugs were employed in a variety of contexts, ranging from staying awake all night, to enhancing memory recall, to sedating victims for human sacrifice. Thus, the golden age of psychopharmacology more deservingly belongs to Aztec empiricism than to the ancient Greeks.

Late Medieval and Renaissance witchcraft marked the next significant developments in psychopharmacology. A number of chroniclers of those times (cf. Harner 1973) noted the specialized use of hallucinogens belonging to the Solanacea order of plants, including Datura, Mandragora (mandrake), Hyoscyamus (henbane), and Atropa belladonna (deadly nightshade). Each of these contains atropine and related tropane alkaloids (hyoscyamine and scopolamine), all of which have hallucinogenic effects. They formed the principal active ingredients of brews, love potions, and narcotic preparations. The European witches made ointments of the drugs, whose content of atropine was absorbed through the skin. The nakedness associated with witches' sabbats facilitated the application of these ointments. The familiar broomstick was "an applicator for the atropine-containing plant to the sensitive vaginal membranes as well as providing the suggestion of riding on a steed, a typical illusion of the witches' ride to the Sabbat" (Harner 1973, p 131).

Romantic History

Romanticism was a literary, artistic, and philosophic movement that began in Europe in the eighteenth century and was characterized by a reaction against the reason and intellect of neoclassism. The movement emphasized the freely individualized expression of emotion and imagination and, in the drug literature, it was marked by introspective autobiographic accounts. Perhaps the most popular drug of this time was opium and many writers of the nineteenth century were addicts, including Crabbe, Coleridge, De Quincey, Wilkie Collins, and Francis Thompson. Other writers experimented with opium, which inspired their work. These include Keats, Edgar Allan Poe, Baudelaire, Walter Scott, Dickens, Elizabeth Browning, and James Thomson among others.

In 1821 De Quincey published *Confessions of an English Opium Eater*, which clearly described the subjective drug effects and has since become a classic in drug addiction. De Quincey described serene euphoria, waking dreams, nightmares, paralyzed will, mental confusion, and discussed the changing effects as the addiction progressed in his own body. Baudelaire's *Paradis Artificiels* (1857) is equally important in the drug literature. The first half of the book analyzes the mental effects of drug addiction, with particular reference to hashish, and the second half, on opium, endorses De Quincey's reports. Baudelaire, like his colleagues in the Club des Haschischins, was more enticed by the romanticism of hashish than by opium.

Some historians (eg, Holmstedt 1967) consider the first systematic experiments with psychoactive drugs to have been started by the French psychiatrist Jacques Moreau (de Tours) in 1845. Moreau (1804–1884) studied under Esquirol at the Charenton mental hospital in France. His numerous publications emphasized the treatment of mental illness with plant hallucinogens. Moreau, like Timothy

Leary some 115 years later, tried to persuade his colleagues to try hashish in order to produce an artificial mental illness which then could be studied. His medical friends were hesitant but the Bohemian artists and writers of nineteenth-century Paris were more receptive. Among them were Baudelaire, Balzac, Dumas, Gautier, and Hugo—all members of the Club des Haschischins. Their writings, like Moreau's, were replete with the excitement that characterized those early drug explorations.

Other historians (eg, Hordern 1968) consider Emil Kraeplin (1856–1926) the father of psychopharmacology. Kraeplin, a student of Wundt, published the first book on the use of psychologic methods in clinical pharmacology. Louis Lewin (1850–1929), a German researcher and teacher of psychopharmacology, influenced many scholars including J.J. Abel (the father of American pharmacology), Sigmund Freud, and Albert Einstein. Lewin (1931) published a major handbook of clinical pharmacology as well as books on toxicology, ocular effects of drugs, and hallucinogens.

Modern History

Psychopharmacology grew rapidly throughout the nineteenth and early twentieth centuries. That history, marked by the development of new drugs and research methodologies, is still being made today. The major events are outlined below:

1800   Publication of Sir Humphrey Davy's monograph on nitrous oxide
1829   Paraldehyde discovered and introduced into medicine in 1882
1830   Chloral hydrate discovered and introduced as a therapeutic depressant in 1869 by Liebreich
1845   *Cannabis* introduced into psychiatry by Moreau
1847-1848   Chloroform and ether inhalation therapy used in psychiatry
1862   Barbiturates discovered and first used clinically in 1903
1880   Cocaine "therapy" for morphine and alcohol addiction introduced into America
1884   *Über Coca*, Freud's first paper on cocaine, is published
1893–1894   Publication of British *Indian Hemp Drugs Commission Report*
1897   Sleep therapy for morphine addiction started with sodium bromide in Shanghai; by 1900 it was used for the treatment of acute mania
1898   Havelock Ellis introduced his mescaline experiences into the literature

1920   Kläsi in Switzerland introduced sleep therapy with morphine
       and scopolamine, and then "Somnifen" barbiturates
1926   Heinrich Klüver begins the experimental analysis of hal-
       lucinosis using mescaline
1929   Sodium amytal introduced and sodium amytal narcosis starts
       in 1930; carbon dioxide inhalation used for psychosis by
       Meduna
1931   Rauwolfia alkaloids used by Sen and Bose in Indian
       psychiatry
1933   Insulin therapy introduced into psychiatry by Sakel and the
       results suggest efficacy of insulin coma which becomes the
       preferred therapy for schizophrenias by 1935
1935–1936   Amphetamines introduced as treatment in narcolepsy
       and depression; metrazol introduced as shock therapy
1938   LSD synthesized by Stoll and Hofmann but the
       psychotomimetic properties were not discovered until 1943;
       LSD introduced as a clinical therapeutic drug in 1947
1944   Publication of Mayor La Guardia's Report on *The Marihuana
       Problem in the City of New York*
1947   Chlordiazepoxide synthesized but its first use in the treat-
       ment of anxiety was in 1958
1949   Cade in Australia introduced lithium for treatment of mania
1950   Promethazine introduced into psychiatry; meprobamate dis-
       covered; chlorpromazine synthesized at the Rhone-Poulenc
       laboratories in Paris by Charpentier and becomes the major
       revolutionary force in modern psychopharmacology; the
       French surgeon Laborit used a "lytic cocktail" of chlor-
       promazine, promethazine, and pethidine for "anesthesia
       without anesthetics" and discovered its unique ability to in-
       duce "pharmacologic lobotomy"; clinical trials by French in-
       vestigators showed potency in alleviating delusions, halluci-
       nations, and disturbed behavior in psychotics
1952   Delay and Deniker foster the acceptance of chlorpromazine
       and propose the term "neuroleptic therapy"
1953   First meeting on psychiatric chlorpromazine therapy held in
       Switzerland and a revolution in psychiatry is heralded;
       rauwolfia therapy gains notice
1957–1958   Imipramine introduced as a major antidepressant
1959   First issue of *Psychopharmacologia* appears
1960–present   Psychopharmacology experiences a tremen-
       dous growth in basic and applied research; the American Col-
       lege of Neuropsychopharmacology briefly reviewed the prog-
       ress from 1957 to 1967 in a volume of more than 1300 pages
       (Efron 1968); the recreational and nonmedical use of drugs

escalated through the 1960s; advances in neurobiochemistry contribute to understanding mechanisms of drug action

Future History

Science fiction writer Robert Heinlein (1973) coined the phrase "future history" to refer to the past as seen from the future. Such speculation concerning future happenings tells us much about current trends as viewed through our expectations and aspirations. Psychopharmacologists themselves have enjoyed engaging in speculative commentaries on their work, forecasting the development of memory pills, antiaging pills, peace pills, a cheap 5-cent intoxicant that is both legal and safe, among others. A study group of the American College of Neuropsychopharmacology produced a monograph on *Psychotropic Drugs in the Year 2000* (Evans and Kline 1971) and the National Commission on Marihuana and Drug Abuse even commissioned a study of drug abuse in the future (Shulgin 1973).

Perhaps the best source of speculation concerning the future history of psychopharmacology can be found in the science fiction genre. Silverberg (1974) showed a shift in science fiction themes over the past decade from a view of drugs as destructive to a view of drugs as a means of growth. Aldous Huxley viewed the drug soma as an instrument of repression in the totalitarian society of his 1932 classic *Brave New World*. However, in Huxley's 1962 *Island*, the drug moksha was described as "the reality-revealer, the truth-and-beauty pill."

In the future, we may speculate that drugs will be used as euphorics, mind expanders, panaceas, mind controllers, intelligence-enhancers, sensation-enhancers, reality-testers, mind-injurers, and as a means of communication. Drugs are envisioned as therapy for major social and physical problems caused by technologic alienation, tension, depression, overcrowding, boredom, and so forth. Some writers predict psychedelic wars, euphoric and escapist journeys from reality, new medicinal drugs discovered on alien planets, and the use of drugs in outer space as tools for hibernation and longevity.

From the flowering of the angiosperms millions of years ago, came the seeds of psychopharmacology. From *Pharmakoi* to pharmacology; from better living through human sacrifice to better living through chemistry; from the first medical text on a Sumerian tablet from the end of the third millennium BC, which equated the word *live* with *intoxicate*, to Huichol Indians in present-day Mexico who use peyote "to find our lives"; from Homeric songs of drugs to the lyrics of the acid-rock culture; from the romantic imagination of the Club des Haschischins to the speculative imagination of science fiction writer Doris Buck (1964) who envisioned pills to escape the stress of future living by mentally transporting the user to the Mesozoic Era as a dinosaur—the history of psychopharmacology, like all history, repeats itself.

References

Abdo Abbasy M: The habitual use of "qat." Int J Prophylak Med Sozialhyg 1:20–22, 1957

Bever O: Why do plants produce drugs? Which is their function in the plants? Q J Crude Drug Res 10: 1541–1549, 1970

Blum RH et al: Society and Drugs. San Francisco, Jossey-Bass, 1969

Buck DP: Come where my love lies dreaming. Fantasy and Science Fiction 26:113–126, 1964

Caldwell AE: History of psychopharmacology. In Clark WG, del Guidice J (eds): Principles of Psychopharmacology. New York, Academic, 1970a, pp 9–30

Caldwell AE: Origins of Psychopharmacology. From CPZ to LSD. Springfield, Ill, Charles C Thomas, 1970b

Del Pozo EC: Empiricism and magic Aztec pharmacology. In Efron DH (ed): Ethnopharmacologic Search for Psychoactive Drugs. Public Health Service Publication No. 1645. Washington, DC, U.S. Government Printing Office, 1967, pp 59–76

Efron DH (ed): Psychopharmacology. A Review of Progress 1957–1967. Public Health Service Publication No. 1836. Washington, DC, U.S. Government Printing Office, 1968

Eisner T. Halpern BP: Taste distortion and plant palatability. Science 172: 1362, 1971

Evans WO, Kline NS (ed): Psychotropic Drugs in the Year 2000. Springfield, Ill, Charles C Thomas, 1971

Flannery KV: The ecology of early food production in Mesopotamia. Science 147: 1247–1256, 1965

Folkard R: Plant Lore, Legends, and Lyrics. London, Sampson Low, Marston, Searle, and Rivington, 1884

Harner MJ: The role of hallucinogenic plants in European witchcraft. In Harner MJ (ed): Hallucinogens and Shamanism. London, Oxford, 1973, pp 125–150

Heinlein RA: Time Enough for Love. New York, Putnam, 1972

Holmstedt B: Historical survey. In Efron DH (ed): Ethnopharmacologic Search for Psychoactive Drugs. Public Health Service Publication No. 1645. Washington, DC, U.S. Government Printing Office, 1967, pp 3–32

Hordern A: Psychopharmacology: Some historical considerations. In Joyce CRB (ed): Psychopharmacology. Dimensions and Perspectives. London, Tavistock, 1968, pp 95–148

Huxley A: Island. New York, Harper & Row, 1962

Levi WM: The Pigeon. Sumter, Levi, 1957

Lewin L: Phantastica: Narcotic and stimulating drugs. London, Kegan Paul, Trench, Trubner, and Co, 1931

Schultes RE: Random thoughts and queries on the botany of cannabis. In Joyce CRB, Curry SH (eds): The Botany and Chemistry of Cannabis. London, J and A Churchill, 1970, pp 11–38

Shulgin AT: Drugs of abuse in the future. In Drug Use in America: Problem in Perspective. Appendix, Vol 1. Washington, DC, U.S. Government Printing Office, 1973, pp 209–236

Siegel RK: An ethologic search for self-administration of hallucinogens. Int J Addict 8: 373–393, 1973

————, Collings PR, Diaz JL: On the use of *Tagetes lucida* and *Nicotiana rustica* as a Huichol smoking mixture: The Aztec "yahutli" with suggestive hallucinogenic effects. Econ Bot (in press)

Silverberg R: Drug themes in Science Fiction. Rockville, Md, National Institute on Drug Abuse, 1974

Swain T: Cold-blooded murder in the Cretaceous. Spectrum 120: 10–12, 1974

Taylor N: Plant Drugs that Changed the World. New York, Dodd, Mead, 1965

psychopharmacology and the family physician

commentary

Dr. Geyman has given us an overview of psychiatric conditions the primary care physician is apt to encounter and describes a useful outline of steps that the physician should take in dealing with these conditions. There is much evidence that the primary care physician will become an increasingly important bulwark of medical treatment in the United States, and his knowledge of psychopharmacology should therefore be adequate to the task before him. Psychopharmacologic agents can be handled without extra special training, but in complicated cases the individual should be referred to a psychopharmacologically oriented psychotherapist.

psychopharmacology and the family physician

John P. Geyman, M.D.

The past 20 years have seen a growing awareness of the importance of psychologic dysfunction of individuals in our growing population and our increasingly complex society. A continuing redefinition of these problems and varied approaches to their treatment have also been seen. Whether viewed as "mental illness," "psychiatric problems," "stress illness," or "functional disorders," these problems, in aggregate, may well be more frequent and more incapacitating than any other disease or disorder. During this same period, a dynamic growth of psychopharmacology as a discipline has been observed. The introduction of massive numbers of psychotropic drugs, however, has been a source of immense confusion to family physicians and others in primary care who provide initial and often definitive care for a large proportion of patients with these problems.

Concurrent with these changes, and despite impressive advances in biomedical technology, increasing disenchantment, both within and outside medicine, with the problems of overspecialization and depersonalization of medical care has been observed. Social attitudes are changing toward greater concern for what Lewis Mumford (1965) calls "the primacy of the person," whom he sees as devitalized and frustrated by the growth of technology. The pendulum in American medicine is now swinging toward the renaissance of the generalist, particularly in the form of the family physician but also in the form of other kinds of primary care physicians with backgrounds in internal medicine and pediatrics. McWhinney (1975) reminds us that "it is no accident that family medicine is

23

emerging at a time when the interrelatedness of all things is being rediscovered, when the importance of ecology is being focused on one's awareness—when human values are being asserted over technology."

Against this background, this chapter will aim to briefly describe the kinds of "psychiatric problems" occurring in primary care, and what the family physician needs to know about the use of psychopharmacologic agents. A conceptual model will be suggested concerning decision making for the selection and use of psychotropic drugs. Finally, some directions will be discussed for future efforts involving psychiatrists, psychopharmacologists, and family physicians.

Psychiatric Conditions in Primary Care

The precise overall incidence of psychiatric conditions in primary care, together with the incidence of specific entities, has been difficult to ascertain due to the relatively recent development of research in primary care, difficulty in arriving at specific and uniform coding methods, and the fact that patients with these conditions frequently do not fall into discrete diagnostic categories. Earlier studies reported an overall incidence in the range of 2 to 5 percent (Densen et al 1960, General Practice 1951, Logan and Cusion 1958, Obstetrics-Gynecology Study 1959, Peterson 1956, Tabenhaus 1955). A subsequent study of the practices of family physicians in Monroe County, New York, showed that 17 percent of their patients had significant emotional disorders, with women having a "psychiatric problem rate" double that of men, and the highest problem rates occurring in patients with digestive disorders, senility, and ill-defined conditions (Locke and Gardner 1969).

The most recent comprehensive and in-depth study of family practice yet done has been conducted by the Department of Family Practice at the Medical College of Virginia. The health care problems of 88,000 patients presenting to 118 family physicians were studied over a period of 18 months. It is interesting that 90 percent of a total of 383,805 health care problems were contained within 172 descriptive problems, using a coding system for primary care developed by the Royal College of General Practice in England. Table 1 shows the rank order and percentage of *total* health care problems represented by the 12 most common "mental and behavioral problems" within the 90 percent of these practice profiles (Marsland et al 1976). It can be seen in Table 1 that these 12 problems comprise 5.27 percent of the 383,805 health problems reported. Although this figure proba-

TABLE 1
MOST COMMON MENTAL AND BEHAVIORAL PROBLEMS
(118 VIRGINIA FAMILY PHYSICIANS)

Rank Order	Problem	Number	Percent of Total
13	Depressive neurosis	5282	1.38
16	Anxiety neurosis	4812	1.25
25	Physical disorders of presumably psychogenic origin	3056	0.80
70	Functional gastric disorders	1132	0.29
73	Tension headache	1083	0.28
83	Debility or fatigue	975	0.25
84	Abuse of alcohol	962	0.25
100	Family relationship problems	825	0.21
114	Schizophrenia	707	0.18
145	Organic psychoses	527	0.14
148	Other psychotropic drugs	520	0.13
168	Malingering	425	0.11
	TOTALS	20,326	5.27

bly provides an *approximate* order of magnitude of these problems, it is clear that more definitive studies are still needed to better delineate the occurrence of psychiatric conditions in family practice.

A recent study by Morrison (1975) has shown that about three-fifths of the annual number of ambulatory, physician visits in the United States are made to general /family physicians, who are responsible for about two-thirds of the estimated 1 billion out-of-hospital acquisitions of prescribed medicines annually. Prescriptions for psychotropic drugs comprise a substantial portion of this total. In a study of drug use in an American community, Stolley and co-workers (1972) have found that psychotherapeutic drugs made up 17 percent of all prescriptions, including "tranquilizers" (7.7 percent), hypnotics and sedatives (3.6 percent), and amphetamines (3.4 percent). In another study of a general medical care clinic, carried out at the University of California at Irvine, 65 percent of all patients were using some kind of psychoactive medication (Gottschalk et al 1971). Further, Balter and Levine (1970) have found that general /family physicians prescribe over 70 percent of all prescriptions for these drugs in the United States.

The family physician's involvement with "psychiatric conditions" is markedly different from the psychiatrist's experience, which frequently involves the management of severe psychiatric disorders in a hospital or crisis intervention setting. The family physician, on the other hand, sees a wide range of less severe and often situational emotional problems in his everyday practice, including anxiety reactions, psychosomatic disorders, depressive reactions, psychoneuroses, grief reactions, hysterical reactions, school problems, sexual and marital problems. Patients with these kinds of problems are frequently troubled in a more general and nonspecific way, thereby rendering decisions concerning their care, particularly the use of psychoactive drugs, especially complex. Patients frequently present with a somatic complaint which they hope will be more acceptable (or taken more seriously) to their physicians, while the actual reason prompting the visit may be an unstated constellation of fears and anxieties (Geyman 1971). As a practicing family physician, Ganz (1961) prefers to view emotional disorders in his practice as "stress illness." "In my practice I see very little imagined illness. But I see lots of physical illness, the cause of which lies in the environment, the personality, or the emotional makeup of the patient. To my way of thinking, 'stress illness' communicates a more acceptable and certainly more proper image to patients. It also indicates to the doctor a truer etiology."

Psychopharmacologic Needs of the Family Physician

In view of the frequency of psychiatric conditions in family practice and the family physician's active role in the recognition and management of most of these problems, he clearly must have a broad base of knowledge in practical psychopharmacology. The acquisition and maintenance of this knowledge base has been difficult for a variety of reasons—the confusing array of psychotherapeutic agents, difficulty in adequately evaluating the therapeutic efficacy of these drugs in vivo, the relative lack of training in psychopharmacology in formal medical education at all levels, and lack of adequate emphasis on this subject in the literature generally read by family physicians. For example, it is ironic that such excellent and definitive material as the article "A Usage Guide for Psychoactive Drugs," published in Diseases of the Nervous System, failed to reach the large audience of prescribing physicians (Appleton 1971).

From a cognitive standpoint, the family physician must have a current working knowledge of the following areas (Appleton 1971, Norris and Yervanos 1973, Wheatley 1973):

1. Obtaining an adequate data base for the patient's problem
2. Assessment and/or specific diagnosis of problems

3. Kinds of psychiatric problems amenable to psychoactive drugs, including role of drug therapy in larger therapeutic plan
4. Kinds of psychiatric problems for which drug therapy is *not* indicated
5. Principles of setting *specific* goals for intervention with psychoactive drugs
6. Major classes of psychoactive drugs:
    a. In-depth knowledge of *two* effective drugs in each major class, including indications, contraindications, dosage, side effects, toxic reactions, basic mechanism of action, dose-response principles, and potential for dependency, if any
    b. Understanding of anticipated level of efficacy of psychoactive drugs for each major condition
    c. Equivalency between comparable drugs
7. Selection of a particular psychoactive drug with consideration of:
    a. Efficacy
    b. Safety
    c. Incidence, nature, and severity of side effects
    d. Dose form and schedule
    e. Cost
    f. Pitfalls of use
8. Principles of monitoring patient during drug therapy with consideration of:
    a. Important parameters to follow (history, physical examination, and /or laboratory studies)
    b. Frequency of follow-up
    c. Signs and symptoms of toxicity
    d. Management of side effects and toxicity
9. Principles of changing dose or drug:
    a. Understanding of adequate therapeutic trial
    b. Increasing or decreasing drug dose
    c. Discontinuance of drug and /or adding another drug
10. Understanding special circumstances, including:
    a. Pediatric patients
    b. Obstetric patients (ie, placental transfer)
    c. Geriatric patients
    d. Maintenance drug therapy following psychiatric hospitalization
    e. Influence of psychoactive drug on patient's individual life style (eg, occupation)
    f. Drug interaction
11. Feasible and available method for updating knowledge of psychopharmacology

12. Understanding of self as therapeutic agent and awareness of own limitations
13. Indications for psychiatric consultation and /or referral

A Conceptual Approach to the Use of Psychoactive Drugs

It is critical that we proceed well beyond the cognitive elements of psychopharmacology if a reasonable level of understanding of the role and use of psychopharmacologic agents in family practice is to be acquired. Intervention with such drugs is only part of a larger therapeutic mileau involving psychosocial factors impinging upon the patient (from both within and outside his family), the doctor–patient relationship, the physician's communication and diagnostic skills, and the physician's own level of self-awareness as a therapeutic agent. Levine (1970) reminds us that it is well documented throughout the scientific community that "the therapeutic response to an administered psychotropic drug is dependent upon pharmacologic as well as nonpharmacologic factors." Tupin and Schuller further point out that "in those clinical situations where psychosocial elements play a significant role, the practitioner with skills in interviewing, history taking, and observation will excel and the patient will benefit. In this situation, the psychologic-mindedness of the physician is the single most important ingredient. One cannot perceive that for which one is blind" (Tupin and Schuller, unpublished data).

Although rapid advances in the technology of psychopharmacology in recent years have certainly led to improved care and /or cure for many patients with psychiatric problems, abuse of psychoactive drugs has likewise become a significant problem. These drugs can afford the busy physician with a "crutch," which can adversely affect his understanding of the patient's problems and delay or prevent their resolution. In a paper entitled "The Overmedicated Society," Muller (1972) suggests that physicians can be both unintelligent and lazy in their excessive use of drug therapy. Based on his studies of repeat prescriptions in family practice in England, Balint and co-workers (1970) expand on this point in these words—"On the basis of our results we think that in reality the repeat prescription (instead of a treatment) is a diagnosis, not of the patient nor of his doctor but of the doctor–patient relationship."

The problem-oriented medical record developed by Weed has become a standard part of practice for many family physicians in recent years. The problem-oriented approach can likewise be applied

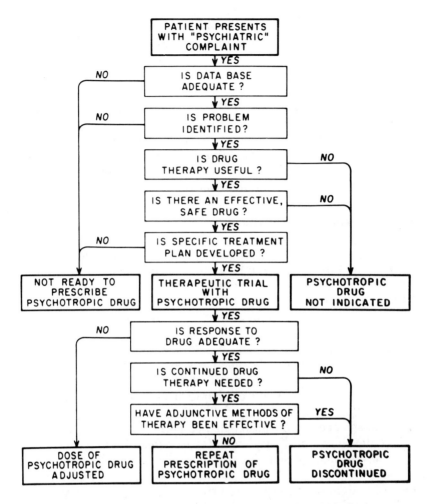

Fig. 1. A conceptual model for use of psychotropic drugs.

to nonorganic problems and help the family physician to identify and understand psychosocial problems in his patients and their families. This is an essential first step before any therapeutic intervention can be considered. In this regard, Freyhan (1962) has recommended that disease-oriented therapeutic indications for psychoactive drugs can be exchanged for symptom-directed criteria (ie, "target symptoms" in identified areas of drug treatable. psychopathology). The family physician's task, then, is to identify the patient's problems as specifically as possible, including aspects of the patient's behavior that require treatment. He must then develop a treatment plan that is realistic, meets the individual patient's needs, and involves repeated measurement of therapeutic response so that therapy can be revised or discontinued as necessary. In this connection, it is also useful for the physician to understand which of the following broad objectives is involved by each treatment plan— (a) cure; (b) rehabilitation; (c) relief of symptoms; (d) maintenance of improvement; (e) prophylaxis against recurrent attacks of a cyclic or periodic disorder; or (f) adjunctive to some other treatment such as psychotherapy (Kline and Lehmann 1962).

These ideas are incorporated in a conceptual model for the use of psychotropic drugs (Fig. 1), which form a basis for managing patients with psychiatric or functional problems.

Some Future Directions

Shifting priorities at all levels toward strengthening primary care in medical education and clinical practice are creating new opportunities for understanding the nature and management of common psychiatric conditions. Greater emphasis is being placed on ambulatory care, the provision of more comprehensive and accessible health care services, and viewing the patient as a whole person instead of a disease in his family and community setting. There is every evidence that family practice will continue to develop as a major field in primary care and that student interest will be sustained at a high level. As the academic discipline of family medicine continues to be more sharply defined, continued emphasis on behavioral science can be anticipated as part of that discipline.

The development of academic departments of family practice in most of our medical schools, together with the application of new research methodologies in primary care, should facilitate more intensive and productive study of primary care problems, which have previously been largely overlooked. In the area of psychopharmacology, it is hoped that active cooperative efforts can be mobilized, involving psychiatrists, clinical pharmacologists, family physicians and their patients in the expansion of research and teaching in this important discipline.

References

Appleton WS: Psychoactive drugs: a usage guide. Dis Nerv Syst 32:607–616, 1971

Balint M, Hunt J, Joyce D, Marinker M, Woodcock J: Treatment or Diagnosis, A Study of Repeat Prescriptions in General Practice. London, Tavistock, 1970, p 145

Balter M, Levine J: The nature and extent of psychotropic drug usage in the United States. Psychopharmacol Bull 5:3, 1970

Densen PM, Balamuth E, Deardorff NR: Medical care plans as sources of morbidity data: prevalence of illness and associated volume of service. Milbank Mem Fund Q 38:48–101, 1960

Freyhan FA: Rationale and indications for biological treatment of psychiatric disorders. In Rinkel M (ed): Biological Treatment of Mental Illness. New York, Page, 1962, p 455

Ganz RH: The family physician as counselor. Physician's Manage 9:68, 1961

General Practice, Internal Medicine and Pediatrics National Disease and Therapeutic Index. Flewrtown, Penn, Lea Associates, 1951

Geyman JP: The Modern Family Doctor and Changing Medical Practice. New York, Appleton, 1971, p 149

Gottschalk LA, Bates DE, Fox RA, James FM: Psychoactive drug use: patterns found in samples from a mental health clinic and a general medical clinic. Arch Gen Psychiat 25:393, 1971

Kline NS, Lehmann H: Handbook of Psychiatric Treatment in Medical Practice. Philadelphia, Saunders, 1962, p 31

Levine F: Drug metabolism and therapeutic response. Psychopharmacol Bull 6:3, 1970

Locke BZ, Gardner EA: Psychiatric disorders among the patients of general practitioners and internists. Pub Health Rep 84:167–173, 1969

Logan WPD, Cusion AA: Studies on medical and population subjects, No. 14. In Morbidity Statistics from General Practice, Vol. 1 London, His Majesty's Stationery Office, 1958

Marsland DW, Wood M, Mayo F: Data for the rational development of curriculum and patient care systems in family practice. J Fam Pract, 1976
McWhinney IR: Family medicine in perspective. New Engl J Med 293:180, 1975

Morrison N: Prescription Drugs and the Physician: An Analysis of the Acquisition, Use, Type and Cost of Prescribed Medicine in the United States. New York, Appleton, 1975

Muller C: The overmedicated society: forces in the marketplace for medical care. Science 176:488, 1972

Mumford L: The Transformations of Man. New York, Harper & Row, 1965

Norris AS, Yervanos N: Pharmacologic agents. In Conn HF, Rakel RE, Johnson TW (eds): Family Practice. Philadelphia, Saunders, 1973, pp 248–258

Obstetrics-Gynecology Study, American Academy of General Practice, Kansas City, Mo, 1959

Peterson OL: Analytical study of North Carolina general practice, 1953–54. J Med Educ (Suppl) 31:12, 1956

Stolley PD, Becker MH, McEvilla FD, Lasagna L, Gainor M, Sloane LM: Drug prescribing and use in an American community. Ann Intern Med 76:537, 1972

Tabenhaus LJ: Study of one rural practice, 1953. GP 12:97–102, 1955

Tupin FP, Schuller AB: The pathophysiology of psychosomatic disorders: psychosocial aspects of GI function. In Bolt RJ, Palmer PES, Ruebner B, Watson DW (eds): The Digestive System. New York John Wiley (in press)

Wheatley D; Psychopharmacology in Family Practice. London, William Heinemann Medical Books, Ltd, 1973, pp 12–15

the chemical structure of drugs

commentary

While the practicing physician rarely has an opportunity to consider the structure of drugs, these are of extreme importance in determining both the actions and toxicity. To have an effect, a drug must somehow resemble a chemical structure already found in the body in some way. It either fits into and blocks the action of or stimulates a receptor. It may also block the transport of normal chemical constituents in the body by changing the permeability of membranes. Thus, drugs like atropine, LSD, and amphetamine compete with physiologic transmitters, such as acetylcholine, serotonin, and dopamine, while drugs like ethyl alcohol and diethyl ether probably impair the normal functioning of membranes, though they may also influence transmitter action (particularly gamma aminobutyric acid). A knowledge of structure-activity relationships is particularly important in the search for new and better drugs. The practitioner may find it useful to know that a family of drugs exists because slight differences in structure produce differences in efficacy and toxicity, and such knowledge may be useful in matching the idiosyncrasies of patients. Differences, whether genetically determined or acquired, in the ability of patients to metabolize drugs must also be taken into account to maximize efficacy and minimize toxicity.

the chemical structure of drugs

Donald J. Jenden, M.D.

The vast amount of data relating pharmacologic activity to the chemical structure of compounds contains a striking anomaly. In some series of drugs, such as opiate analgesics and antihistamines, very similar pharmacologic properties are exhibited by compounds showing great disparity of structure; in other cases an apparently minor change can completely alter the pharmacologic spectrum and even eliminate the properties entirely. As long ago as 1868, Crum Brown, and Fraser reported that addition of an N-methyl group to morphine and other alkaloids led to a total disappearance of their characteristic pharmacologic activity and replaced it with a uniform paralytic effect. More recently, substitution of a chlorine atom for hydrogen in the antihistamine promazine led to the discovery of the first synthetic compound with antipsychotic activity, chlorpromazine, although promazine itself is totally lacking in this property. A great deal of effort has been directed toward the interpretation of these and related phenomena over the past few decades, and while many now have rational explanations, others remain enigmatic.

One of the principal difficulties in relating structure to pharmacologic activity lies in the oversimplified view of molecular structure, which the conventional two-dimensional formula conveys. For example, morphine, methadone, and meperidine appear in Figure 1 to have very dissimilar structure. Their common pharmacologic properties become much easier to understand when three-dimensional molecular models are constructed from which common structural features can readily be discerned (Beckett and Casey

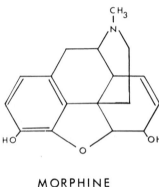

METHADONE   MEPERIDINE

MORPHINE

Fig. 1.   Structures of methodone, meperidine, and morphine as conventionally represented.

1965). It is important, however, to visualize drug molecules not as fixed arrangements of atoms in space, but as entities that are flexible to varying degrees and can assume quite different conformations by rotation of groups about the axes of certain (but not all) interatomic bonds. P. Pauling and his colleagues (1975) have recently postulated, on the basis of x-ray crystallographic evidence, that the muscarinic and nicotinic properties of acetylcholine depend on the ability of the molecule to adopt similar conformations, but the nicotinic properties require that the functional groups be planar. Projections of the structures of acetylcholine and oxotremorine obtained by x-ray crystallography are more informative than the conventional representations in Figure 2, but do not necessarily correspond with their conformations in aqueous solution.

The arrangement of atoms in space is not the only structural ele-

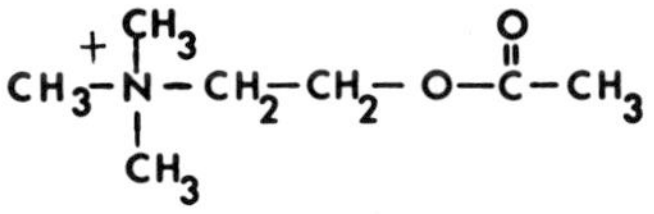

$$CH_3-\overset{+}{\underset{CH_3}{\overset{CH_3}{N}}}-CH_2-CH_2-O-\overset{O}{\overset{\|}{C}}-CH_3$$

ACETYLCHOLINE

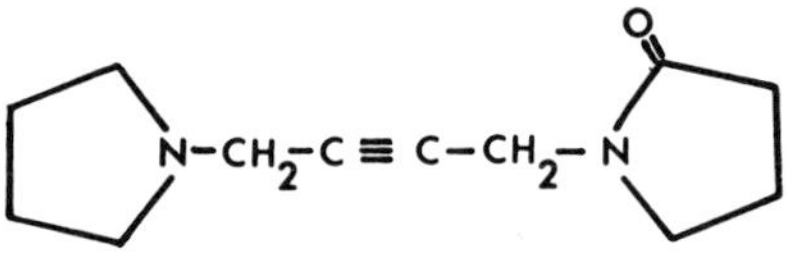

OXOTREMORINE

Fig. 2. Structure formulas of acetylcholine and oxotremorine.

ment of significance in determining pharmacologic properties. The charge distribution throughout the molecule is not uniform, and the net charge on certain atoms or groups is very important in determining chemical (eg, stability, base strength, and partition coefficient) and pharmacologic properties (distribution, selectivity, and potency). Unfortunately, there is no way to construct a simple model of this feature, which is comparable to the useful atomic models in visualizing shape. Theoretical calculations based on quantum mechanics can provide approximations of charge distribution in simple molecules, if the conformation is known or assumed (Kier 1971), and the conformation of compounds in crystals can be calculated from x-ray crystallographic data. There is no presently available method to assess either the conformation or charge distribution of drug molecules in aqueous solution, except by indirect inference from their physicochemical properties or pharmacologic activity. A further complication arises from the fact that the steric arrangement of atoms in a molecule and the charge distribution among them are closely interdependent; changes in both can be induced by adjacent molecules, including solvent and receptor molecules in close proximity. The steric flexibility and polarizability, ie, the ease with which the conformation and charge distribution can be deformed by the microenvironment, are both potentially important factors in determining pharmacologic activity.

A bleak picture has been presented of our present ability and future hope for relating chemical structure to pharmacologic activity. Nevertheless there are well-established principles and even more empirical generalizations that may help not only in understanding the pharmacology of psychoactive drugs but in the search for more potent and specific agents.

To be psychoactive a drug must, of course, be capable of reaching the brain—ie, it must cross the blood-brain barrier (see p 167). Structural characteristics that permit this are well understood. In general compounds with a markedly nonuniform charge distribution or a net positive or negative charge—so-called polar compounds —penetrate the blood-brain barrier slowly if at all, and hence are unlikely to have any psychopharmacologic effect. For this reason N-methylmorphine, referred to above, lacks analgesic activity when administered conventionally. If it is placed directly in certain areas of the brain in animals, its analgesic effects are apparent (Foster et al 1967).

Another factor that may obscure the relation between structure and pharmacologic activity is drug metabolism, an area currently receiving a great deal of attention because of the enormous advances that have recently taken place in analytic methodology. It has been known for some time that certain drugs have a very short duration of action because they are rapidly converted, usually in the liver, to inactive metabolites. Many cases are now known, and others almost certainly remain to be discovered, in which the parent drug is pharmacologically inert or less active than one or more of its metabolites. Attempts to fit the structure of the parent compound into a hypothetical scheme of structure-activity relationships are then likely to be futile.

Some years ago a new synthetic compound was discovered by Everett and named tremorine because of its remarkable ability to reproduce in experimental animals a syndrome resembling Parkinson's disease (Everett et al 1956). This compound was subsequently shown to owe its pharmacologic properties entirely to its biotransformation to an oxidation product, oxotremorine (Cho et al 1961). This finding has been very valuable in screening new compounds for their potential value in treating Parkinson's disease (Jenden 1967). Elucidation of the structure of oxotremorine led to a search for chemically related compounds that might antagonize it, an approach that has proved successful for several other groups of drugs. Several potent antagonists have now been described, some of which appear to be potentially useful in treating Parkinson's disease and other extrapyramidal disorders (Karlen et al 1970). The mechanism by which oxotremorine produces these peculiar effects and its analogs antagonize them is not known with certainty but appears to depend on a subtle structural resemblance to acetylcholine, which is certainly not obvious from a superficial inspection of their formulas (Fig. 2) but can be rationalized in terms of its three-dimensional structure and charge distribution (Cho et al 1962, Bebbington et al 1966).

Metabolic transformation of an inert compound to a pharmacologically active product is not simply an experimental curiosity. There is evidence that the hepatotoxic effects of halogenated hydrocarbons may be due to their conversion in the liver to highly reactive and toxic products that destroy the cells in which they are formed (Brodie et al 1971). Their toxic properties may be suppressed by inhibiting their transformation and enhanced by accelerating it. Many therapeutically useful and interesting compounds have been shown to owe part or all of their actions to metabolic products. These compounds include imipramine, diazepam, thioridazine, tetrahydrocannabinol, phenylbutazone, and chloral hydrate. Others have been deliberately designed to achieve this; for example, a dopamine defect in the nigrostriatal pathway is believed to be responsible for many of the features of parkinsonism. This disease cannot be treated effectively by administering dopamine because the drug cannot reach its intended site of action. Levodopa, on the other hand, can pass through the blood-brain barrier, and is decarboxylated in the brain (and elsewhere) to yield dopamine at the site to which it must be delivered.

These examples serve to illustrate that there may be no obvious relationship between pharmacologic activity and structure because structure is visualized too superficially or because an inactive precursor is mistaken for the active compound. Many psychoactive compounds, however, bear a rather obvious structural resemblance to biogenic amines, leading to the conclusion that their effects may be due to interference with the metabolism or function of these endogenous compounds. The nature of this interference and its relevance to the therapeutic or toxic effects of a drug are not easy to establish, and some of the current hypotheses are extrapolations from results of experiments on simpler structures from the autonomic nervous system or even from invertebrates. These allow better experimental control than an intact brain and permit distinctions to be made between effects on neurotransmitter metabolism or transport, mimicking or blocking the effects of neurotransmitters, or incorporation of the drug itself into the metabolic pathway of a neurotransmitter, where it may interfere with neurotransmitter release or be relessed in its place.

Central stimulants of the amphetamine type bear an obvious resemblance to catecholamines, and amphetamine and some of its metabolites and analogs have been shown to interfere with

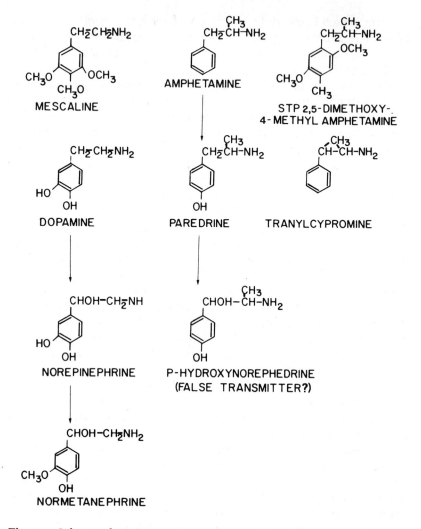

Fig. 3. Scheme showing some structural relationships in psychoactive compounds related to catecholamines.

catecholaminergic function in a number of specific ways. The relation between psychotropic and toxic properties and these cellular actions is somewhat more controversial; a structural resemblance or even a specific cellular effect is no guarantee that this underlies the clinical effect seen (Fig. 3).

The tricyclic antidepressants, while having little structural similarity to norepinephrine or serotonin, are potent inhibitors of the reuptake of these transmitters by the neurons that release them. It is generally believed that one of these effects underlies their antidepressant properties, but a great deal of work must be done before their mechanism is completely understood.

Perhaps the most remarkable group of drugs in regard to apparent structural inhomogeneity are the antipsychotic phenothiazines and butyrophenones. Despite their differing structures, these drugs block dopamine receptors, an action that is believed to underlie both their antipsychotic properties and perhaps their extrapyramidal side effects as well. However, at least some of the phenothiazines are converted metabolically to other compounds, which may well contribute to both the therapeutic and toxic effects by mechanisms still to be discovered. Many of these compounds are also capable of antagonizing the effects of norepinephrine in the brain and in the periphery. The complexity of the problems of identification of these metabolites in man and their pharmacologic evaluation can scarcely be overstated. As in other areas, there is reason to hope for rapid progress as our knowledge of basic neurobiology expands and more powerful means become available for understanding molecular structure (Forrest et al 1974).

References

Bebbington A, Brimblecombe RW, Shakeshaft D: The central and peripheral activity of acetylenic amines related to oxotremorine. Br J Pharmacol 26:56–67, 1966

Beckett AH, Casey AF: Analgesics and their antagonists: biochemical aspects and structure-activity relations. Prog Med Chem 4:171–218, 1965

Brodie BB, Reid WD, Cho AK, Siper G, Krishna G, Gillette JR: Role of metabolism in hepatotoxicity of halobenzene. Proc Natl Acad Sci 68:160–164, 1971

Cho AK, Haslett WL, Jenden DJ: The identification of an active metabolite of tremorine. Biochem Biophys Res Commun 5:276–279, 1961

———, Haslett WL, Jenden DJ: The peripheral action of oxotremorine, a metabolite of tremorine. J Pharmacol 138:249–257, 1962

Crum Brown A, Fraser TR: On the connection between chemical constitution and physiological action: on the physiological action of the salts of ammonia, of tri-methylamine and of tetramethylammonium; of the salts of tropia and of the ammonium bases derived from it; and of tropic, atropic and isatropic acids and their salts. Trans R Soc Edin 25:151, 1868

Everett GM, Blockus LE, Shepperd IM: Tremor introduced by tremorine and its antagonism by anti-Parkinson drugs. Science 124:79, 1956

Forrest IS, Carr CJ, Udin E (eds): Phenothiazines and Structurally Related Drugs: Advances in Biochemical Psychopharmacology, Vol 9. New York, Raven, 1974

Foster RS, Jenden DJ, Lomax P: A comparison of the pharmacological effects of morphine and N-methyl morphine. J Pharmacol 157:185–195, 1967

Jenden DJ: Testing of drugs for therapeutic potential in Parkinson's disease. In Burger A (ed): Methods of Pharmacological Testing. New York, Dekker, Inc, 1967, p 337–361

Karlen B, Lindeke B, Lundgren S, Svensson KG, Dahlbon R, Jenden DJ, Giering JR: Acetylene compounds of potential pharmacological value. XIV. N-(t-amino-alkynyl)-substituted succinimides and maleimides. A class of central anticholinergic agents. J Med Chem 13:651–657, 1970

Kier LB: Molecular Orbital Theory in Drug Research. New York, Academic, 1971

Pauling P: The shapes of cholinergic molecules. In Waser PG (ed): Cholinergic Mechanisms. New York, Raven, 1975, p 241

part II
experimental
psychopharmacology
drugs as tools

Introduction

Although much more is known about the brain and behavior than was known 50 or even 10 years ago, we still have to depend a great deal upon inference to guess at the contents of the "black box." Psychotropic drugs can help bridge this gap because they get into the "black box" and their influence upon behavior can be observed. Because they are chemicals, drugs are easy to manipulate, weight, and measure. Also, the same drugs that are given to patients can be studied in animals (in vivo) and in the test tube (in vitro). Thus, for example, schizophrenia can be thought of as a disease caused by excess dopamine in the limbic system because drugs that are effective in this disease also block dopaminergic neurones in rats and block the activation of limbic adenylate cyclase in the test tube (Clement-Cormier et al 1974). Also, drugs like amphetamine, which exacerbate schizophrenia, will stimulate dopaminergic pathways.

Even in clinical practice, drugs can be used as diagnostic tools. If a patient fails to respond to an antipsychotic drug, the diagnosis of schizophrenia can be reconsidered. To be sure, psychotropic drugs are not as specific as antibiotics, but they can be an additional factor in diagnosis. A test dose of quinine will ameliorate myotonia and exacerbate myasthenia and can help to establish the nature of the disease. A positive response to lithium can tell the physician that the patient very likely is manic.

Drugs can also help to reveal mechanisms underlying the components of mental life, such as consciousness, perception, learning, and mood. Ordinarily portions of a living human brain cannot be extirpated nor probed with electrodes, especially in these days of strict control of human experimentation. But drugs whose actions are reversible can be given to patients and may influence one or another of these functions. The same drugs can be examined in vivo and in vitro and extrapolations made to effects in humans.

In the section that follows major symptoms and functions dealt with every day by the practitioner will be discussed from a psychopharmacologic point of view. Thus the nature of pain and why it should be modifiable by drugs will be considered. How drugs may affect sleep, conditioning, and the electrical activity of the brain will also be shown. The fact that drugs can change these normal functions means that a chemical link resembling the drug must be involved in brain mechanisms controlling these functions.

References

Clement-Cormier YC, Kebabian JW, Petzold GL, Greengard P: Dopamine-sensitive adenylate cyclase in mammalian brain: a possible site of action of antipsychotic drugs. Proc Natl Acad Sci 71:1113–1117, 1974

contemporary studies of placebo phenomena

commentary

The degree of relief afforded by drugs through their placebo action is substantial. Indeed there is a common view that 35 to 40 percent of the effectiveness of most psychoactive agents is due to placebo action. There is considerable individual variability and the true figures may range anywhere from zero to 80 percent, depending upon the suggestibility of the individual, the nature of the disorder, and the persuasiveness of the therapist. Although the physician may have qualms about administering saline injections or lactose placebos, the quasiplacebo effects of questionably effective agents, such as vitamins, analgesics, and antianxiety agents, should be kept in mind. There appears to be no medical condition for which patients may not receive some relief from a placebo. Since there are many medical conditions for which no truly effective specific agent exists, the importance of placebo medication is obvious. The physician should always be aware of what he is doing, and the ethical and legal considerations, though complex, should be carefully weighed. Placebos are useful drugs when properly used, especially when administered with warmth and reassurance.

contemporary studies of placebo phenomena

Ronald G. Gallimore, Ph.D.
Jim L. Turner, Ph.D.

Although the healing potentials of faith, treatment ritual, and the physician–patient relationship have been recognized since the days of Hippocrates, it wasn't until 1945 that the ancient word *placebo* first appeared in the title of a medical journal (Pepper 1945, Shapiro 1960). The evolution of scientific interest in placebo effects during the last century parallels the three-stage progression of ignorance, coping, and exploitation, outlined by McGuire (1969) in his analysis of the natural history of artifacts (ie, misleading or error-producing factors).

During the *ignorance stage* of any type of investigation, researchers and practitioners alike are oblivious to a variable or effect that becomes eventually identified as a methodologic artifact. During the *coping stage*, the heretofore ignored factor is viewed as a methodologic nuisance, and increasingly sophisticated efforts are made to eliminate the contamination of investigations by the unwanted artifact. The final stage is *exploitation*; during this stage the artifact is recognized as a variable worthy of study in its own right. Such a progression may be occurring in placebo studies.

The first of McGuire's stages in the case of the placebo is represented by much of medical history, which can be viewed as an archival testimonial to placebo therapy. The physicians of the day remained largely unaware of the artifactual basis of their successes. Until this century, the prevailing conception of placebo was that of an inert drug "given more to please than to benefit the patient." The general tendency was to underestimate or deny the saliency and pervasiveness of nonspecific factors in treatment. Deliberate administration of inert substances was considered a form of quackery, which fostered the "nostrum evil" (Cabot 1906).

For the past several decades, the placebo effect has been viewed primarily as a potentially powerful contaminating influence, which must be controlled in order to conduct objective and scientific evaluations of therapies. This period represents the second of McGuire's stages. Double-blind placebo control studies have become standard in psychopharmacologic research and efforts have been made to identify "placebo reactors" to eliminate them from subject populations. During the coping stage, widespread clinical use has continued, while deliberate administration of placebos in research is seen mainly as a methodologic tool and the placebo effect as a conceptual nuisance.

Finally, the view has emerged that the pervasive and reliable phenomenon of placebo should be exploited rather than treated as a nuisance. The secondary information gained as drug researchers sought to cope with placebo effects has led some investigators to regard the phenomenon as having considerable clinical and theoretical significance in its own right. For instance, the finding that placebos are proportionately more effective with increasing stress was noted by Beecher (1955) as implicating a fundamental new principle of drug action. Weil (1972) cites the placebo literature as evidence that researchers studying psychoactive drugs should consider shifting their theoretical focus from "the chemical basis of mental events" to the "mental basis of chemical events." Clinical and social psychologists have begun trying to specify "nonspecific" or placebo processes as part of the general study of behavior-influence processes (Krasner and Ullmann 1973).

In this paper contemporary research on the placebo and its effects is summarized. We recently collected a comprehensive bibliography on placebo and its effects and found nearly 1500 books and articles. Despite this large body of literature, it remains that placebo effects, though widely observed and documented, have yet to be explained in any comprehensive fashion. Many theories have been proposed or developed, but to date no one of them is sufficient to integrate available data. Most commonly, explanations simply invoke another construct, which itself is not well understood or validated, eg, transference, suggestion, expectation, and so forth.

Range of Placebo Phenomena

As scientific study of the placebo effect expanded, it became clear that the question of what is specific and nonspecific is not uniquely applicable to drug therapy. Contemporary definitions have thus broadened to include "any therapy, or that component of any therapy, that is deliberately used for its presumed specific effect on a patient, symptom, or illness, but which, . . . is without specific activity for the condition being treated" (Shapiro 1968).

Nondrug Placebos

Inclusion of nondrug therapies in the above definition is supported by a number of studies. Beecher (1961), for example, notes that the surgical enthusiast gets better results than the skeptic, and reviews, as an instance of placebo surgery, the brief history of internal mammary artery ligation in the treatment of angina pectoris. Angina patients treated by sham surgery reported equal or greater relief than a comparison group on whom artery ligation was actually performed.

In addition to surgery a variety of treatment modes can produce placebo effects. For example, Greene and Laskin (1972) reported that 40 percent of patients suffering myofascial pain dysfunction exhibited remission or noticeable symptom reduction with use of a placebo appliance that did not directly modify occlusal contact or alter mandibular placement. Machines may also function as placebos. Placebo apparatus has also been shown to significantly reduce hallucinating in hospitalized schizophrenics (Weingartner 1971) and cure some children of bedwetting (Collins 1973).

All forms of psychotherapy probably include a substantial placebo component. Over the past decade it has become increasingly common practice to include a "pseudotherapy" placebo control group in studies of various psychotherapeutic procedures based on learning and conditioning techniques. Treatment has focused on weight loss, alcoholism, insomnia, smoking, and various types of phobic anxiety. Overall, approximately 40 percent of the patients receiving pseudotherapy show gains equivalent or superior to those receiving theoretically active treatment. Since virtually none of these studies have employed a double-blind design and there is reason to believe that the pseudotherapies utilized are often less credible (McGlynn and McDonell 1974), it appears likely that the saliency of placebo processes is still being underestimated in this literature.

Placebo Responsive Disease and Functions

The variety of diseases, psychiatric disorders, and assorted mental and physical conditions that have been shown to yield partially or entirely to placebo treatment preclude easy generalization as to what is , and is not, a placebo-responsive symptom or function. One point of view is that placebo effects are mainly associated with subjective complaints and /or subjective assessment procedures. While such an argument has some validity, it would also hold true for many "active" treatment procedures, and there is considerable evidence that placebos do produce objective change on various somatic and psychic functions, which can be measured more objectively.

Our review of the literature yielded over 65 different treatment foci in which a certain percentage of the patients showed a significant placebo effect. A representative sample of placebo-responsive conditions being treated would include acne, allergy, angina pectoris, arthritis, asthma, behavior disorders, common cold, diabetes, depression, gastrointestinal disorders, migraine, post-operative pain, radiation sickness, rheumatism, stuttering, and warts. Although the average degree of effectiveness of placebo across these various conditions has not been computed, earlier reviews have reported that around 35 percent of those treated obtain satisfactory relief (Beecher 1968). Meaningful statements about the effectiveness of placebo treatment of various conditions are difficult because of extreme variability in patient response, both within and across treatment modalities. The percentage of patients with angina pectoris reported as responding to placebo therapy, for example, may range from 0 to 57 percent and for rheumatism from 4 to 84 percent. Such variability is characteristic (Lehmann 1964).

Other studies have focused on the placebo responsivity of specific psychologic (Lehmann 1960, Cleghorn 1949) and physiologic functions. In general, of the more complex psychologic functions, the components concerned with accuracy of performance are relatively placebo resistant, while those related to speed of performance tend to be placebo prone (Eldred 1960). Some physiologic functions have also been reported to be responsive to placebo. These include adrenal cortical activity (Abramson 1967), blood chemistry changes (Frankenhaeuser 1963), gastric acid secretion (Abbot 1952), and blood pressure (Rickels 1968).

Correlates of Placebo Responsivity

Placebo response is not consistently related to age, sex, education, race, or social class. Children, healthy adults, college students (including medical, nursing, and pharmacy students) have all been shown capable of a placebo response. To this list could be added psychotics, neurotics, drug addicts, the mentally retarded, and assorted animal species. Selected studies have linked various demographic characteristics (Rickles 1968), severity of illness (Nicolis 1967, Shapiro 1968), duration of illness (Rickels 1966), and type of psychiatric diagnosis (Rossi 1968) to differential rates of placebo responsivity. However, there is no convincing evidence that such findings can be generalized beyond the particular samples studied or that a fixed level of placebo responsiveness is associated with membership in specific patient groups or classes.

Throughout the 30-year history of interest in placebo, there has been a relatively unsuccessful but persistent effort to identify the so-called *placebo reactor* (Fisher 1967, Liberman 1967). The bulk of this research has been based on a personality trait theory approach, and the results are less than impressive. Our survey revealed that over two dozen distinct personality traits have been entertained as possible correlates. Only a few studies report significant correlations between personality traits and placebo responding, most have not been replicated, and, in any case, the degree of correlation is usually minimal, accounting for less than 10 percent of the variance. In short, research to date does not support the concept of "placebo reactor" as a unitary personality type or cluster of personality traits.

A case in point is the concept of suggestibility—presumably a trait more characteristic of some persons than others—which is often invoked to account for different rates of placebo reactivity (Conn 1959). There are a variety of different measures of suggestibility, most being either measures of primary (ie, hypnotic suceptibility) or secondary suggestibility (ie, general susceptibility to social influence). Virtually all of these tests have been employed in one or more studies to explore the relationship between suggestibility and placebo responsiveness. Occasionally it will be reported that one particular test had a low, but positive and significant, correlation with placebo reactivity (Duke 1964, Hornsby 1967). The cumulative evidence, however, is persuasive that neither primary nor secondary suggestibility is a reliable or effective predictor of placebo response (Bentler 1963, Steinbook 1965).

The one personality trait found to correlate with placebo responsivity frequently and reliably is generalized chronic anxiety. This relationship appears to be most clearly established for chronically anxious patients treated for pain (Evans 1974). Chronic anxiety has also been linked to placebo-induced symptom reduction for a variety of other psychiatric and somatic complaints. The well-established effects of anxiety on susceptibility to social influence may account for the observation that patient "suggestibility" is associated with placebo responsiveness (Walters and Parke 1964). Perhaps it is the role of anxiety-induced influence susceptibility—secondary suggestibility—that affects placebo response rather than hypnosis-related suggestibility.

Influence of Treatment Agent on Placebo Response

Evidence now available suggests that attitudes and characteristics of the physician rather than those of the patient may be more critical in producing the placebo response (Shapiro 1969). In drug research it is almost axiomatic that double-blind studies produce significantly greater placebo response than those in which the physician knows (or is able to guess) which patients are receiving a placebo (Tetreault 1970). This is consistent with the common finding that physicians' attitudes toward chemotherapy play a significant role in the effectiveness of active drugs (Foreyt 1973, Honigfeld 1963, Lipman 1967, Sheard 1963).

A somewhat more subtle demonstration of the physician's role in placebo effects is the mimicking by placebos of the comparison drug. The analgesic effectiveness of a placebo, for example, averages around 55 percent of the active agent, regardless of whether the analgesic is aspirin, propoxyphene hydrochloride, or morphine (Evans 1974). Apparently, when the administering physician knows or discovers that a powerful analgesic is being used (eg, morphine), the placebo is correspondingly strong. When the analgesic is considered to be less effective (eg, aspirin), the placebo's effects are weaker. In both cases, however, the placebo is about half as effective as the agent tested, thus suggesting that the physician's perception of the active drug has a profound impact on the degree of placebo efficacy. Of similar import is the frequency with which placebos are reported to induce negative side effects equivalent in type and intensity to those associated with the active comparison drug (Pogge 1963). As a result of such findings researchers are beginning to focus more on the physician's contribution to placebo effects and its implications for research design and treatment assessment procedures.

The notion that the physician may be the more crucial placebo component in the doctor–patient relationship is of particular significance to those interested in exploiting the clinical potential of this phenomenon (Gelbman 1967). As long as the patient was assumed to be primarily responsible, the use of placebo as a reliable clinical tool was more limited. A shift of emphasis from patient to physician, however, offers considerably more opportunity for developing and improving placebo therapy techniques and for understanding and teaching the appropriate role of placebo therapy in medical and psychiatric practice.

Among the examples of placebo therapy described in the medical literature is Hollender's (1958) recommendation that the physician adopt a psychologic frame of reference when treating with placebos. Placebo therapy can thus be viewed as a psychologic form of treatment using a physical substance, and may be properly regarded as a form of psychotherapy or behavior-influencing procedure. The selection of patients for treatment with a placebo should be based on the usual criteria employed by the physician for selection of one or another psychologic procedure. Some patients may be relieved of suffering by a physician's reassurance; others may profit from a bit of medical education. Some may need a chance to discuss their problems, and others may be best helped by placebo therapy. All of these constitute recognition of the role of patient psychology in medical practice and of the substantial influence of the physician as a psychologic influence agent.

Once the potency and pervasiveness of the placebo effect are appreciated, steps can be taken by individual physicians to make more systematic use of it as a tool in medical practice and enhance the efficiency with which other remedies are used (Glass 1962). All of these suggestions merely involve making explicit and taking advantage of what is already, and inevitably, a part of physician–patient relationships.

Another practical use of placebos was suggested by Bakke (1960). He recommended use of placebos and the double-blind method in office practice as a means of evaluating the necessity for long-term use of expensive and dangerous medications. He restricted his proposal to treatment of subjective complaints and highly variable objective disorders.

Placebos and Ethics

The literature abounds with controversy over the use of placebos in medical practice. Over the past 30 years, virtually every imaginable point of view has been published at one time or another. A more systematic assessment of practitioner attitudes suggests there are considerable misgivings among some physicians about the propriety of placebo therapy. One interesting fact is that the more frequent use of placebos is attributed to others rather than to one's self (Shapiro 1960). Another study found that physicians with negative attitudes toward placebo use tend to be older, have spent more time in private practice, have engaged in little research, and were defensive about treatment preferences.

At a time when there is growing appreciation of users of placebo therapy, the medical profession is being challenged to be more candid and disclosing with patients about problems and limitations of current medical knowledge and practice. If placebo therapy is regarded as a form of deception, then, of course, an ethical dilemma arises. However, we believe the evidence currently available strongly supports the idea that placebo therapy is a reliable and safe form of treatment for many conditions, if administered with appropriate caution and concern for patient welfare. It may not always be the most effective for most patients, but clearly any treatment that averages 35 percent effectiveness, and more in many cases, cannot be dismissed as merely an unethical deception. The problem is one of definition. Contemporary research supports a definition of placebo therapy as an important and valuable treatment method as well as a methodologic strategy. What is needed is a redefinition of placebo or nonspecific effects in psychologic or psychotherapeutic terms. Of course it follows that physicians must accept a role as psychologic influence agent. The evidence suggests they may have little choice, and that the medical profession has, in fact, relied heavily on psychologic techniques throughout history. However, the future of placebo therapy depends more on public attitudes than on scientific findings. Very likely it will take many years for the public to appreciate the vital and inevitable role of psychologic factors in medical practice.

References

Abbot FK, Mack M, Wolf S: The action of Banthine on the stomach and duodenum of man, with observations on the effects of placebos. Gastroenterology 20:249–261, 1952

Abramson E, Arky RA: Treatment of the obese diabetic. A comparative study of placebo, sulfonylurea and phenformin. Metab Clin Exp 16:204–212, 1967

Bakke JL: Use of the placebo in tests and in treatment. Northwest Med 59:1134–1141, 1960

Beecher HK: The powerful placebo. JAMA 159:1602–1606, 1955

————: Surgery as placebo: a quantitative study of bias. JAMA 176:1102–1107, 1961

————: Placebo effects of situations, attitudes and drugs: a quantiatative study of suggestibility. In Rickels (ed.): Nonspecific Factors in Drug Therapy. Springfield, Ill, Charles Thomas, 1968, pp 27–39

Bentler PM, O'Hara JW, Krasner L: Hypnosis and placebos. Psychol Rep 12:153–154, 1963

Cabot RC: The physician's responsibility for the nostrum evil. JAMA 47:982–983, 1906

Cleghorn RA, Graham BF, Campbell RB, et al: Anxiety states: their response to ACTH and to isotonic saline. In Mote JR (ed): Proceedings of the First Clinical ACTH Conference. Philadelphia, Blakiston, 1949, pp 561–565

Collins RW: Importance of the bladder-cue buzzer contingency in the conditioning treatment for enuresis. J Abnorm Psychol 82:299–308, 1973

Conn JH: Cultural and clinical aspects of hypnosis, placebos and suggestibility. Int J Clin Exp Hypn 7:175–185, 1959

Duke JD: Placebo reactivity and tests of suggestibility. J Pers 32:227–235, 1964

Eldred SH, Bell NW, Sherman LJ: A pilot study comparing the effects of pineal extract and a placebo in patients with chronic schizophrenia. N Engl J Med 263:1330–1335, 1960

Evans FJ: The placebo response in pain reduction. In Bonica JJ (ed): Advances in Neurology, Vol 4. New York, Raven, 1974, pp 289–296

Fisher S: The placebo reactor: thesis, antithesis, synthesis and hypothesis. Dis Nerv Syst 28:510–515, 1967

Foreyt JP, Hagen RL: Covert sensitization: conditioning or suggestion? Abnorm Psychol 82:17–23, 1973

Frankenhaeuser M, Jarpe G, Svan H, Wrangsjo B: Psychophysiological reactions to two different placebo treatments. Scand J Psychol 4:245–250, 1963

Gelbman F: The physician, the placebo and the placebo effect. Ohio State Med J 63:1459–1461, 1967

Glass AJ: Significance of the therapeutic effect of placebos. J Oral Surg, Anesth Hosp Dent Serv 20:25–34, 1962

Greene CS, Laskin DM: Splint therapy for the myofascial pain-dysfunction (MPD) syndrome: a comparative study. Am Dent Assoc 84:624–628, 1972

Hollender MH: Observations on the use of the placebo in medical practice. Am Pract Dig Treat 9:214–217, 1958

Honigfeld G: Physician and patient attitudes as factors influencing the placebo response in depression. Dis Nerv Syst 24:343–347, 1963

Hornsby LD, Bishop MP, Gallant DM: Suggestibility and placebo response: further positive findings. Curr Ther Res 9:46–47, 1967

Krasner L, Ullmann LP: Behavior Influence and Personality. New York, Holt, 1973

Lehmann HE: The placebo response and the double-blind study. In Hoch PH, Zubin J (eds): The Evaluation of Psychiatric Treatment. New York, Grune, 1964, pp 75–93

Liberman R: The elusive placebo reactor. In Brill H, Cole JO, Deniker P, Hippiuf S, Bradley PB (eds): Neuropsychopharmacology, Vol 5. Excerpta Medica Foundation, 1967, pp 557–566

Lipman RS: Differential results of pharmacotherapy in clinics following an identical protocol. In Brill H, Cole JO, Deniker P, Hippiuf S, Bradley PB (eds): Neuropsychopharmacology, Vol 5. Excerpta Medica Foundation, 1967, pp 525–535

McGlynn FD, McDonell RM: Subjective ratings of credibility following brief exposure to desensitization and pseudotherapy. Behav Res Ther 12:141–146, 1974

McGuire WJ: Suspiciousness of experimenter's intent. In Rosenthal R, Rosnow RL (eds): Artifacts in Behavioral Research. New York, Academic, 1969, pp 13–57.

Nicolis FB, Silvestri LG: Hypnotic activity of placebo in relation to severity of insomnia: a quantitative evaluation. Clin Pharmacol Ther 8:841–848, 1967

Pepper OH: A note on the placebo. Am J Pharm 117:409–412, 1945

Pogge RC: The toxic placebo. Part I—Side and toxic effects reported during the administration of placebo medicine. Med Times 91:1–6, 1963

Rickels K: Antineurotic agents: specific and nonspecific effects. In Efron DH (ed): Psychopharmacology—A Review of Progress—1957–1967. Public Health Publication No. 1836. Washington, DC, US Government Printing Office, 1968, pp 231–247.
————, Lipman R, Raab E: Previous medication, duration of illness and placebo response (Librium). J Nerv Ment Dis 142:548–554, 1966

Rossi R, Gilberti F, Conforto C: Autonomic response to intravenous injection of inactive fluid in mental patients. Comp Psychiatry 9:209–217, 1968

Shapiro AK: A contribution to a history of the placebo effect. Behav Sci 5:109–135, 1960

————: Attitudes toward the use of placebos in treatment. J Nerv Ment Dis 130:200–211, 1960

————: Semantics of the placebo. Psychiatr Q 42:653–695, 1968

————: Iatroplacebogenics. Int Pharmacopsychiatr 2:215–248, 1969

————, Wilensky H, Struening E: Study of the placebo effect with a placebo test. Compr Psychiatry 9:118–137, 1968

Sheard M: The influence of doctor's attitude on the patient's response to antidepressant medication. J Nerv Ment Dis 136:6, 1963

Steinbook RM, Jones, MB, Ainslie JD: Suggestibility and the placebo response. J Nerv Ment Dis 140:87–91, 1965

Tetreault L, Bordeleau JM: use of placebo and of the double-blind technique for the evaluation of psychotropes. Encephale 59:5–24, 1970

Walters RH, Parke RD: Social motivation, dependency and susceptibility to social influence. In Berkowitz L (ed): Advances in Experimental Social Psychology, I. New York, Wiley, 1964

Weil A: The Natural Mind. Boston, Houghton Mifflin, 1972

Weingartner AH: Self-administered aversive stimulation with hallucinating hospitalized schizophrenics. J Consult Clin Psychol 36:422–429, 1971

learning and psychopharmacology

commentary

Both patients and practitioners experience behavioral conditioning in their interaction with one another. Drug use also involves conditioned responses, both of the instrumental or operant variety (Skinner) and of the classical variety. Sometimes these conditioning effects may be desirable, as with placebo effects, and sometimes undesirable, as in the persistence of drug habits. Dr. Siegel provides a readable, though erudite, discussion of how conditioning may be of interest to the medical practitioner.

learning and psychopharmacology

Shepard Siegel, Ph.D.

The Experimental Study of Learning

Historically, one of two strategies has generally been adopted in the experimental study of learning. One is to use the paradigm described by the American psychologist Thorndike, and the other is to use the paradigm described by the Russian physiologist Pavlov.

In the Thorndikian (or instrumental) conditioning situation a contingency is arranged such that a designated response, usually skeletal, is instrumental in leading to reinforcement or punishment. The study of instrumental conditioning involves analysis of the modification of monitored behavior as a function of the consequences of the behavior. This approach to the interaction of learning and pharmacology involves the evaluation of behavior change when drug administration is made contingent upon the behavior, and is the method of Skinnerian or operant conditioning.

In the Pavlovian (or classical) conditioning situation, events are presented to the organism without regard to its behavior. A contingency is simply arranged between two environmental events, or stimuli, such that one stimulus reliably predicts the occurrence of a second stimulus. Using the usual terminology, the second of these stimuli is termed the *unconditional stimulus*. The unconditional stimulus, as the name implies, is selected because it elicits relevant activities from the outset—unconditionally—prior to any pairings. The stimulus signaling the presentation of the unconditional stimulus is selected because it is "neutral," ie, it elicits little relevant activity prior to its pairing with the unconditional stimulus, and is termed the *conditional stimulus*. The conditional stimulus, as the name implies, becomes capable of eliciting new responses as a function, ie, conditional upon its pairing with the unconditional stimulus.

In Pavlov's original observations, the conditional stimulus consisted of preparations for feeding (including the sight and smell of the food); the unconditional stimulus was the ingested food. In Pavlov's later and better-known conditioning work (Pavlov 1927), the conditional stimulus was some conveniently manipulated exteroceptive stimulus (bell, light, and so on), and the unconditional stimulus was either food or orally injected dilute acid, both of which elicited a conveniently monitored salivary response.

Classical Conditioning and Psychopharmacology

It was Pavlov who first demonstrated that drugs can be effective unconditional stimuli in the classical conditioning paradigm:

> A dog was given a small dose of apomorphine subcutaneously and after one or two minutes a note of a definite pitch was sounded during a considerable time. While the note was still sounding the drug began to take effect upon the dog: the animal grew restless, began to moisten its lips with its tongue, secreted saliva and showed some disposition to vomit. After the experimenter had reinforced the tone with apomorphine several times it was found that the sound of the note alone sufficed to produce all the active symptoms of the drugs, only in a lesser degree. . . . (Pavlov 1927, p 35)

Additional research by Krylov (reported by Pavlov 1927, pp 35–37), using morphine as the unconditional stimulus, suggested that even if there is no explicit conditional stimulus, such as a tone, the mere preparations for the injection of the drug (the presence of the experimenter, opening the box containing the hypodermic syringe, cropping the fur, and so forth) could stimulate many of the effects of the narcotic. Similar phenomena have been reported in humans with a history of opiate administration (eg, Levine 1974).

Subsequent research (Bykov 1959, Thompson and Pickens 1971) demonstrated that a wide variety of drugs are effective unconditional stimuli in the classic conditioning paradigm, and that a host of visceral and behavioral responses can be affected by initially neutral cues that signal the systemic effects of these drugs. Since, in the absence of special precautions, drug administration is invariably preceded by a set of cues (the administration procedure, or ritual), which have the potential of functioning as conditional stimuli, an analysis of drug effects must include not only the central effects of the chemicals (ie, the unconditional response to the drug) but also responses evidenced in anticipation of the actual pharmacologic assault (ie, conditional responses).

Assessment of Conditional Pharmacologic Response

There are several ways of determining whether the organism has learned the association between predrug environmental cues and the systemic effects of the drug:

1. The conditional response may be detected in the interval between the presentation of the conditional stimulus and the presentation of the unconditional stimulus. For example, in experiments by Yakovlevich (described by Genes 1955, p 213), dogs were brought into a distinctive room (the conditional stimulus) before they were injected with insulin (the unconditional stimulus). After a number of such pairings, merely bringing the dog into the room where it had previously been injected induced the motor behavior, salivation, respiratory changes, and other responses initially elicited by the insulin. Similarly, Rikki (research described by Bykov 1959) placed a dog on a table to administer a choleretic agent on two or three occasions when "a sudden and dramatic increase in bile formation was observed when the animal was placed on the experimental table, preparatory to receiving the cholagogue" (Bykov 1959, p 61).

2. The association between predrug cues and drug may be seen on a test session in which a subject with a history of drug administration is presented with the usual drug administration cues, but either no substance is administered or the subject is injected with a placebo. For example, in rats made morphine-dependent by a regimen of morphine injections, each injection signaled by a bell, the hypothermia symptomatic of morphine withdrawal occurring some hours after the last morphine injection, which is typically relieved by administration of the narcotic, could be reversed by the bell and a physiologic saline placebo (Roffman et al 1973).

   Many other examples of such "placebo effects" in animals are presented by Bykov (1959).

3. Conditional responses evidenced just prior to (or almost simultaneously with) unconditional responses would be expected to interact with the unconditional reflexive effects of a drug, and thus pharmacologic conditioning may be evidenced by modula-

tion of the unconditional effects of the drug. For example, Tatarenko (1954) reported that psychiatric patients who underwent a regimen of insulin shock therapy not only evidenced insulinoid behaviors in anticipation of the central effects of the hormone, but that these conditional responses summated with the unconditional effects of the drug such that it became possible to induce comas with a fraction of the insulin dose initially required. Interestingly the investigators reported that these small doses were effective only if the patients did not see that they were being administered a smaller-than-usual amount of insulin.

The modulation of behavioral activation effects of amphetamine over the course of repeated administrations of the stimulant provides another example of unconditional response alteration by classical conditioning. Amphetamine unconditionally elicits an increase in activity, and such hyperactivity becomes conditioned to drug administration cues (Pickens and Dougherty 1971). In a subject repeatedly injected with amphetamine, the unconditional activity-inducing effect of the drug becomes more pronounced, and this unconditional response modification can be interpreted as a summation of the conditional anticipatory response with the unconditional effects of amphetamine (Tilson and Rech 1973).

The Form of the Conditional Pharmacologic Response

Pavlov's theory of the neurologic basis of conditional response formation exerted a tremendous influence on researchers in the area for many years. The theory demands that the conditional response mimick the unconditional response, and, indeed, much research on pharmacologic conditioning has demonstrated a similarity between learned and reflexively elicited response (Bykov 1959).

However, there is evidence that, depending upon the details of the conditioning situation (not as yet well specified), the conditional response appears to be a preparation for the unconditional response, rather than a replica of it (eg, see Seward 1970, pp 59–60). Perhaps the first example of a preparatory conditional pharmacologic response was provided by Subkov and Zilov (1937). They demonstrated that in dogs repeatedly injected with epinephrine (each injection unconditionally eliciting an increase in heart rate), injection of a placebo elicited a compensatory decrease in heart rate. These investigators cautioned against "the widely accepted view that the external modifications of the conditional reflex must always be identical with the response of the organism to the unconditional stimulus" (Subkov and Zilov 1937, p 296).

Subsequent research has provided many additional examples of compensatory-type conditional drug responses (see summary by Siegel 1975b): in addition to its tachycardiac effect, epinephrine elicits hyperglycemia, and rats with a history of epinephrine administration display a conditional decrease in blood glucose concentration. Compensatory hypoglycemic conditional responses have also been reported if the hyperglycemic unconditional response is elicited more directly by intragastric or intravenous administration of glucose. Similarly, if an unconditional depression in blood glucose is repeatedly induced by injections of a small dose of insulin, injection of a placebo reveals a conditional compensatory increase in blood glucose concentration. In animals repeatedly administered anticholinergic drugs, such as atropine or Ditran (each administration inducing antisialosis), the administration procedure alone, without the drug, leads to excessive salivation.

Although it is traditional to speak of the unconditional (or conditional) response in the classic conditioning situation, it is obvious that the conceptualization of a single, reflexively elicited (or learned) response is a gross oversimplification. Stimuli in general, and pharmacologic stimuli in particular, initiate a complex of responses and homeostatic counter-responses. However, typically only one, or at most a few, of these responses are monitored during the course of conditioning. When multiple components have been measured during the course of conditioning, marked divergencies in the form of conditional and unconditional responses have frequently been noted, with some components of the conditional response mimicking the unconditional response, and some components opposite in direction to the unconditional response. Research by Siegel (1972, 1975a) indicates that the conditional response in rats with a history of insulin injections (and ensuing hypoglycemia and insulinoid behaviors) consists of an insulin-like pattern of motor behavior (decreased activity, convulsions, and nonresponsiveness to peripherally applied stimulation), but simultaneously a compensatory hyperglycemic response; in dogs with a history of anticholinergic drug administration the conditional response consists of a druglike mydriatic but a compensatory hypersalivary response (Lang et al 1966); as indicated earlier, Pavlov (1927) reported that the conditional response following training with morphine consists of morphine-like behavioral symptoms; however Siegel (1975b) reported a compensatory conditional response with respect to pain sensitivity.

There have been attempts to relate the form of the conditional

66   Experimental Psychopharmacology: Drugs as Tools

response to its adaptive significance (Schneiderman 1974) or physiologic pathways involved in the expression of the unconditional response (eg, Wikler 1973). However, the scarcity of data concerning pharmacologic conditioning makes any generalizations about the relationship between the forms of conditional and unconditional responses very tentative.

Significance of the Conditional Pharmacologic Response

Since the central unconditional effects of a drug are almost always signaled by environmental cues associated with the drug administration procedure, the administration of a drug constitutes a Pavlovian conditioning trial, and the psychopharmacologist must be cognizant not only of the unconditional effects of a drug, but also of the potential conditional effects.

Most of us have some familiarity with pharmacologic phenomena, readily interpretable as conditional drug effects. The late-arriving guest at a party may prematurely evidence symptoms of inebriation; the social drinking environment, because of its past association with the central effects of alcohol, may elicit alcohol-like behaviors in an individual before he imbibes sufficiently for these behaviors to be attributable to the systemic effects of alcohol. Similarly the patient with a history of drug administration, when presented with the usual drug administration ritual but now given an inert substance, frequently evidences either druglike (Wolf 1959) or drug-compensatory (Valins and Nisbett 1971) responses. Although there is a tendency to attribute such positive and negative placebo effects to complex cognitive processes involved in the patient–doctor interaction, they are, as has been indicated previously, demonstratable in the experimental animal. It would be difficult to underestimate the role of placebo effects in clinical pharmacology, and the role of Pavolovian conditioning in such phenomena appears well documented (for example, Gliedman et al 1957). Indeed, the clinician can use conditioning principles to therapeutic advantage. To cite just one example, Rubenstein (1931) reported that morphine-addicted patients could be treated by the gradual substitution of conditional stimuli for the opiate.

Conditional drug responses are also relevant to the phenomena of tolerance and sensitization. Therapists and experimental pharmacologists have long known that many of the effects of drugs change over the course of their successive administrations. The drug effect may become less than it was originally (tolerance) or more pronounced than it was originally (sensitization). Most theories of altered drug responsiveness as a function of repeated experience with the drug postulate some systemic change within the organism as a result of the initial drug experience, which either modifies receptor sensitivity to the drug, changes the metabolism of the drug, or induces some immunifacient effect. However, recent research suggests a role for Pavlovian conditioning processes in understanding changes in the effect of a drug over the course of repeated administrations (ie, repeated pairings of the environmental conditional stimuli and pharmacologic unconditional stimuli).

Many instances of drug tolerance may be due to compensatory conditional responses. Such a conditional response, evidenced in anticipation of the actual pharmacologic assault, should serve to attenuate the effects of the drug. As predrug environmental stimuli are paired with increasing frequency with the systemic effects of the drug, the magnitude of the compensatory conditional response would be expected to increase, hence the degree to which the pharmacologic unconditional response is attenuated should become more marked, producing tolerance. Many studies (see review by Siegel 1975b) have demonstrated the importance of environmental cues in the acquisition of tolerance in the rat. That is, the magnitude of tolerance to the analgesic effect of morphine depends upon the number of pairings of a distinct drug administration ritual with the systemic effects of the drug, rather than merely the frequency with which the drug has been systemically introduced. Subsequent research (Siegel 1975b) demonstrated that when rats with a history of morphine administration are presented with the usual drug administration procedure but are actually administered a placebo, they respond with a conditional, heightened sensitivity to nociceptive stimulation, and analgesic tolerance can be understood as resulting from attenuation of the unconditional analgesic effect of the narcotic by this conditional, compensatory, hyperalgesic response.

Another phenomenon associated with repeated morphine administration further suggests that conditional responses serve to modulate the unconditional effects of a drug over the course of repeated administrations. Small doses of the opiate in rats cause an enhancement of general motor activity, and this hyperactivity becomes more pronounced over the course of successive administrations of morphine (Babbini and Davis 1972). The conditional activity response in rats with a history of injections of such small doses of morphine is a drug like increase in activity (Kamat et al 1974). Thus, it appears likely that sensitization to the activity-inducing effects of morphine is due to augmentation of the unconditional activation effects of the drug by conditional hyperactivity elicited by the injected procedure. Research has been described previously (Tilson and Rech 1973), which similarly suggests that sensitization of the activity inducing effects of amphetamine is readily interpretable as a conditioning phenomenon.

There is a substantial body of clinical literature which, in agreement with experimental evidence, indicates that pharmacologic conditioning is an important determinant of pharmacologic responsivity. For example, it has been frequently noted (Schuster and Villarreal 1968) that the effects of opioids are quite different if they are passively received (as in the case of a patient undergoing medical treatment) or self-administered following a distinctive ritual (as in the case of drug abuse by medical professionals). Furthermore, both evidence from the laboratory with animal subjects (eg, Thompson and Ostlund 1965) and clinical observations of human patients and addicts (eg, Levine 1974, Wikler 1973) strongly suggest that Pavlovian conditioning principles are relevant to drug dependence phenomena. This is discussed more fully in Wikler's chapter in this volume.

References

Babbini M, Davis WM: Time-dose relationships for locomotor activity effects of morphine after acute or repeated treatment. Br J Pharmacol 46:213–224, 1972

Bykov KM: The cerebral cortex and the internal organs. Moscow, Foreign Languages Publishing House, 1959

Genes SG: The nervous system and internal secretion (Nervnaya sistema i veotrennyaya sekretsiya). Moscow, Gosudarstvennoe Isdatelistvo Meditsinskoi Literaturii Medgiz, 1955 (Read in translation parepared by Shein LJ, Department of Russian, McMaster University.)

Gliedman LH, Gantt WH, Teitelbaum HA: Some implications of conditional reflex studies for placebo research. Am J Psychiatry 113:1103–1107, 1957

Kamat KA, Dutta SN, Pradhan SN: Conditioning of morphine-induced enhancement of motor activity. Res Commun Chem Pathol Pharmacol 7:367–373, 1974

Lang WJ, Brown ML, Gershon S, Korol B: Classical and physiologic adaptive conditioned responses to anticholinergic drugs in conscious dogs. Int J Neuropharmacol 5:311–315, 1666

Levine DG: "Needle freaks": compulsive self-injection by drug users. Am J Psychiatary 131:297–300, 1974

Pavlov IP: Conditioned Reflexes (Translated by GV Anrep). London, Oxford, 1927 (Reprinted, New York, Dover, 1960)

Pickens R, Doughterty J: Conditioning the activity effects of drugs. In Thompson T, Schuster C (eds): Stimulus Properties of Drugs. New York, Appleton, 1971

Roffman M, Reddy C, Lal H: Control of morphine-withdrawal hypothermia by conditional stimuli. Psychopharmacologia 29:197–201, 1973

Rubenstein C: The treatment of morphine addiction in tuberculosis by Pavlov's conditioning method. Am Rev Tuberc 24:682–685, 1931

Schneiderman N: The relationship between learned and unlearned cardiovascular response. In Obrist PA, Black AH, DiCara LV (eds): Cardiovascular Psychophysiology: Current Issues in Response Mechanisms, Biofeedback and Methodology. Chicago, Aldine, 1974

Schuster CR, Villarreal JE: The experimental analysis of opiod dependence. In Effron DH, Cole JO, Levine J, Wittenborn JR (eds): Psychopharmacology: A Review of Progress. Washington, DC, U.S. Government Printing Office (Public Health Service Publication Number 1836), 1968

Seward JP: Condition theory. In Marx M (ed): Learning: Theories. New York, Macmillan, 1970

Siegel S: Conditioning of insulin-induced glycemia. J Comp Physiol Psychol 78:233–241, 1972

————: Conditioning insulin effects. J Comp Physiol Psychol 89:189–199, 1975a

————: Evidence from rats that morphine tolerance is a learned response. J Comp Physiol Psychol 89:498–506, 1975b

Subkov AA, Zilov GN: The role of conditioned reflex adaptation in the origin of hyperergic reactions. Bull Biol Med Exp 4:294–296, 1937

Tatarenko NP: Pathophysiology of schizophrenia. Zhurnal Neuropatologii i Psikhiatrii Imeni S.S. Korsakova 54:710–714, 1954 (Available as Technical Translation 1720 from the National Research Council of Canada.)

Thompson T, Ostlund W Jr: Susceptibility to readdiction as a function of the addiction and withdrawal environments. J Comp Physiol Psychol 60:388–392, 1965

————, Pickens R (eds): Stimulus Properties of Drugs. New York, Appleton, 1971

Tilson HA, Rech RH: Conditioned drug effects and absence of tolerance to d-amphetamine induced motor activity. Pharmacol Biochem Behav 1:149–153, 1973

Valins S, Nisbett RE: Attribution processes in the development and treatment of emotional disorders. In Jones EE, Kanouse DE, Kelley HH, et al: Attribution: Perceiving the Causes of Behavior. Morristown, NJ, General Learning Press, 1971

Wikler A: Dynamics of drug dependence. Arch Gen Psychiatry 28:611–616, 1973

Wolf S: The pharmacology of placebos. Pharmacol Rev 11:689–704, 1959

drug state-dependent learning

commentary

Certain psychoactive drugs produce a state of intoxication characterized by a change in consciousness, thinking, and other cognitive activities. The question frequently arises as to whether the intoxicated state is dissociated from the sober state, so that in effect the individual is a different person. Frequently, even though a patient seems to be able to communicate while intoxicated, he cannot remember what happened to him when he becomes sober. This one-way amnesia is frequently encountered, but we cannot be sure whether the last memories were never acquired or simply cannot be retrieved. More rarely, one finds a two-way dissociation in which the individual is able to recover his lost memories if he is again intoxicated. In this case there is an obvious error of retrieval, and the memory storage must be intact.

Drug discrimination occurs when an individual is sophisticated enough to recognize a particular drug. It can be expected that drug-dependent individuals should be able to recognize the drugs to which they are addicted. The cues that individuals use in distinguishing drugs have not been carefully studied as yet, and for the untrained subject they are often difficult to describe. In addition to the primary sensory effects of drugs, there is the pleasantness (eg, of sedative hypnotics or amphetamines) as compared with the unpleasantness (the phenothiazines and various antihypertensive drugs). More research is needed to characterize the acceptability of drugs.

drug state-dependent learning*

Donald A. Overton, Ph.D.

Amnesia and Dissociation

This chapter concerns drug effects on memorization and memory retrieval, especially the amnesias produced by drugs. The term *amnesia* refers to a situation in which something cannot be remembered that might reasonably be expected to be remembered. Hence, if a person is unable to recall his name or what he did yesterday, the term amnesia is appropriate. However, the word amnesia is not used to describe normal forgetting or the elimination of responses through experimental extinction.

Some amnesias are permanent. A patient who suffers a head injury may never be able to recall events that occurred just before the injury. It is commonly assumed that the head injury somehow disrupted the process of memory consolidation so that memories of the few minutes prior to injury were not permanently recorded in the brain. Other amnesias are temporary and reversible. At one point in time a patient may show extensive amnesia for events that occurred during the preceding year, and two weeks later he may show good recall for the same events. Obviously, the memories were in the brain all the while, but were temporarily irretrievable.

The term *dissociation* is sometimes used in cases where memories are irretrievable but still present in the brain. The word dissociation is used quite concretely to indicate that various memories in the brain have somehow detached from one another, leaving some

*Supported in part by DA-00301 and MH-25136.

memories retrievable and others not. Striking examples of dissociation, such as fugue states and cases of multiple personality, are infrequent. However, dissociation also occurs in everyday life. For
example, Evans et al (1970) report a dissociation between the waking state and the REM sleep state. This may contribute to the
difficulty people have in recalling their dreams. Dissociations of
memory can also be induced by drugs that produce an effect called
state-dependent learning (Overton 1968). This drug effect makes
memory retrieval depend on reinstatement of the drug condition
that existed during memorization. If a different drug state is present,
then memories will be dissociated, ie, irretrievable. Drug-induced
dissociation and other drug effects on memory are the primary subject of this chapter.

Drugs have several different effects on memory, and Table 1 describes four common effects of drugs on the memory process. The
table shows the possible outcomes of a test for retention of a memory
(or response) that has previously been learned. There are four possible pairs of drug conditions; the subject may be either undrugged or
drugged during initial learning and during retention testing. The
four columns in the table represent the four possible combinations of
drug treatments.

A very common drug effect on memory is impairment of the process of memorization by the drug so that memories are not formed
(Row A in Table 1). Groups 3 and 4 did not form permanent
memories because they were drugged during the learning experience; Groups 1 and 2 did form memories and recall them during
testing. The drug does not prevent retrieval of memories in Group 2.
The drugged subjects resemble senile persons who can remember
events that happened earlier in life even though they have great
difficulty in forming new memories. Row B of the table illustrates
the case in which drug prevents adequate retrieval of memories,
even though it did not prevent initial consolidation. Groups 1 and 3
both show good recall as they are undrugged during retention testing; Groups 2 and 4 show that the drug impairs retrieval; Group 3
shows that memories could be formed under the influence of drug.
Drug effects on retrieval have not been studied extensively and may
not occur frequently in humans. Row C of Table 1 illustrates a state-
dependent learning effect. Retention occurs whenever testing takes
place under the same drug condition that was present during initial
learning. Groups 1 and 4 remember well, and the unimpaired recall
by Group 4 illustrates that material can be both learned and recalled
under the influence of drug; neither Groups 2 nor 3 remember, because the drug state during retention testing differs from that present
during training. It can be demonstrated that the amnesias in Groups

TABLE 1
COMMON EFFECTS OF DRUGS ON MEMORIZATION
AND RETRIEVAL*

	Group			
	1	2	3	4
Independent variables				
Drug state during learning	N	N	D	D
Drug state during retention	N	D	N	D
Inferred effect of drug				
A. Defect in memorization	+	+	−	−
B. Defect in retrieval	+	−	+	−
C. State-dependent learning	+	−	−	+
D. Asymmetrical dissociation	+	+	−	+

N = No drug; D = drug
+ = indicates normal performance during testing.
− = indicates impaired performance during testing.

*Good performance during testing indicates that both memorization and memory retrieval were unimpaired.

2 and 3 are based on dissociation of memory by showing that Group 2 will remember when undrugged (the training state) and Group 3 will remember when drugged. The memories are actually present in the brain in all four groups but are irretrievable in Groups 2 and 3 under the changed-state test conditions. As can be seen, the so-called state-dependent learning effect actually involves a state-dependent defect in retrieval. Finally, Row D in the table illustrates an effect called "asymmetrical dissociation." Responses learned while undrugged can be remembered with or without drug. However, responses learned while drugged can be recalled only when the subject is again drugged and are irretrievable in the nondrug state. This effect has been frequently observed in animal experiments, but is poorly understood.

Clinical Significance of Memory Dissociation

The clinical significance of dissociation of memory induced by drugs has not been adequately explored. There have been virtually no studies thus far using clinical doses of therapeutic agents in a medical context. However, nonclinical human and animal experiments allow us to make rather educated guesses about the probable clinical significance of drug dissociation (Overton 1972). First, strong dissociative effects are observed only when high doses of a drug are used. These doses must be sufficient to produce obvious behavioral toxicity (eg, drunkenness, ataxia, confusion, disorientation, or loss of judgment). It follows that dissociation would not occur with normal doses of minor tranquilizers used for outpatient treatment of neurotic anxiety. Second, drugs differ markedly from one another in their ability to dissociate learning; even at toxic doses some drugs produce little dissociation (eg, phenothiazines). Third, a particular change in drug state will often dissociate one type of learning while leaving another type virtually unaffected. For example, Bliss (1974) used monkeys to show that a learned color discrimination response was dissociated by pentobarbital but a position discrimination was not. This finding places some limitations on our ability to extrapolate from experimental materials to clinical learning situations, and it emphasizes the importance of confirming basic research by further studies in clinical settings. However, such studies will not be easy to conduct due to some serious methodologic problems (Overton 1974).

Although drug-induced dissociations will not be observed with low doses of most drugs, there are clinical situations where dissociated learning is likely. For example, learning may occur at certain stages of surgical anesthesia, and such learning may be dissociated (Levinson 1965). In this case the patient will report amnesia after he recovers from anesthesias, but nonetheless memories may have been formed. Fortunately, it is becoming customary to restrict conversation in the operating arena to statements that might be uttered if the patient were conscious. Another situation in which state dependency may occur is that in which intoxicating doses of minor tranquilizers are used as adjuncts to conditioning of desensitization therapy. Drugs reduce anxiety and hence may facilitate new learning. However, the patient's subsequent recall of the new learned responses may be somewhat impaired by dissociation after the drug wears off, thus reducing the overall effectiveness of the treatment. Third, partially dissociated learning is reported to occur when people get drunk with alcohol or very "high" with other abused drugs (Goodwin et al 1969, Rickles et al 1973). Hence, patients' reports of their behavior during episodes of drug intoxication may be inaccurate.

Drug Discrimination

Drug discrimination is a phenomenon closely related to state-dependent learning. Rats can learn to respond differentially, depending on whether or not they are drugged; eg, turn right in a maze when drugged and turn left when undrugged. Drugs differ in their ability to control such discriminative behavior, and Table 2 shows the ease with which rats can discriminate a number of common drugs. With most drugs, repeated training sessions are required be-

TABLE 2
RELATIVE DISCRIMINABILITY OF VARIOUS DRUGS*

Easy to discriminate	Moderately discriminable	Difficult to discriminate
Anesthetics	*Stimulants*	*Phenothiazines*
Alcohol	Amphetamine	Chlorpromazine
Barbiturates	Cocaine	Perphenazine
Meprobamate	Methylphenidate	
Methyprylon		*MAO inhibitors*
Ether	*Narcotic analgesics*	Parnate
	Morphine	Phenelzine
Dissociative Anesthetics	Codeine	
Ketamine	Meperidine	*Muscarinics*
Phencyclidine		Physostigmine
	Hallucinogenics	Carbachol
Minor Tranquilizers	Mescaline	
Chlordiazepoxide	LSD	*Convulsants*
Diazepam		Bemegride
Flurazepam	*Muscle relaxants*	Picrotoxin
	Carisprodol	
Nicotinics	Methocarbamol	*Anticonvulsants*
Nicotine		Dilantin
	Antinicotinics	Trimethadione
Antimuscarinics	Mecamylamine	
Artane	Pempidine	*Narcotic antagonists*
Atropine		Naltrexone
Scopolamine	*Antihistamines*	Naloxone
Ditran	Benadryl	
	Dramamine	*Analgesics*
Miscellaneous		Aspirin
Dextromethorphan	*Serotonin blockers*	Antipyrine
Nikethamide	Cyproheptadine	
	Methysergide	*Miscellaneous*
		Lithium
	Tricyclics	Curare
	Imipramine	
	Doxepin	

*Highly discriminable drugs produce state-dependent retrieval.

fore the animals eventually learn the discrimination. However, with some "easily discriminated" drugs, increases in dose produce more and more rapid discrimination, until at high doses only two training sessions are required to produce criterion performance (Overton 1974). In this case, the behaviors can reasonably be called *state dependent*. For example, suppose that a monkey is trained to press a red lever while drugged. Then, on another day while undrugged, it is trained to press a blue lever. After the second training session the monkey has mastered both habits and will regularly press the red lever when drugged and press the blue lever when undrugged (Bliss 1974). In each condition the monkey is unable to recall one response due to dissociation and performs exclusively the other nondissociated response. His behavior is controlled by the imposed drug state. Hence we see that discriminative drug effects produce state-dependent learning if they are sufficiently strong.

Three facts about drug discriminations are most salient: (a) they can develop with doses of drug much lower than those required to produce obvious dissociative amnesias; (b) almost all drugs that act on the brain are discriminable to some degree, but some are more readily discriminated than others (Table 2); and (c) drug discriminations generally develop only after repeated exposures to drug, except in the case of drugs with strong dissociative effects.

Drug discriminations in man have not yet been investigated. However, they occur reliably in several animal species, and it appears almost certain that they will occur in humans and have appreciable clinical relevance. Drug abuse appears to provide the conditions necessary for the development of drug discriminations; drugs are repeatedly administered and drug users are typically exposed to consistently different reinforcement contingencies while drugged than while undrugged. Reinforcement theory suggests that drug abusers should eventually develop a repertoire of drug-state responses that differs from their normal undrugged behavior. As another example, suppose that a patient consistently takes Librium only when he expects to be exposed to an anxiety-provoking situation. It is conceivable that some of the patient's "anxious" behaviors may become associated with the drug state, thus reducing the utility of the drug and perhaps eventually causing it to trigger rather than allay anxiety. Finally, and less speculatively, repeated experience with various drugs apparently increases a person's ability to make discriminations between drug states.

This chapter has dealt with two drug effects: state-dependent learning and drug discriminations. State-dependent learning has been repeatedly demonstrated in human subjects. However, since it is only produced by high (toxic) doses of drugs, its clinical relevance may be restricted to a smaller number of situations than has sometimes been suggested (Heistad 1957). Drug discriminations in humans have not been studied as yet. However, they are reliably produced by low doses of drugs in other species; thus it seems likely they will also be significant in human subjects.

References

Bliss DK: Theoretical explanations of drug-dissociated behaviors. Fed Proc 33:1787–1796, 1974

Evans FJ, Gustafson LA, O'Connell DN, Orne MT, Shore RE: Verbally induced behavioral responses during sleep. J Nerv Ment Dis 150:171–187, 1970

Goodwin DW, Powell B, Bremer D, Hoine H, Stern J: Alcohol and recall: state dependent effects in man. Science 163:1358–1360, 1969

Heistad GT: A bio-psychological approach to somatic treatments in psychiatry. Am J Psychiatry 114:540–545, 1957

Levinson BW: States of awareness during general anesthesia—preliminary communication. Br J Anaesthesiol 37:544–546, 1965

Overton DA: Dissociated learning in drug states (state-dependent learning). In Efron DH, Cole JO, Levine J, Wittenborn R (eds): Psychopharmacology, A Review of Progress, 1957–1967, Public Health Service Publication 1836 U.S. Government Printing Office, Washington, DC, pp 918–930, 1968

———: State-dependent learning produced by alcohol and its relevance to alcoholism. In Kissen B, Begleiter H (eds): The Biology of Alcoholism Vol 11: Physiology and Behavior. New York, Plenum Press, 1972, pp 193–217

———: Experimental methods for the study of state-dependent learning. Fed Proc 33:1800–1813, 1974

Rickles WH, Jr, Cohen MJ, Whitaker CA, McIntyre KE: Marijuana induced state-dependent verbal learning. Psychopharmacologia 30:349–354, 1973

anesthesia
and the brain

commentary

The neural basis of consciousness is a subject of inestimable importance. Almost all drugs in sufficient doses influence consciousness and arousal, but the anesthetics and sedative-hypnotics have a particular ability to influence this function. Sedative drugs are used to allay anxiety in doses that have only a minimal effect upon consciousness (see p 309, 327). But the widespread use of drugs such as phenobarbital, meprobamate, and diazepam for the treatment of anxiety must be related to their usefulness in larger doses for the induction of sleep (see p 105). The volatile anesthetics, because of their physical characteristics, are not used in the daily practice of medicine, although chloral hydrate and ethyl alcohol do share some features with the more potent anesthetic agents.

The reticular activating system, whose function was first elucidated by Dr. Magoun, maintains its importance as a site of action for drugs that influence states of consciousness. It would pay the practitioner to study this chapter, even though he may be unfamiliar with some of the terminology, because he would learn about some of the basic research in neuropharmacology.

anesthesia and the brain

Horace W. Magoun, Ph.D.

The Reticular Formation of the Brain Stem and General Anesthesia

Over the past quarter century, considerable attention has been directed to the reticular formation of the brain stem for its role in the initiation and maintenance of wakefulness, and conversely in the suppression of sleep. During arousal of a sleeping animal by peripheral stimulation, the same conversion of large-amplitude slow waves and spindle bursts to low-voltage fast activity in the EEG was obtained by direct electrical stimulation of the brain stem reticular formation. On recording from the reticular formation, all modalities of afferent stimulation (sound, sight, smell, touch) evoked potentials in this region and appeared to exert their arousing influence through its diffuse projections to the cortex (Morillo and Baylor 1963) (Fig. 1). Moreover, experimental destruction of this region was followed by chronic unresponsiveness, even though major afferent pathways to the cortex were spared and viable.

Against this background it was natural to explore the possible involvement of the reticular formation in general anesthesia. In Figure 2 light doses of barbiturates, which eliminated electroencephalographic arousal during afferent stimulation, were seen also to block arousal evoked by direct stimulation of the reticular formation. Similarly, in recording experiments, responses elicited in the reticular formation by somatic afferent stimulation were progressively diminished or eliminated during deepening barbiturate anesthesia;

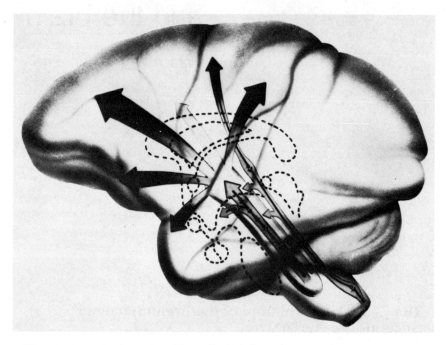

Fig. 1. Lateral view of monkey's brain, showing ascending reticular system in the brain stem, receiving spino-reticular and paralemniscal afferents, and projecting widely to the cerebral cortex. Reproduced by permission from Magoun HW: The ascending reticular system and wakefulness. In Delfresnaye JF (ed): Brain Mechanisms and Consciousness Oxford, Blackwell, 1954, p. 1

while those recorded from the cortical sensory areas were unattenuated or increased in amplitude in their initial phases, although later components were typically reduced. From these pioneering studies in the early 1950s, it appeared that a reversible pharmacologic blockade of ascending arousing influences of the reticular formation contributed significantly to the induction of general anesthesia induced by barbiturates and ether (Fig. 3).

Over the intervening period to the present, the observations pertaining to barbiturate anesthesia have repeatedly been confirmed and extended (Borbely 1973); those involving ether have been opposed by some and supported by others (Lindsley and Adey 1961); and a range of new insights and concepts have become available from the application of increasingly sophisticated investigative techniques. A brief review of their highlights may now be presented.

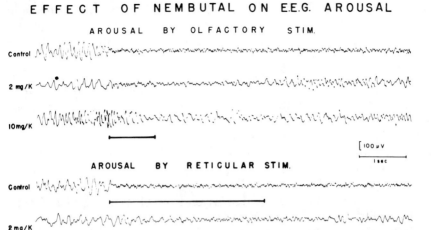

Fig. 2. EEG of curarized rabbit, showing effects of doses of pentobarbital upon EEG arousal induced by olfactory (above) and midbrain RF (below) stimulation (heavy line). Reproduced by permission from Arduini A, Arduini MG: J Pharmacol Exp Ther 110:76, 1954

Somatic Afferent Excitation (Sensory Stimulation) of the Reticular Formation

In 1957 Davis et al investigated the effects of several anesthetics on the amplitude of somatic afferent-evoked responses in the midbrain reticular formation and the sensory relay nucleus of the thalamus. Nitrous oxide, a poor hypnotic but potent analgesic, had the least effect on either system. Barbiturates, potent hypnotics but poor analgesics, markedly depressed the reticular formation potential, but left thalamic potentials relatively intact. Cyclopropane, both a strong hypnotic and analgesic, affected both systems appreciably, the reticular formation earlier and more profoundly. These results were considered to support the concept that the general anesthetic state is associated with reversible suppression of the midbrain reticular formation activating system.

In 1966 Boyd and Meritt showed that barbiturates depressed the recovery cycle of afferent evoked responses, both in the thalamic sensory relay nucleus and the midbrain reticular formation, the more dramatic and marked effects occurring in the latter. It was concluded that depression of the reticular formation by barbiturates could be a significant factor in the production of sedation. In 1968 Gyermeck indicated that evoked potentials and electroencephalographic arousal, induced by corticifugal excitation of the reticular formation by stimulating the opposite internal capsule, were also highly vulnerable to barbiturate anesthesia.

In 1969 with implanted electrodes, Olds and Olds demonstrated that unit (single cell) discharges evoked in the reticular formation by somatic afferent stimulation, in freely moving rats, were significantly more depressed at lower doses of barbiturates and at an earlier time than were responses in the preoptic area of the hypothalamus and hippocampus. Blockade of conduction of impulses within the reticular formation, of electroencephalographic arousal in the cortex, and of theta rhythms in the hippocampus,

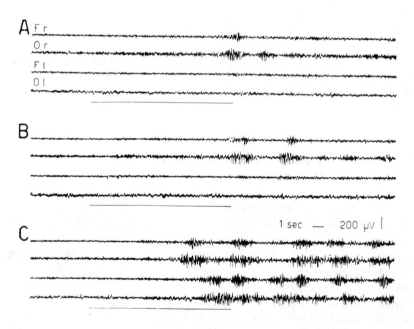

Fig. 3. EEG changes in encephale isole cat induced by injection of 0.1 mg (A), 0.3 mg (B), and 0.6 mg (C) of thiopental directly into right carotid circulation. Channels record from right (r) and left (1), frontal (F) and occipital (O) cortical areas. Reproduced by permission from Magni F, Moruzzi G, Rossi CF, Zanchetti A: Arch Ital Biol 97:33, 1959

induced by stimulation of the reticular formation, were attributed to the direct action of barbiturates on drug receptors in the reticular formation before other structures were influenced.

In 1971 Golovchinsky and Plehotkina observed that barbiturates caused marked depression of activity in the midbrain reticular formation, responses evoked by somatic stimulation, and electroencephalographic arousal induced by stimulation of the reticular formation. Barbiturates had no effect, however, on cortical transcallosal responses, which provided a direct test of cortical excitability. By contrast, ether caused early and marked depression of transcallosal cortical responses, and although it caused early depression of afferent input to the reticular formation, it displayed only weaker influences upon the intrinsic excitability of the reticular formation. These observations indicated that mechanisms of general anesthesia were not identical for different anesthetic agents. Barbiturate anesthesia was attributable to depression of the reticular formation, whereas the anesthetic action of ether was attributed to depression of cortical activity.

Auditory Excitation of the Reticular Formation

To examine the role of the auditory system in drug-induced sedation, Winters et al (1967) and Mori et al (1968), recorded the cortical electroencephalogram, click-evoked responses in the cochlear nucleus, and multiple unit activity in the midbrain reticular formation during progressively deepening stages of anesthesia induced by barbiturates, ether, halothane, and nitrous oxide. All records during Stages I and II, when the latter occurred, were characteristic of central neural excitation; whereas those of Stage III were typical of central neural depression. During Stage III, responses of the cochlear nucleus (the first relay nucleus in the auditory system) remained unchanged, whereas those of the reticular formation and auditory cortex were progressively reduced. Levels of unit activity in the reticular formation dropped rapidly in Stage III. In general the reticular formation was markedly depressed by anesthesia when auditory input was only minimally affected. These findings agreed with the original observations of French et al (1953), and other reviewed above, that ascending conduction in the reticular formation evoked by afferent stimulation is blocked by anesthetic agents when activity is classic sensory pathways is relatively intact; depression of activity in the reticular formation leads to loss of consciousness and induction of the general anesthetic state (Figs. 4 through 6).

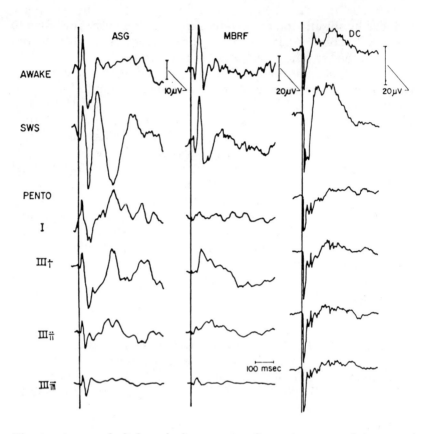

Fig. 4. Averaged click-evoked responses of anterior suprasylvian cortex (ASG), midbrain RF (MBRF) and dorsal cochlear nucleus (DC) of chronic implanted cats during wakefulness (Awake), slow wave sleep (SWS), and the stages of pentothal anesthesia indicated at left. Reproduced by permission from Mori K, Winters WD, Spooner CE: EEG Clin Neurophysiol 24:242, 1963

Visual Excitation of the Reticular Formation

In 1969 Bonnet and Briot investigated the late components of the visual cortical response evoked by stimulation of the optic nerve or lateral geniculate nucleus. An initial component, limited to the visual area, represented discharge of the specific visual cortical projection. It was followed by two later, more widely distributed waves—T1 and T2—considered to be nonspecific projections—T1 from the thalamus and T2 from the midbrain reticular formation. T1 was preserved but T2 was eliminated by precollicular transection of the brain stem. Although the initial component was unaffected, both

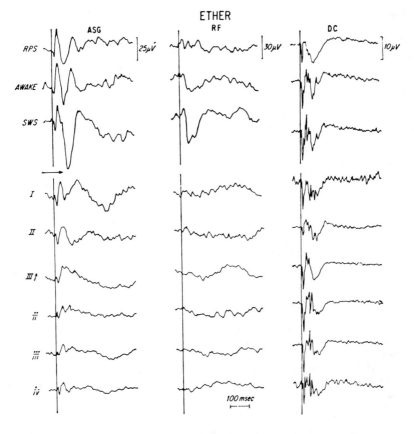

Fig. 5.   As Figure 4, but during stages of ether anesthesia. Reproduced by permission from Mori K, Winters WD, Spooner CE: EEG Clin Neurophysiol 24:242, 1968

of these latter elements were eliminated by barbiturate anesthesia.

In 1969 Nakai and Domino observed that barbiturates markedly depressed both cortical visual responses and influences of the reticular formation on them, the former more than the latter. Their results indicated that barbiturates had a somewhat greater depressive effect on the neocortex than on the midbrain reticular formation.

Synaptic Organization and Susceptibility of the Reticular Formation to Anesthetic Agents

In the original study identifying blockade of the reticular formation in anesthesia, French et al (1963) noted that, upon afferent stimula-

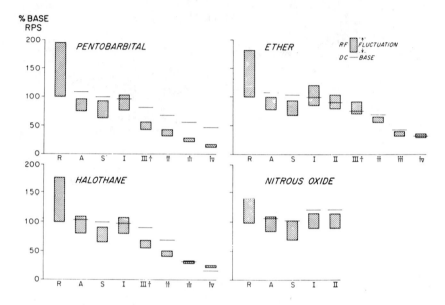

Fig. 6. Bar-graphs representing multiple unit activity of midbrain RF during rhombencephalic sleep (R), wakefulness (A), slow wave sleep (S) and Stages (I-) of pentobarbital, ether, halothane, and nitrous oxide anesthesia. Height of bar indicates neuronal excitability expressed as percent of level during rhombencephalic sleep (percent base RPS). Reproduced by permission from Mori K, Winters WD, Spooner CE: EEG Clin Neurophysiol 24:242, 1968

tion, the brief, short-latency, spikelike potential of the lemniscal pathway was known to be paucisynaptic and, without any direct evidence, the reticular formation pathway was inferred to be multisynaptic, a feature that was proposed to account for its susceptibility to anesthetics.

Contrary evidence was not long in accumulating, however. In 1956 King reported that electroencephalographic arousal induced by stimulation of the reticular formation was blocked selectively, not only by small doses of barbiturates but also by anesthetic doses of chloralosane and ether. In analogous experiments, however, nonanesthetic interneuron-depressant agents, such as mephenesin and the benzothiazoles, had no influence upon the excitability of the electroencephalographic arousal system. Although the results clearly eliminated a proposed multisynaptic organization accounting for the sensitivity of the reticular formation to anesthetic agents, they provided additional support for the hypothesis that selective depression of the reticular formation might account for the loss of wakefulness and the blockade of arousal to afferent stimulation during anesthesia (see also Killiam 1962, 1968).

In a related direction, in 1961, the exquisite silver-impregnation studies of the Scheibels identified the absence of true short-axoned, Golgi Type II cells in the reticular formation of the brain stem and revealed instead an extensive overlap and arborization of the many collaterals of long ascending and descending processes of reticular neurons. In the immediate neighborhood of each reticular soma (cell body), they found hundreds of heterogenous dendrites of near and distant cells. The terminals of as many as six or more separate fiber systems might converge upon and contribute to the terminal array on any single reticular neuron.

In the same year Yamoto and Schaeppi (1961) analyzed modifications in the patterns of unit firing in the midbrain reticular formation and sensory cortex during barbiturate anesthesia. In commenting on the findings they suggested that neurons with looser or less dense synapses might be more sensitive to anesthetic agents, both in the cortex and in the reticular formation. Units dominated by a single afferent system were more resistant to anesthesia than others activated from several sources. In the reticular formation each neuron received converging impulses from different peripheral receptors and central origins. The anesthetic action of barbiturates, they proposed, might not be due to any special affinity of the drug for the reticular formation but to the more complicated and weaker synaptic organization of this region.

In 1966 Mannen classified the gray matter of the central nervous system into nuclei with extrafocal dendrites, called *open nuclei*, and those lacking such terminals, called *closed nuclei*. The dendrites of open nuclei extended beyond the limits of the nucleus and penetrated neighboring regions. In the brain stem, the reticular formation constituted a vast such open system. It included several cellular masses, the dendrites of which overlapped one another extensively. A prime example was the gigantocellular nucleus, the limits of which were almost impossible to define. The Scheibels had calculated that there were about 4125 neurons in a territory occupied by the soma and dendrites of a single neuron in the gigantocellular nucleus. In the reticular formation each large cell had an average of 61 dendritic branches, a surface of 68,600 μm^2 and a volume of 78,700 μm^3 with 90 percent of its surface and volume in a sphere 600 μm in diameter.

The functional implications of these differential synaptic organizations have most recently been elaborated by Albe-Fessard et al (1970). They point out that, in specific relays, conservation of a point-to-point organization all along the pathway means that a large

number of axon terminals converge upon, and make powerful connections with, a small number of postsynaptic neurons so that spatial summation is maximal. This results in a high safety factor for
synaptic transmission as well as resistance to anesthetic blockade.

By contrast divergence and dispersal is the rule in nonspecific
relays, and terminals of a single axon are distributed to a very large
number of postsynaptic elements. Spatial summation is minimal,
and temporal summation, requiring the coincidental discharge of
terminals from a variety of sources, is required for impulse transmission. The inherently low safety factor of such an arrangement reduces the probability that a signal, arriving by any single axon, will
be transmitted to the next neuron. Precisely timed convergence of
signals from several sources is necessary for transmission in this
type of synaptic organization. In the view of Albe-Fessard et al this
feature, and not some nonexistent multiplicity of synapses, makes
nonspecific or "open" relays more susceptible to certain anesthetics
than specific or "closed" relays.

Postsynaptic Potentials and General Anesthesia

With possible relevance to features of the synaptic organizations just
discussed, Brazier, in 1970, recalled attention to the earlier studies
of Somjen and Gill (1963) on the mechanism of anesthetic blockade
of synaptic transmission in the spinal cord. They recorded ventral
(motor) root potentials evoked transsynaptically by stimulation of
the corresponding dorsal (sensory) root. In the control state the excitatory postsynaptic potential rose rapidly to the level required for
initiation of a conducted spike potential. During barbiturate or ether
anesthesia, there was no delay in the onset of the excitatory postsynaptic potential, but its rise-time was markedly slowed and the
level to which it rose was reduced, so that its build-up to the
threshold required for conducted depolarization of the motor neuron
was prevented. Alternatively, because the excitatory postsynaptic
potential is a graded, rather than an all-or-none process, its failure to
reach the threshold for transmitted depolarization may have been
due to some impairment or inadequate amount of neurotransmitter
substance liberated by the presynaptic neuron into the synaptic cleft
to induce the excitatory postsynaptic potential.

Whether or not these anesthetic effects upon synaptic transmission in spinal reflexes are applicable to loss of consciousness in
general anesthesia remains to be determined. With intracellular mic-
roelectrode recording, however, Albe-Fessard et al (1970) confirmed
the existence of hyperpolarization of cerebral cell membranes dur-

ing different types of anesthesia. Additionally they pointed out that
relatively short-latency activities evoked in the brain do not provide
satisfactory tests of anesthetic actions, which have to be made on
longer-lasting phenomena better correlated with pain, analgesia,
and consciousness.

In a series of studies, summarized in 1969 by Krnjevic, Shute and
Lewis (1963), Kanai and Szerb (1965), Celesia and Japser (1966),

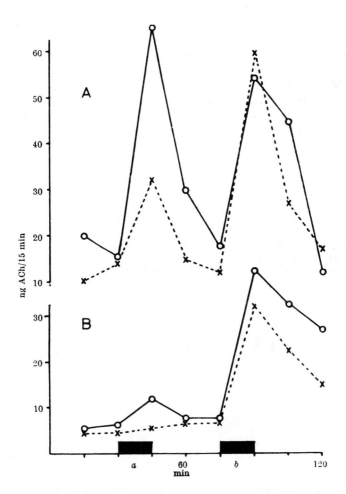

Fig. 7. Graph of acetylcholine output from postcruciate (solid line) and
medial ectosylvian (dotted line) gyri of cat's cortex, during stimulation of
forepaw (a) and midbrain RF (b), under light (A) and deep (B) halothane
anesthesia. Reproduced by permission from Kanai T, Szerb JC: Nature 265:
80, 1965

and others have attributed electroencephalographic arousal to an acetylcholine/mediated influence of the midbrain reticular formation on the cerebral cortex (Fig. 7). As Krnjevic has pointed out, a general facilitatory action on the cortex seems an appropriate function for the slowly acting excitatory effect of acetylcholine, which can influence the general responsiveness and duration of firing of cortical neurons in a manner that may be important both for the development of conscious processes and memory traces. On stimulation of the exposed sensory cortex of waking human subjects, Libet (1973) has pointed out that direct cortical stimulation must be maintained for 0.5 to 1.5 seconds before a subjective sensation is elicited.

In 1971 Shimoji and Bickford presented their elegant analyses of the differential impact of anesthetics on the more prolonged, as well as earlier, features of spontaneous activity and evoked discharge of units in the midbrain reticular formation. During wakefulness, the mean interspike interval of spontaneously firing reticular formation units

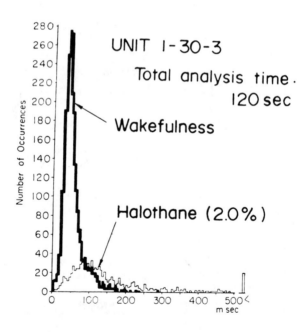

Fig. 8. Histograms showing duration of interspike intervals during spontaneous firing of a single unit in the midbrain RF, in a chronic implanted cat, during wakefulness (heavy line) and halothane anesthesia (light line). The mean interval was 52 msec during wakefulness and 149 msec during anesthesia. Reproduced by permission from Shimoji K, Bickford RG: Anesthesiology 35:76, 1971

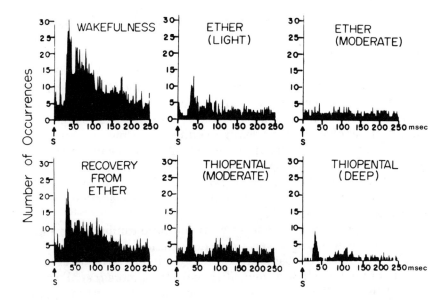

Fig. 9. Poststimulus histograms of midbrain RF units showing short- and long-latency discharges evoked by somatosensory stimulation, during wakefulness, ether and thiopental anesthesia in a chronic implanted cat. Reproduced by permission from Shimoji K, Bickford RG: Anesthesiology 35:76, 1971

was about 50 msec (Fig. 8) and, on somatosensory stimulation, an early burst of firing occurred at 30 to 40 msec, while later prolonged discharge continued, with declining intensity, for as long as 250 msec (Fig. 9). The impact of halothane, ether, and thiopental anesthesia on these patterns of reticular formation unit discharge was striking. Under halothane, the mean interspike interval during spontaneous firing increased to about 150 msec (Fig. 8). Ether anesthesia eliminated both the early and late discharge evoked by afferent stimulation and, while these responses could still be identified during thiopental anesthesia, their amplitude was markedly reduced (Fig. 9).

Excitatory Influences During Induction of Anesthesia

The pronounced depression of central neural excitability characteristic of fully developed Stage III anesthesia is, in the case of a

number of agents, prefaced during earlier stages by excitatory manifestations. As long ago as 1955, in a study of ether and barbiturates,
Domino presented evidence for an ascending deactivating or inhibitory system in the brain stem. In 1961 Brazier called attention to
an exaggeration of electrocortical responses during lighter levels of
anesthesia and proposed that the increment might result from disinhibition. In 1971 Liebeskind and Mayer observed that barbiturate
anesthesia abolished late negative components, but not an early
positive phase, of responses evoked in the mesencephalic central
gray matter by stimulating the tail of the rat. Light doses enhanced
the early phase of the response, possibly by release from tonic inhibition, since the increment coincided with an exaggeration of the
animal's stimulus-elicited agressive behavior.

Major support for the concept of disinhibition induced by anesthesia came earlier, however, from the experiments of Magni et al
(1959), who injected a barbiturate directly into the vertebral arterial
supply of the lower brain stem, after preventing more rostral extension of the anesthetic by ligation of the basilar artery at midpons.
Ongoing electroencephalographic patterns of slow waves and spindle bursts were promptly supplanted by maintained electroencephalographic arousal. Contrasting injection of the agent directly into
the upper brain stem and cerebrum, through the carotid circulation,
promptly converted ongoing electroencephalographic arousal patterns to those of slow waves and spindle bursts (Fig. 3). Such inverse results were also obtained by experimental cooling of the exposed floor of the fourth ventricle at bulbar or pontile levels respectively (Berlucchi et al 1964).

In 1966 these studies were followed up by Rosina and Mancia in
chronic animals with midpontile ligation of the basilar artery. Injection of a barbiturate into the vertebral artery during slow-wave sleep
was promptly followed by the electroencephalographic, elec-
tromyographic, and behavioral features of rapid eye movement
(REM), as activated sleep. The results indicated that during slow-
wave sleep, more caudal synchronizing structures exerted an inhibitory control upon pontile components responsible for electroencephalographic desynchronization during REM sleep. When
these lower brain stem structures were selectively anesthetized,
REM sleep appeared as a release phenomenon. More generally the
findings provided additional indication of the sensitivity of the
brain stem reticular formation to barbiturate anesthesia. In addition
if the manifestations of central neural excitement during lighter
stages of anesthesia are actually attributable to disinhibition, central
inhibitory mechanisms of the brain stem appear even more sensitive
to anesthetic agents than do excitatory ones.

A Synthesis of Neurophysiologic Correlates of the Anesthetic State

Winters (1973) has recently presented a synthesis of neuropharmacologic correlates of surgical anesthesia, which he defines as a
drug-induced state in which the patient is relatively unresponsive to
painful stimulation and amnestic. Such a state can be achieved
either by central neural excitation or depression, and a multidirectional schema of the stages involved is shown in Figure 10. The
schema indicates that most anesthetics induce an initial excitation
(Stage I), characterized by increased motor activity. Some anesthetics then proceed directly to surgical anesthesia (Stage III), characterized by central depression and a loss of responsiveness. Further
depression to Stage IV, with reduced respiration and /or cardiovascular function, leads to medullary paralysis and death.

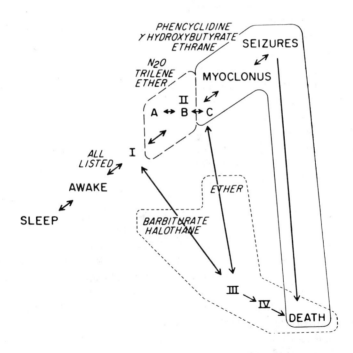

Fig. 10. Multidirectional schema of reversible CNS excitation or depression during stages or states induced by the several anesthetic agents indicated. Reproduced by permission from Winters WD: Neurophysiological
correlates of the Anesthetic state. In Brechner VL (ed): Pathological and
Pharmacological Considerations in Anesthesiology. Springfield, Ill, Charles
C Thomas, 1973

Following Stage I, other anesthetics induce Stage II, characterized first by bizarre hallucinatory and then cataleptoid behavior. Some then remain at this latter level of Stage II, during which the subject is also relatively unresponsive. Others progress to heightened levels of central excitation, leading to myoclonic jerking followed by generalized seizures. Still other anesthetics, having proceeded from Stage I to II, then go on to induce Stage III.

As regards neurophysiologic correlates, multiple-unit records of activity in the brain stem reticular formation vary with changes in the electroencephalogram and behavior, during these stages of excitation or depression, as shown earlier in Figure 6. During Stage I, the level of reticular formation unit activity is slightly elevated over the waking control (Fig. 6A). During Stage II, the level is first equal to or slightly less than Stage I; and later clearly lower than Stage I. During myoclonus and seizures, reticular formation unit responses are increased. By contrast, agents inducing Stages III and IV cause a marked fall in reticular formation unit excitability.

Further comparison of central excitability with these stages is demonstrated by the responses of the reticular formation to clicks. In control states the click-evoked reticular formation response is smallest during REM or activated sleep, larger when awake, and largest during slow-wave sleep (Figs. 4 and 5). With excitatory agents, during Stage I and II, the response of the reticular formation is larger than that of the waking control and markedly larger during myoclonus. By contrast, during State III, the response of the reticular formation to clicks is essentially eliminated. Clearly the progression from Stage I to Stage II reflects central nervous system excitation, while Stage III reflects central nervous system depression.

The reticular activating system of the brain stem is influenced by all anesthetic agents; some depress or eliminate its excitability during Stage III, while others render it hyperexcitable, resulting in disorganization of its function during Stage II. Some agents, such as ether, first induce excitation and then depression, depending on their concentration. Some induce only the cataleptoid level of Stage II; other provoke further excitation leading to seizure discharge. Still other agents, such as halothane and barbiturates, do not induce Stage II but progress directly from Stage I to Stage III.

Both the cataleptoid level of Stage II and the depressed level of Stage III—each of which is characterized by analgesia, loss of responsiveness, and amnesia—satisfy the basic requirements for surgical anesthesia. Since both excitant and depressant drugs can induce general anesthesia, Winters (1973) concludes that the concept of a single or holistic anesthetic state or mechanism is no longer tenable.

Brazier (1972) has similarly concluded a recent monograph on the neurophysiologic background for anesthesia as follows: "As research continues and knowledge grows, generalizations about the neural basis of anesthesia prove more and more risky. Not only do species differences crop up, but the very agents themselves show differences of effect that point away from a unitary theory of brain mechanisms concerned with the obtunding of conscious awareness. ... What emerges from these studies is that pain, memory and consciousness still hide secrets to lure the neurophysiologist and the anesthesiologist into this field of research."

References

Albe-Fessard D, Besson JM, Abdelmoumene M: Action of anesthetics on somatic evoked activities. In Yamamura H (ed): Anesthesia and Neurophysiology, Boston, Little Brown, 1970, p 129

Arduini A, Arduini MG: Effect of drugs and metabolic alterations on brain stem arousal mechanism. J Pharmacol Exp Ther 110:76, 1954

Berlucchi G, Maffei L, Moruzzi G, Strata P: EEG and behavioral effects elicited by cooling of medulla and pons. Arch Ital Biol 102:372, 1964

Bonnet V, Briot R: Etude des composantes intracorticales tardives de la response de l'aire visuelle du chat a une volee d'influx afferents. Arch Ital Biol 107:105, 1969

Borbely AA: Pharmacological Modifications of Evoked Brain Potentials. Bern, Hans Huber, 1973.

Boyd ES, Meritt DA: Effects of barbiturates on recovery cycles of medial lemiscus, thalamus and reticular formation. J Pharmacol Exp Ther 151:376, 1966

Brazier MAB: Some effects of anesthesia on the brain. Br J Anesthesiol 33:194, 1961

————: Effect of anesthesia on visually evoked responses. In Yamamura H (ed): Anesthesia and Neurophysiology. Boston, Little Brown, 1970, p 103

————: The Neurophysiological Background for Anesthesia. Springfield, Ill, Charles C Thomas, 1972

Celesia GG, Jasper HH: Acetylcholine released from cerebral cortex in relation to state of activation. Neurology 16:1053, 1966

Davis HS, Collins WF, Randt CT, Dillon WH: Effect of anesthetic agents on evoked CNS responses. Anesthesiology 18:634, 1957

Domino EF: A pharmacological analysis of the functional relationship between the brain stem arousal and diffuse thalamic projection systems. J Pharmacol Exp Ther 115:449, 1955

French JD, Verzeano M, Magoun HW: A neural basis of the anesthetic state. Arch Neurol Psychiat 69:519, 1953

————, King EE: Mechanisms involved in the anesthetic state. Surgery 38:228, 1955

Golovchinsky VB, Plehotkina SI: Difference in the sensitivity of cerebral cortex and midbrain reticular formation to action of ether and thiobarbital. Brain Res 30:37, 1971

Gyermek L: Anesthesia and descending influences on brain stem reticular formation. Arch Int Pharmacodyn 175:28, 1968

Kanai T, Szerb JC: Mesencephalic reticular activating system and cortical acetylcholine output. Nature 205:80, 1965

Killam EK: Drug action on the brain stem reticular formation. Pharmacol Rev 14:175, 1962

————: Pharmacology of the reticular formation. In Efron DH (ed): Psychopharmacology, A Review of Progress, 1957–67. Public Health Service Publication 1836, 1968

King EE: Differential action of anesthetics and interneuron depressants upon EEG arousal and recruitment responses. J Pharmacol Exp Ther 116:404, 1956

Krnjevic, K: Central cholinergic pathways. Fed Proc 28: 113, 1969

Liebeskind JC, Mayer DJ: Somatosensory evoked responses in the mesencephalic gray matter of the rat. Brain Res 27:133, 1971

Libet B: Electrical stimulation of cortex in human subjects and conscious sensory aspects. In Iggo, A. (ed): Somatosensory system, Handbook of Sensory Physiology, Chap 14, Vol 2. Springer 1973, p 743

Lindsley DF, Adey WR: Availability of peripheral input to the midbrain reticular formation. Exp Neurol 4:358, 1961

Magni F, Moruzzi G, Rossi CF, Zanchetti A: EEG arousal following inactivation of lower brain stem by selective injection of barbiturate into vertebral circulation. Arch Ital Biol 97:33, 1959

Magoun HW: The ascending reticular system and wakefulness. In Delafresnaye JF (ed): Brain Mechanisms and Consciousness. Oxford, Blackwell, 1954, p 1

Mannen H: Contribution to the morphological study of dendritic arborization in the brain stem. Prog Brain Res 21A:131, 1966

Mori K, Winters WD, Spooner CE: Comparison of reticular and cochlear multiple unit activity with auditory evoked responses during various stages induced by anesthetic agents. EEG Clin Neurophysiol 24:242, 1968

Morillo A, Baylor D: Electrophysiological investigation of lemniscal and paralemniscal input to the midbrain reticular formation. EEG Clin Neurophysiol 15:455, 1963

Nakai Y, Domino EF: Differential effects of pentobarbital, ethyl alcohol and chlorpromazine in modifying reticular facilitation of visually evoked responses in cat. Int J Neuropharmacol 8:61, 1969

Olds ME, Olds J: Effects of anxiety-relieving drugs on unit discharges in hippocampus, reticular midbrain and preoptic area in freely moving rat. Int J Neuropharmacol 8:87, 1969

Rosina A, Mancia M: Electrophysiological and behavioral changes following selective and reversible inactivation of lower brain stem structures in chronic cats. EEG Clin Neurophysiol 21:157–167, 1955

Scheibel ME, Scheibel AB: On circuit patterns of the brain stem reticular core. Ann NY Acad Sci 89:857, 1961

Shimoji K, Bickford RG: Differential effects of anesthetics on mesencephalic reticular neurons. I. Spontaneous firing patterns. Anesthesiol 35:68, 1971; II. Responses to repetitive somatosensory electrical stimulation. Anesthesiology 35:76, 1971

Shute CCD, Lewis PR: Cholinesterase-containing systems in the brain of the rat. Nature 199:1160, 1963

Somjen GG, Gill M: Mechanism of blockade of synaptic transmission in mammalian spinal cord by diethylether and by thiopental. J Pharmacol Exp Ther 140:19–30, 1963

Winters WD, Mori K, Spooner CE, Bauer RD: The neurophysiology of anesthesia. Anesthesiology 28:65, 1967

Winters WD: Neurophysiological correlates of the anesthetic state. In Brechner VL (ed): Pathological and Pharmacological Considerations in Anesthesiology. Springfield, Ill, Charles C Thomas, 1973

Yamoto S, Schaeppi U: Effects of pentothal on neural activity in somatosensory cortex and brain stem in cat. EEG Clin Neurophysiol 13:248, 1961

drugs
and
sleep

commentary

Drugs have two main influences upon sleep: (a) they can induce it or (b) they can prevent it. During the past two decades, our knowledge of the phases and functions of sleep has increased tremendously. Many specialized laboratories have been studying the way in which drugs can influence sleep phases and also the way in which sleep can influence drug action. The result is a more rational approach to the use of drugs to control sleep. Hypnotic drugs are the most commonly used to induce sleep; frequently stimulant drugs, like amphetamine and caffeine, are used to forestall sleep.

Sedative hypnotic drugs are used to induce sleep (see also p 327), although antipsychotic, antidepressant, antimanic, and other psychoactive drugs do influence sleep. The role of neurotransmitters and of drugs that influence them in the control of sleep is becoming clearer. Thus, 5-hydroxytryptamine (5HT) seems necessary for slow-wave sleep, and lack of 5HT results in total insomnia. Norepinephrine apparently is needed for REM sleep. Acetylcholine, particularly in the cerebral cortex, plays an important role in maintenance of arousal. Most drugs appear to suppress REM sleep with subsequent rebound. A few agents have been shown to increase REM sleep, but these results are very preliminary and need confirmation. Flurazepam is said to spare REM sleep, unlike most hypnotics (see p 110). Relatively few laboratories are equipped to do sleep studies with drugs in a parametric fashion, and thus it takes years to collect comparative information on drugs.

drugs
and
sleep

Jon F. Sassin, M.D.
Robert Rubin, M.D.

Sleep and dreams have long been a state of curiosity to man, but serious interest in sleep as an object of scientific investigation has arisen relatively recently, flourishing only since the 1950s. Perhaps the lack of enthusiasm for studying sleep was due partly to the necessity that the investigator himself stay awake all night, inverting his own diurnal sleep-waking cycle. In addition through much of man's history there appears to have been a conceptual framework in which sleep was viewed as a passive or inactive state. Discovery of the physiologic correlates of dreaming, that is, rapid-eye-movement (REM) sleep, by Dr. Nathaniel Kleitman and his colleagues (Aserinsky and Kleitman 1953, Dement and Kleitman 1955) spurred the flurry of investigation into the mechanisms and functions of sleep. More recently a great deal of interest has also arisen in the investigation of clinical disorders of sleep, such as insomnia and hypersomnia. Despite the intensity of recent sleep research, with literally thousands of publications in the field, the functions and biologic significance of this ubiquitous state remain unclear.

The experimental attack on sleep has been interdisciplinary, so that at present, sleep researchers are derived from nearly every field of biologic science. Pharmacology has contributed to our present understanding of sleep in two ways: (a) the manipulation of central nervous system mechanisms underlying sleep and waking by the use of both clinically applicable and research drugs and (b) the use of drugs in the treatment of disorders of sleep.

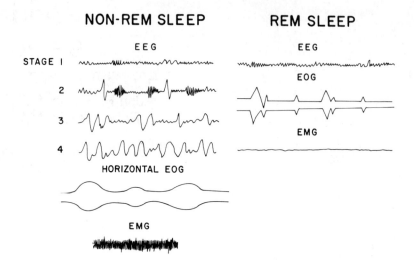

Fig. 1   Graphic representation of EEG, EOG, and EMG patterns during the stages of sleep. *Left*, non-REM sleep; *right*, REM sleep. EEG = electroencephalogram; EOG = electroculogram: EMG = electromyogram.

The Phenomenology of Sleep

Electrophysiologic recordings of normal nocturnal sleep in humans yield the dramatic finding that sleep is not a unitary state but consists of two distinct phases. The nomenclature for these phases has been a matter of considerable dispute, but most investigators accept a general division into REM and non-REM stages (Fig. 1). The definition of these stages depends on three parameters: electroencephalogram, electromyogram, and electrooculogram. Using these criteria, it is also possible to divide non-REM sleep into numbered stages, 1, 2, 3, and 4. The two latter stages (3 and 4) are defined by the presence of a certain amount of synchronized slow-wave activity in the electroencephalogram, giving rise to the names *S state* or slow-wave sleep (Freemon 1972, Williams 1974).

Stages of Non-REM sleep

In most normal adult humans, the waking electroencephalogram is dominated by alpha rhythm (8–12 Hz) and the transition between waking and sleep, Stage 1, is characterized by the disappearance of greater than 50 percent of this rhythm. There still is debate as to whether this stage is actually a part of sleep or of waking. The appearance of sleep spindles, a characteristic 12 to 14 cps activity, defines the onset of Stage 2 sleep. Stages 3 and 4 are marked by the further development of high voltage, synchronized slow waves, which, when in moderate amount, constitute Stage 3, and when dominant, Stage 4. During these stages of sleep there are frequently slow, rolling eye movements and muscle tone at a level slightly below that of waking.

Normal sleeping subjects pass regularly through Stages 1, 2, 3, and 4 at the onset and through the first 1 to 2 hours of sleep. There then occurs a shift to stage REM in which the electroencephalogram shows desynchronized low-voltage activity, in general resembling waking more than slow-wave sleep. In addition bursts of rapid eye movements and a dramatic, persistent decrease in muscle tone occur. Although considerable mental activity can be elicited during the non-REM stages of sleep, during REM sleep the great bulk of what is considered to be dreaming occurs. Through the rest of sleep, non-REM and REM stages alternate rhythmically in cycles having a periodicity of approximately 100 minutes (Fig. 2). As sleep progresses, Stages 3 and 4 (slow-wave sleep) become progressively less prominent in the recording, and REM sleep becomes more prominent. By the latter portions of normal sleep, stage REM occupies about half of the sleep time and Stage 2 the rest. The percentage of time spent in each of these sleep stages is relatively constant, under normal conditions, from night to night and from subject to subject, with Stage 2 comprising nearly half of the total sleep time, stage REM, 20 to 25 percent, Stages 3 and 4 together, 20 to 25 percent, and

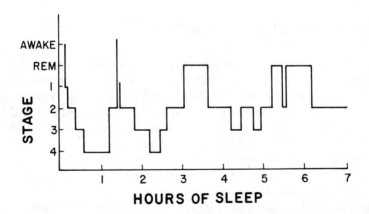

Fig. 2. A histogram of a night's sleep in a normal human subject demonstrating rhythmic alternation on non-REM and REM stages. Note the tendency for REM to increase as sleep proceeds and for non-REM Stages 3 and 4 to decrease.

Stage 1 occupying only 4 to 5 percent of total sleep time. Thus, sleep researchers have available a number of quantifiable variables with which to measure the effects of various agents on sleep. These variables include total sleep time, latency to sleep onset, percentages of stages, body movements, density of eye movements, descriptions of mental activity, the quality of sleep, and the number of awakenings.

The Function(s) of Sleep

It is to some extent disappointing that after a number of years of research little more is known about the biologic significance of sleep than has been known for centuries, ie, it "knits up the ravelled sleeve of care," as Shakespeare put it. A number of theories of the function of sleep have been proposed, none of which incorporates all of the presently known data. The most tempting of these theories has been that sleep serves an anabolic function, first recognized through the universally experienced restorative value of a "good night's sleep." It is the basis of these theories that repair and restoration occur during this time period, especially during the phases of slow-wave sleep. Many attempts at delineating function have centered around sleep deprivation, either total or partial, that is, *stage* deprivation. Despite widespread publicity to the contrary, results to date indicate that while *sleep* is necessary to normal waking function, the *type* of sleep does not appear to be as critical (Hartmann 1973).

The Pharmacology of Sleep Stages

Converging lines of evidence from many areas reveal the importance of *biogenic amines* in the production and maintenance of sleep and its stages, work pioneered by Professor Michel Jouvet (Jouvet 1972, Fuxe 1973). Pharmacologic as well as direct biochemical and histochemical data have indicated the various roles in sleep for the transmitters norepinephrine, 5-hydroxytryptamine (5HT), dopamine, and their metabolites, along with the earlier discovered influence of acetylocholine in arousal.

The development of compounds more or less specifically enhancing or inhibiting the metabolism of these transmitters greatly stimulated investigation into their role in sleep, as well as into the other central nervous system functions now known to be mediated by them. Of special usefulness, particularly in animal investigations of sleep mechanisms, have been the drugs parachlorphenylalanine

(PCPA), an inhibitor of 5HT; alpha-methylparatyrosine, and 6-hydroxydopamine, agents interfering with catecholamine metabolism; levodopa, the precursor of dopamine; the tricyclic antidepressants and monoamine-oxidase inhibitors; and atropine, the well-known anticholinergic drug that produces a sleeplike slow electroencephalographic pattern. PCPA produces nearly total insomnia in cats, reversed by the administration of 5HT, while the other agents affect REM sleep.

The use of these agents combined with stereotaxic lesions in animals and histofluorescent techniques have revealed distinct roles in the production of sleep states for each of the biogenic amines mentioned. 5HT appears to be the dominant neurotransmitter in producing slow-wave sleep through neuronal systems located along the midline raphe of the brain stem and projecting rostrally. 5HT or one of its metabolic products also seems to be important in the induction of REM sleep and is inhibitory to the production of the pontogeniculooccipital spikes, characteristic electrophysiologic correlates of REM sleep (studied best in cats and other subprimate mammals). Pharmacologic lesions, such as that of PCPA, and anatomic lesions depleting 5HT result in marked or total insomnia reversible by administering of 5HT or its precursors.

REM sleep, like wakefulness, appears to be dependent on noradrenergic and perhaps cholinergic neuronal pathways. The pathways for REM sleep begin in the brain stem, especially in the region of the locus coeruleus, and project rostrally. Functioning norepinephrine systems are necessary for the production of pontogeniculooccipital spikes and the tonic inhibition of muscle tone seen in REM. The important finding correlating catecholamines and REM sleep is that the amount of REM sleep is inversely related to the availability of catecholamines to the central nervous system. Much evidence indicates that cortical arousal is dependent on cholinergic systems as well as ascending dopaminergic pathways.

Effects of Drugs on Human Sleep

The results of the study of drug effects on human sleep have been at times contradictory and misleading, partly because of experimenter bias as well as the fact that many drugs affect sleep differently in different doses and that many lose their effectiveness over repeated administration (Kales 1974, Oswald 1973). Even so, the ubiquity and intolerability of sleep disorders, especially insomnia, have led to the development of more potent and safe agents for their treatment. This applied research has also yielded basic information on drug effects on sleep and sleep cycles and some insight into sleep mechanisms. An extensive list of the actions of various clinical and research drugs on sleep is provided by Freemon in his review of recent sleep research (Freemon 1972). It would appear that no drug developed to date reduces the need for sleep. There has been, however, one clear and reproducible effect of nearly all drugs tested on human sleep: the reduction of REM sleep with its attendant rebound for 2 or 3 days after discontinuance of the drug. It is this effect which is central to the problems involved in the chronic use of hypnotic drugs (Kales 1974). To the patient REM rebound means more dreaming activity and waking during unpleasant dreams. To avoid this the patient requests more sleeping medication, often resulting in a cycle leading to habituation. Two of the most commonly used psychopharmacologic agents, alcohol and barbiturates, produce this clear depression of REM sleep with attendant rebound.

Only a few agents have been shown to increase REM sleep: reserpine, chlorpromazine, tryptophane, 5-hydroxytryptophane, methyldopa, and, in animals, growth hormone, a polypeptide pituitary hormone released during sleep as described in another chapter. LSD increases REM sleep only early in the night, without a marked effect on total REM time. Drugs such as amphetamines and levadopa heighten arousal, reduce sleep, and reduce REM. In clinical situations, such as a variety of medical and psychiatric illnesses in which a decrease in total sleep time is a symptom, many sleep-promoting compounds will increase REM sleep by increasing the overall amount of sleep.

Slow-wave sleep is less affected by clinically useful pharmacologic compounds. A notable example is the benzodiazepine, flurazepam, which significantly decreases slow-wave sleep (Stages 3 and 4). Detrimental effects of this diminution of slow-wave sleep have not been demonstrated to date.

Insomnia

Insomnia is undoubtedly the most significant disorder of sleep, perhaps afflicting as much as 30 percent of the population of this country and accounting for the prescription of literally billions of sleep-inducing compounds yearly, many of which have significant detrimental effects on performance and a high probability of abuse (Williams 1974). In the past 5 years a number of sleep disorder clinics have been established to deal with this problem, resulting in better description and definitions of insomnia and the discovery of a variety of causes, many of which cannot be adequately treated by pharmacologic agents at present. A leading example is the syndrome of sleep-apnea, a condition in which nocturnal insomnia and subsequent daytime *hypersomnia* is caused by a cessation of respiration each time the patient falls asleep. Other forms of insomnia described by this so-called medical model include drug dependency as noted above; disruptions of normal circadian sleep-waking cycles by a variety of environmental factors; and the syndrome of nocturnal myoclonus, spontaneous movements of the legs with accompanying arousal. Insomnia is also a constant concomitant of numerous medical and psychiatric disturbances. Thus, before amelioration of a patient's complaint of sleeplessness is approached by the use of drugs, an evaluation should be undertaken to uncover one or more of these possible specific causes. When it is necessary to intervene by means of hypnotic drugs, it should be done for limited time periods, such as 1 to 2 weeks only and employing a drug with as low abuse potential as possible that preferably will not result in REM rebound on discontinuance. At present flurazepam is the most widely used drug fulfilling these requirements.

Amphetamines and tricyclic antidepressants have been found of value in sleep disorders of an opposite nature, such as narcolepsy, a disorder characterized by episodic, irrepressible attacks of sleep during normal waking hours. The associated symptoms of narcolepsy (cataplexy, sleep paralysis, and hypnagogic hallucinations) can be controlled by the use of moderate doses of imipramine, while the sleep attacks in this illness seem resistant to all medications but amphetamines.

Summary and Conclusions

While the mechanisms and functions of sleep and sleep stages remain obscure, pharmacologic agents have been widely useful in the manipulation of various aspects of sleep, both from the basic scientific and clinical point of view. Drugs that affect biogenic amine metabolism have been used to demonstrate the importance of noradrenalin, serotonin, and dopamine in the production and maintenance of sleep states. Despite significant drawbacks, drugs affecting sleep have been found useful in the management of various sleep disorders.

References

Aserinsky E, Kleitman N: Regularly occurring periods of eye motility and concomitant phenomena during sleep. Science 118:273–274, 1953

Dement W, Kleitman N: The relation of eye movements during sleep to dream activity. J Exp Psychol 53:339–346, 1957

Freemon J: Sleep Research: A Critical Review. Springfield, Ill, Charles C Thomas, 1972

Fuxe K, Lidbrink P: Biogenic amine aspects of sleep and waking. In Sleep: Physiology, Biochemistry, Psychology, Pharmacology, Clinical Implications. First European Congress on Sleep Research, Basel, 1972, pp 12–26

Hartmann E: The Functions of Sleep. New Haven, Yale University Press, 1973

Jouvet M: The role of monoamine and acetylcholine-containing neurons in the regulation of the sleep-waking cycle. Ergebn Physiol 64:166–307, 1972

Kales A, Bixler E, Tan T -L, Scharf M, Kales J: Chronic hypnotic drug use. JAMA 227:513–517, 1974

Oswald I: Drug research and human sleep. Ann Rev Pharmacol 13:243–252, 1973

Williams RL, Karacan I, Hursch CJ: Electroencephalography of Human Sleep: Clinical Applications. New York, Wiley, 1974

drugs and sexual functioning

commentary

The importance of sexual functioning in the etiology of psychopathologic conditions, and indeed in normal psychology, has been expounded and interpreted
by Freud and his followers. However, only in recent years has there been a
growth of explicit sex therapies, some highly reputable and others of dubious
background. Clearly, rapid progress in understanding sexual psychophysiology
is occurring; pharmacologic factors will play an increasingly important role in
such developments. What follows is a brief survey of drugs that facilitate or
impair various aspects of sexual functioning. The brevity of the following chapter reflects the relative underdevelopment of scientific sexual psychopharmacology. Perhaps in another decade a truly effective armamentarium of agents will evolve.

drugs and sexual functioning

Murray E. Jarvik, M.D., Ph.D.

Sexual pharmacology is a relatively neglected field. Taboos and restrictions have limited research in this area, and until recent years, instruction in the subject in medical schools has been virtually nonexistent. The daring pioneer studies of Kinsey (1948) and Masters and Johnson (1966) lent respectability to investigations of explicit human sexual behavior and opened the door to clinical sexual pharmacology. Today sex therapy is a variegated thriving specialty (Kaplan 1974) and at least one symposium on sexual pharmacology has been published (Sandler and Gessa 1975).

Without question one pharmacologic development has played a key role in the evolution of contemporary sexual mores. This was the worldwide adoption by women of the oral progestational agents for the control of conception. Once the fear of pregnancy was removed, the only effective deterrent to promiscuous sexual activity was the fear of venereal disease. Here too another pharmacologic agent, penicillin, has reduced the fear from this danger. Thus, because of drugs, legal, moral, and religious strictures are the main deterrents to indiscriminate sexual activity, and their effectiveness for the vast majority of mankind is doubtful.

Today patients, both married and unmarried, are more apt to request therapy for sexual dysfunction. Among the more common complaints in the male are impotence and premature ejaculation and in the female frigidity, orgastic dysfunction, and vaginismus. Although there is controversy over whether homosexuality is a disease, there is no question that when patients are unhappy with their sexual orientation they should be helped to make a better adjustment. In extreme cases patients with gender identity problems may require surgery for sexual reversal. However such radical irreversible procedures should always be preceded by pharmacotherapy with sex hormones to determine whether a satisfactory adjustment will be made to a sex reversal.

Sexual dysfunction can occur secondary to another disease, such as myocardial infarction, hypertension, diabetes, benign prostatic hypertrophy, parkinsonism, and a host of others. Therapy of the basic disease if successful will improve the sexual adjustment but even if the basic disease is untreatable some sexual counselling is useful. Many drugs used for the treatment of medical conditions have side effects that impair sexual functioning (Money and Yankowitz 1967, Mann 1968, Story 1974). For example, guanethidine impairs erectile potency and ejaculatory ability in men. Similar effects have been noted from thioridazine and other phenothiazine and, in fact, all agents that have sympathetic blocking actions. But all agents that produce nonspecific dysphoric toxic effects can be expected to reduce sexual desire and impair sexual performance.

Aphrodisiacs

Throughout history there has been a search for aphrodisiacs, drugs purported to enhance sexual activity. When demand exceeds supply, entrepreneurs will attempt to meet the demand by hook or crook. Not surprisingly, most aphrodisiacs have been obvious placebos, including substances such as powdered rhinoceros[1] horn and ginseng root.

One of the best known pharmacologically active aphrodisiacs is cantharides or Spanish fly. It is prepared from a species of beetle, which is dried and powdered and then may be taken orally. Components ultimately reach the urinary tract and produce irritation, particularly of the urethra. It has rubefacient vesicant properties when applied to the skin. Although its use has been widespread, its efficacy is questionable, it is hazardous, and deaths have occurred from its use (Sollmann 1936, Goodman and Gilman 1975).

Yohimbine, an alkaloid obtained from West Africa, has complex pharmacologic actions including adrenergic and serotonergic blocking effects. There are no controlled studies confirming its long reputation as an ingredient in nux vomica where it has been promoted as an aphrodisiac. Again there are no controlled studies; however, there might be some rationale for its use. Strychnine has a disinhibiting action on the spinal cord, which could indeed result in enhanced sexual performance. However, to date, it has been used in

humans in homeopathic doses and effects are due solely to suggestion. More research is needed before it could be safely prescribed to
man (McGaugh 1973). Other analeptic drugs have been noted to
result in convulsions, which often are accompanied by erection and
ejaculation. Obviously subconvulsive preparations would have to be
used, even though convulsive-type brain activity has recently been
measured in the human electroencephalogram during sexual orgasm.

The actions of representative drugs on sexual behavior, for which
there is some information in the literature, even though very scanty,
will now be considered.

Effects of Drugs on Sexual Function

Opioids

The opioids in general have been found to depress sexual functioning. Such drugs as morphine, heroin, and methadone almost universally produce a depression in sexual activity. However, under special circumstances they may enhance certain aspects of sexual activity. For example, in India opium has been used as a means of prolonging erection and delaying orgasm. Many of the opioids have
been noted to reduce testosterone levels. This may have a deleterious effect upon sexual activity as well as sexual anatomy (Mendelson et al 1974a). There is some controversy over whether tolerance
develops to the sexually depressing effects of opioids.

Sedative-Hypnotic Drugs

Shakespeare in Macbeth noted that alcohol "provokes the desire but
takes away the performance." Other sedative agents, such as the
barbiturates, the benzodiazepines, and meprobamate, can depress
the sexual reflex while at the same time their central disinhibiting
actions, so useful in treating anxiety, may allow the individual to
take sexual actions he would otherwise suppress. There is ample
evidence in animals that alcohol impairs sexual reflexes (Beach
1967, Merari et al 1973). Alcoholics are frequently impotent and the
anxiety from such impotency often leads to a vicious cycle of drinking to reduce the anxiety.

Many of the sedative-hypnotic drugs in the low-dose excitement
stage have a paradoxical effect that could conceivably stimulate sexual performance (Winters 1975). There are anecdotal reports among
street users of drugs that methaqualone (quaalude) has sexually arousing effects, but these reports are unconfirmed and implausible.

Centrally Acting Sympathomimetics

Cocaine and amphetamine effects are discussed in another portion of this book (see p 467). There is considerable controversy as to whether either class produces facilitation of sexual performance in man. Residents of the Haight-Ashbury district in San Francisco gave high grades to both amphetamine and cocaine as aphrodisiacs, but needless to say these were uncontrolled reports (Gay and Sheppard 1973). There is no question that both of these families of drugs relieve fatigue, and by this action can facilitate sexual performance. One might guess that other central stimulants, such as caffeine, might have similar effects. The brightening of mood produced by these drugs may have a secondary facilitating action on sexual performance.

Tobacco

Smoking cigarettes and other tobacco products has a wide variety of effects on physiologic functioning and health, which may influence sexual performance. The chronic health-impairing properties of cigarette smoking will surely reduce sexual activity. Individuals suffering from cancer, emphysema, or heart disease will obviously have impaired sexual responses. The main pharmacologic acute effects developing from smoking can be attributed to nicotine, with perhaps a small effect from carbon monoxide. The sexual reflexes certainly involve nicotinic synapses as well as postganglionic adrenergic endings, which can both be stimulated or depressed by nicotine. When heavy smokers stop smoking there are frequent reports of increased well-being due to improved respiratory function, increased appetite, diminished susceptibility to infection, and often increased sexual responsiveness. Heavy smokers will precede and follow sexual activity with smoking. One of the appeals to teen-agers to stop smoking is that smoking impairs sexual ability. However, there is, as yet, no valid evidence for such claims.

LSD-Like Drugs

Many of the hallucinogens resembling LSD (lysergic acid diethylamide), such as psilocybin, dimethyltryptamine, and mescaline have been used as aphrodisiacs, but their use is not entirely rational. There have been conflicting reports about the sexual effects of LSD. In some users it may be aphrodisiac and in others the opposite (Gay and Sheppard 1973). Since the use of LSD as a street drug has declined and its use in research has become practically nonexistent, it will be difficult to determine what sexual effects it has, if any. Since it appears that 5-hydroxytryptamine (serotonin, 5HT) does play some role in sexual functioning and since LSD both mimics and blocks 5HT there is a theoretical basis for its action (Chase and Murphy 1973). In one animal study LSD was reported to enhance sexual activity (Bignami 1966).

Cannabis (Marihuana and Hashish)

There is no question that marihuana is the drug that has the widest reputation for improving sexual performance (Gay and Sheppard 1973, Klein 1972). Opinion surveys indicate that most marihuana users report that it improves sexual performance and enjoyment (Robbins and Tanck 1973, Koff 1974). Both sexes report that marihuana seems to improve orgasmic experience, and some women claim that they never had an orgasm until they started using marihuana (Lewis 1970). Again, as with other drugs, objective studies of the effects of marihuana are lacking. Marihuana has a street reputation for enhancing sexual activity (Gay and Sheppard 1973), so it is hard to find a naive subject to test it on. There are several reports that marihuana use lowers testosterone (Kolodny et al 1974), whereas Mendelson (1974b) failed to find an effect on serum testosterone. Marihuana is still an illegal drug. The practicing physician could not legally advocate its use for sexual dysfunction, even if the evidence for its effectiveness were better.

Amyl Nitrite

Amyl nitrite is a vasodilator used to alleviate the pain of angina pectoris. Its use as an aphrodisiac is not listed in the standard textbooks of pharmacology. In recent years it has achieved popular use for this purpose. It supposedly potentiates the orgasm or produces an orgasm in individuals unable to have one without it (Hollister 1975, Everett 1972). These reports have not been verified in controlled studies. The drug produces marked tachycardia and may be dangerous because of its ability to produce orthostatic hypotension.

Local Anesthetics

Local anesthetics such as cocaine and procaine and its congeners have been applied to the genital region in creams or ointments with the aim of reducing sensation and therefore prolonging the preorgasmic phase of sexual activity. Again, although there appears to be some rationale to this theory, controlled studies have not been done.

Hormones

It has long been known that the sex hormone testosterone is necessary for adequate sexual functioning in the male. It is perhaps less well-known that androgens of adrenal origin are also necessary for adequate sexual functioning in the female. Castration in the male results in marked diminution in serum testosterone levels and in sexual excitability, and causes atrophy of the penis. Nevertheless castrated male animals and humans do have some sexual functioning and may be able to produce an erection. Again, it is likely that the adrenal adrogens play an important role in such behavior. The use of testicular extracts to enhance sexual performance dates back to 1889 when Brown-Sequard reported his self-experiment (McGrady 1968). Modern endocrinologists feel that his injections were probably pharmacologically ineffective but had a strong placebo effect. Another famous (or infamous) dispenser of rejuvenation through testicular extracts was Voronoff (see McGrady 1968) whose "monkey glands" preparation became very popular and was certainly a placebo.

A great deal of well-controlled work in animals shows that testosterone regulates not only gonadal functioning but also influences the brain (Carter 1974). The androgens have virilizing and anabolic effects. Even in individuals with emaciating illness they may produce weight gain and renewed interest in sex.

There is also evidence that estrogens may be useful in enhancing sexual activity in castrated or postmenopausal women (Jarvik and Brecher 1975; see Chapter 24).

Anaphrodisiacs

The use of drugs to depress sexual functioning may have some applicability when sexual behavior is impossible or undesirable. Saltpeter (potassium nitrate) has had the reputation for hundreds of years of depressing sexual desire and was added to the diets of schoolboys, prisoners, sailors, and other institutional inmates. However, there is no evidence that it had any effect whatsoever upon libido. It does produce diuresis, and contrary perhaps to the expected effect, in some individuals a full bladder has a sexually stimulating effect.

Many of the antipsychotic drugs appear to produce decreased libido as a side effect. They have been tried in sexual criminals as an alternative to surgery or incarceration. Thioridazine has a greater reputation for producing impotence, due to inhibition of ejaculation, than do the other antipsychotic drugs.

The estrogens have been used as anaphrodisiacs. Competition occurs with the endogenous androgens, perhaps through an effect upon the hypothalamus and pituitary. Feminization is perhaps the most distressing side effect, although nausea and vomiting may occur.

The antiandrogenic drug, cyproterone, is very effective in antagonizing the actions of testosterone. It has demasculinizing and libido-reducing effects. It has been used therapeutically to treat sex offenders with some success and a great deal of controversy (Cooper et al 1972). However, it does not suppress sexual activity of adult male rats (Bloch and Davidson 1967).

The Role of Neurotransmitters

Increasing knowledge about the roles of neurotransmitters is also throwing some light on their action in sexual functioning. The automatic nervous system controls the activity of the sexual organs, including secretion, tumescence, and ejaculation and orgasm. Ganglionic blocking agents with their antinicotinic actions have long been known to produce impotence. Muscarinic blocking agents may impair secretions and prostatic functioning. Nicotine in low doses may facilitate sexual behavior and inhibit it in high doses (Soulairac and Soulairac 1975).

Dopamine seems to be a basic facilitator of sexual function though it inhibits lordosis in female rats. On the other hand, 5HT inhibits sexual activity, especially when an increase in brain serotonin is induced (Gessa and Tagliomonte 1974, Everett 1975). Based on these observations a number of substances have been suggested as sexual facilitators; these include levodopa, parachlorophenylalanine (PCPA), apomorphine, and monoamine oxidase inhibitors. Dopamine blocking agents, such as pimozide, have been shown to be sexual inhibitors. However, Whalen et al (1975) have cautioned investigators not to draw hasty conclusions about the role of neurotransmitters in sexual behavior.

Prostaglandins, first discovered in semen, have been found to have an amazing variety of effect upon diverse organ systems. Although they have important roles in reproductive physiology, there is as yet no evidence that they directly influence sexual behavior. Various other polypeptides, such as fragments of adrenocorticotrophic hormone (ACTH) and posterior pituitary hormones, may be potentially useful in the treatment of sexual dysfunction, but much more research needs to be done before these substances will be ready for clinical use.

References

Beach FA: Cerebral and hormonal control of reflexive mechanisms involved in copulatory behavior. Physiol Rev 47:289–316, 1967

Bignami G: Pharmacologic influences on mating behavior in the male rat. Psychopharmacologia 18:44, 1966

Bloch GJ, Davidson JM: Behavioral and somatic responses to the antiandrogen cyproterone. Hormon Behav 2:11–25, 1971

Carter CS: Hormones and Sexual Behavior. Stroudsburg, Penn, Dowden, Hutchinson and Ross, 1974

Chase TN, Murphy DL: Serotonin and central nervous system function. Ann Rev Pharmacol 13:181–197, 1973

Cooper AJ, Ismail AAA, Phanjoo AL, Love DL: Antiandrogen (cyproterone acetate) therapy in deviant hypersexuality. Br J Psychiat 120:59–63, 1972

Everett GM: Effects of amyl nitrite ("poppers") on sexual experience. Med Aspects Hum Sexual 6:146–151, 1972

———: Role of biogenic amines in the medulation of aggressive and sexual behavior in animals and man. In Sandler M, Gessa GL (eds): Sexual Behavior: Pharmacology and Biochemistry. New York, Raven, 1975

Gay GR, Sheppard C: "Sex-crazed dope fiends"—myth or reality? Drug Forum 2:125–140, 1973

Gessa GL, Tagliomonte A: Possible Role of Brain Serotonin and Dopamine in Controlling Male Sexual Behavior. In Costa E, Gessa GL, Sandler M (eds): Advances in Biochemical Psychopharmacology, Vol. 2. New York, Raven, 1974, pp 217–228

Goodman LS, Gilman A (eds): The Pharmacological Basis of Therapeutics, 5th ed. New York, Macmillan, 1975

Hollister LE: The Mystique of Social Drugs and Sex. In Sandler M, Gessa GL (eds): Sexual Behavior: Pharmacology and Biochemistry. New York, Raven, 1975, pp 85–92

Jarvik ME, Brecher EM: Sexual effects of drugs. In Musaph H, Money J (eds): Textbook of Sexology. Amsterdam, Elsevier, Excerpta Medica, 1976

Kaplan HS: The New Sex Therapy. New York, Brunner /Mazel, 1974

Kinsey AC, Pomeroy WB, Martin CE: Sexual Behavior in the Human Male. Philadelphia, Saunders, 1948

Klein D: Everything You Always Wanted to Know about Marijuana, Chap 7. New York, Tower Publications, 1972, pp 147–162

Koff WC: Marijuana and sexual activity. J Sex Res 10:194–204, 1974

Kolodny R, Masters W, Kolodner R, Toro G: Depression of plasma testosterone levels after chronic intensive marihuana use. N Engl J Med 290:872–874, 1974

Lewis B: The Sexual Power of Marijuana. New York, Peter H. Wyden, 1970

Mann T: Effects of pharmacological agents on male sexual functions. Reprod Fertil Suppl 4:101–114, 1968

Masters WH, Johnson VE: Human Sexual Inadequacy. Boston, Little, Brown, 1970

McGaugh JL: Drug facilitation of learning and memory. Ann Rev Pharmacol 13:229–241, 1973

McGrady P: The Youth Doctors. New York, Coward-McCann, 1968

Mendelson J, Mendelson JE, Patch V: Effects of heroin and methadone on plasma testosterone in narcotic addicts. Fed Proc 33:232, 1974a (abstr)

Mendelson JH, Kuehnle J, Ellingboe J, Babor TF: Plasma testosterone levels before, during, and after chronic marijuana smoking. N Engl J Med 291:1051–1055, 1974b

Merari A, Ginton A, Heifez T, Lev-Ran T: Effects of alcohol on mating behavior of the female rat. Q J Stud Alcohol 34:1095–1098, 1973

Money J, Yankowitz R: The sympathetic-inhibiting effects of the drug ismelin on human male eroticism, with a note on mellaril. J Sex Res 3:69–82, 1967

Robbins PR, Tanck RH: Psychological correlates of marijuana use: an exploratory study. Psychiatr Rep 33:703–706, 1973

Sandler M, Gessa GL: Sexual Behavior: Pharmacology and Biochemistry. New York, Raven, 1975

Sollmann T: A Manual of Pharmacology and Its Applications to Therapeutics and Toxicology. Philadelphia, Saunders, 1936

Soulairac ML, Soulairac A: Monoaminergic and cholinergic control of sexual behavior in the male rat. In Sandler M, Gessa GL (eds): Sexual Behavior: Pharmacology and Biochemistry. New York, Raven, 1975, p 111

Story N: Sexual dysfunction resulting from drug side effects. J Sex Res 10:132–149, 1974

Whalen RE, Gorzalka BB, DeBold JF: Methodologic considerations in the study of animal sexual behavior: In Sandler M, Geser GL (eds): Sexual Behavior: Pharmacology and Biochemistry. New York, Raven, 1975, pp 33–44

Winters WD: The continuum of CNS excitatory states and hallucinosis. In Siegel R, West LJ (eds): Hallucinations. New York, Wiley, 1975

drugs and motor behavior

commentary

Drug-induced movement disorders are extremely important to the primary care practitioner as well as to the psychiatrist, because so many psychiatric drugs affect the motor system. Naturally occurring movement disorders frequently seen by the physician include tremor, dyskinesia, dystonia, ataxia, incoordination, and convulsions. In psychotic disorders it is important to differentiate drug-induced motor dysfunction from those of the disease under treatment. There has been great progress during the past two decades in our understanding of parkinsonism, and a review of the important developments is covered in this chapter. Other movement disorders, including Huntington's chorea, are influenced by drugs and must be dissociated from one another. The treatment of these disorders sometimes results in psychiatric complications. Dopamine plays an important role in the etiology of dyskinesia and also apparently in major psychoses. Movement disorders, such as tardive dyskinesia, are particularly disturbing to the patient and to the physician and require special attention (see p 205). This chapter is a succinct summary of the movement disorders a practitioner is apt to encounter and how drugs may exacerbate or ameliorate them.

drugs and motor behavior

Charles H. Markham, M.D.
Robert D. Ansel, M.D.

The term *movement disorder* refers to disorders of coordination or motor control secondary to brain dysfunction. Convulsive disorders are not included. The regions of the brain usually involved are the cerebellum, cerebral cortex, caudate nucleus, and putamen (together called the striatum), globus pallidus, substantia nigra, and subthalamic body of Luys. The disturbed region can usually be identified by a gross or microscopic pathologic defect, by a biochemical change, or by specific characteristics of the movement disorder itself. The locus of abnormality is unknown in a few naturally occurring disorders such as dystonia musculorum deformans and Gilles de la Tourette's disease.

Naturally Occurring Movement Disorders

Parkinson's Disease

This is a fairly common disease of the nervous system, two prevalence figures in the United States being 114 and 188 per 100,000. For much of this century it has been thought that this disease was due to abnormalities in the basal ganglia. Yet the main change demonstrated by classic neuropathologic techniques, loss of the large pigment-containing cells in the substantia nigra, seemed inadequate to explain this symptom complex of tremor, rigidity, and akinesia. However, a new view was given by the nearly simultaneous demonstration, in the early 1960s, that the nigra, and especially the

127

striatum, contained very large amounts of dopamine; and that dopamine in these sites was much reduced in Parkinson's disease (Ehringer and Hornykiewicz 1960). The striatum had not previously been recognized as being abnormal in any way in Parkinson's disease. The link between these two areas was made when a new histofluorescent technique demonstrated dopamine in large pigmented cell bodies in the nigra, in their ascending axons smaller than the resolving power of ordinary light microscopes, and in their branching, irregular synaptic terminations in the striatum (Hillarp et al 1966). It seems dopamine in the synaptic terminals is released on nigral stimulation, and that it influences many striatal neurons. It is not clear whether dopamine acts as an inhibitory transmitter at these sites, or whether it is excitatory. However, as will be detailed below, therapeutically administered dopa, the precursor of dopamine, markedly benefits symptoms of Parkinson's disease.

Acetylcholine is also present in high concentration in the striatum, but unlike dopamine most of it seems to be contained in neurons, with both cell bodies and terminations within the striatum, ie, interneurons. While neither acetylcholine nor its forming or inactivating enzymes have been shown to be abnormal in Parkinson's disease, the ratio of acetylcholine relative to dopamine may be increased, since anticholinergic drugs reduce certain parkinsonian symptoms.

Two other neurohumors should be mentioned. Serotonin (5-hydroxytryptamine) is somewhat reduced in the striatum (globus pallidus, thalamus, and hypothalamus), in Parkinson's disease (Bernheimer et al 1961). It is contained in synaptic terminals whose cell bodies lie in the raphe nuclei of the pons and midbrain, not far from the substantia nigra. Neither serotonin nor its precursor, 5-hydroxytryptophane, which crosses the blood-brain barrier, significantly influences parkinsonian symptoms (Lee et al 1968). Lastly, gamma aminobutyric acid is highly concentrated in the striatum. It appears to be contained in many interneurons and in some efferent neurons as well. Gamma aminobutyric acid is apparently not altered in Parkinson's disease, but it is markedly reduced in Huntington's chorea, a disease with massive loss of striatal neurons.

The major motor manifestations of Parkinson's disease are those of tremor, rigidity, and akinesia. These symptoms are present in varying degrees and are usually accompanied by impairment of postural reflexes. Other symptoms may include a voice with a low volume and disturbed rhythm, seborrhea, drooling of saliva, as well as depression and slowly progressive dementia. The tremor is usually most obvious with the extremity at rest and is decreased during movement. The tremor frequency varies from 3 to 6 per second and is present to some degree in 80 percent of the Parkinson patients. Rigidity is an increased resistance of the flexor and extensor muscles to either active or passive movement. The patient feels an aching heaviness in his extremities and slowed movement. The physician detects rigidity as increased muscular resistance as the relaxed extremity is moved. When rigidity becomes prominent, a gradually progressive flexed posture usually develops. Akinesia consists of a lack of movement and also a hesistancy or interruption in the performance of certain movements. Akinesia causes a loss of facial movement (masklike facies). The gait becomes awkward and hesitant, and the patient may have many falls. Akinesia almost always appears in Parkinson's disease.

Clinical trials of levodopa soon followed the biochemical evidence of dopamine deficiency in Parkinson's disease. Initially different preparations and modes of administration were used with mixed results. In the late 1960s the presently recognized form of therapy evolved (Treciokas et al 1971). This consists of giving levodopa orally in doses that are small initially and increased slowly over a period of time until a plateau of approximately 3 to 6g is reached. The optimal dose is usually determined by a balance between clinical response and side effects.

The major side effects of levodopa therapy include nausea and vomiting. Recently, the use of about one-fifth the previous dose of levodopa plus dopa decarboxylase inhibitors, which act at therapeutic doses predominantly outside the nervous system, has been most effective in controlling these gastrointestinal problems (Markham et al 1974). Probably the nausea and vomiting are due to a direct effect of levodopa on the stomach or duodenum, and the much lower therapeutic dose of levodopa permitted by the peripherally acting decarboxylase inhibitor reduces the gastrointestinal symptoms. Another major side effect of levodopa is the development of abnormal involuntary movements, which is clearly the action of levodopa within the central nervous system. This problem will be discussed under *Drug-Induced Motor Disease.*

About two-thirds of patients with Parkinson's disease have striking improvement in motor symptoms with significant decrease or even disappearance of rigidity and akinesia. Tremor may be helped or may progress in spite of levodopa. As the motor symptoms improve, preexisting depression, although not necessarily worsening, may assume greater importance. Further, as patients have lived longer because of their improved motor status (Markham et al 1974), some have had worsening of their preexisting organic dementia.

Anticholinergic drugs have been used for the treatment of parkinsonian symptoms for many years. They offer a clear, modest reduction in tremor and rigidity in many cases when used alone, and also give an additive improvement when used with levodopa. Centrally acting anticholinergic agents include trihexyphenidyl (Artane), biperiden (Akineton), cycrimine (Pagitane), procyclidine (Kemadrin), ethopropazine (Parsidol), benztropine (Cogentin), chlorphenoxamine (Phenoxene), and orphenardrine (Disipal). In addition, antihistamines, such as diphenhydramine HCl (Benadryl), seem to work by virtue of a mild anticholinergic effect. An additional drug, amantadine HCl (Symmetrel), originally used for prophylaxis of influenza A2 (Asian) respiratory illness, has also proved valuable in reducing parkinsonian symptoms. The mode of action of amantadine is uncertain but probably is unrelated to its antiviral effect. Clinical observations of side effects, such as decreased salivation and urinary hesitancy, suggest it has a mild anticholinergic action. However, experimental evidence shows it releases dopamine from synaptic storage sites (Grelak et al 1970), and it also increases gamma aminobutyric acid in the striatum and substantia nigra (Bak et al 1972).

While many problems are still poorly understood and new questions are being raised regarding the pathophysiology and biochemistry of Parkinson's disease, it is important to appreciate that recent work has opened up a new door in the research of cerebral disorders in general and, in particular, has once again brought out the role of centrally active biogenic amines.

Huntington's Chorea

This is an hereditary disease with a prevalence in the United States of 4 to 5 per 100,000. The clinical onset is usually in adult life. Pathologically there is widespread loss of neurons, with particularly severe loss in the striatum. The latter degeneration of specific species of interneurons is apparently responsible for marked reduction of striatal choline acetylase, and also gamma aminobutyric acid and glutamic acid decarboxylase. On the other hand striatal dopamine content, which is contained in synaptic terminations of nigral cells, is little altered. However, several lines of evidence suggest heightened dopamine activity, either by denervation hypersensitivity or by aberrant sprouting of dopamine terminals onto remaining striatal neurons. These data include accentuation of the choreiform and athetoid movements of Huntington's chorea (and even their production in preclinical cases) by orally administered levodopa (Klawans et al 1972); the similarity between dopa-induced choreoathetosis in parkinsonian patients and the naturally occurring movements in Huntington's chorea; and the reduction of choreiform and athetoid movements in Huntington's chorea by reserpine, which depletes dopamine (and other cerebral monoamines), and a similar effect by phenothiazines, such as chlorpromazine, and butyrophenones, such as haloperidol, which block dopamine receptors. These last mentioned measures are often good treatments for the abnormal movements in Huntington's chorea.

Hepatolenticular Degeneration (Wilson's Disease)

This rare disease, with recessive inheritance, has two chief forms, both with severe movement disorders. Pseudosclerosis occurs in adults and is characterized by a flapping tremor at the wrists and "wing-beating" tremor at the shoulders; and by dysarthria. Dementia is mild, if present at all. The neurologic symptoms progress very slowly, as does the invariably present hepatic insufficiency. Progressive lenticular degeneration starts in late childhood and progresses more rapidly. The main neurologic symptoms are dystonia, with trunk or limb distortion, and resting or intention tremor and organic dementia. Hepatic insufficiency is more severe and rarely children may die in hepatic coma before the first neurologic symptom appears.

The biochemical defect is the same in both forms of Wilson's disease, consisting of a disorder in copper binding. Copper is normally absorbed in the gut, loosely attached to serum albumin, and then forms a tightly bound complex with ceruloplasmin, an alpha-2-globulin. Ceruloplasmin is much reduced in Wilson's disease, and the copper preferentially collects in the liver, kidney, basal ganglia, and cornea. It is also taken up faster from the gastrointestinal tract. Present therapy consists of oral administration of chelating agents, especially penicillamine, and potassium sulfide. The latter renders copper in the food less soluble. These treatments, if started early enough in the course of the disease, can virtually eliminate symptoms and extend life expectancy to near normal.

Essential (Heredofamilial) Tremor

Essential tremor has a prevalence not unlike Parkinson's disease. It is inherited as a recessive trait, has a frequency of six to eight per second, is enhanced by maintained posture or movement of the involved limb, and involves arms, legs, head, or even vocal cords. Its frequency is similar to normal or physiologic tremor. There is no rigidity or akinesia as seen in Parkinson's disease. The tremor may start in the 20s and very slowly progress over the next 50 years. When it starts late in life, it is sometimes called senile tremor. The tremor is incapacitating for the younger individuals only if they are doing fine skilled mechanical tasks, such as electronic parts assembly. By the 70s, it may make feeding oneself very difficult and writing becomes impossible.

Alcohol may temporarily reduce the tremor, but it returns with renewed force a few hours later. Phenobarbital, diazepam (Valium), and chlordiazepoxide (Librium) may help. Levodopa is no help at all. Propranolol (Inderal), a beta-adrenergic blocking agent, has been tried because essential tremor is similar to physiologic tremor and the latter is increased by epinephrine. Whether or not this rationale is valid, we have found propranolol to be very effective in reducing the severity of essential tremor in many patients. Other investigators have been less impressed (Sweet et al 1974). However, we have often found prompt and long-term improvement with daily doses of 80 to 240 mg, with few if any side effects, even with these large doses.

Spasticity

This is a state in which the "deep" or myotatic reflexes are increased, and muscle tone is increased in a special way such that a quick passive stretch will evoke greater resistance than a slow or gradual one. In man this phenomenon predominates in the extensor muscles of the leg and trunk, but is about equal in flexors and extensors of the arm. It is due to injury to fibers descending from the premotor cortex (area 6 especially) to the brain stem and spinal cord, or to fibers descending from the brain stem in close proximity to the corticospinal tract in the cord. It may be most disabling.

There is no satisfactory treatment, although two drugs may be of some help. The benzodiazepines, especially diazepam (Valium) and chlordiazepoxide (Librium), occasionally reduce human spasticity, possibly because they depress transmission in polysynaptic reflex pathways (Greenblatt and Shader 1974). Dantrolene sodium (Dantrium) is a new agent said to reduce spasticity by acting directly on the skeletal muscle, probably by interfering with release of calcium from the sarcoplasm. It appears that released calcium is the first step in muscular contraction. Too much dantrolene causes weakness. Some cases of chronic spasticity have been much improved (Chyatte et al 1973); other have not been helped (Gelenberg and Poskanzer 1973). Our own limited experience has included a few patients who were mildly benefitted, and more who were not.

Paroxysmal Choreoathetosis

This unusual disorder consists of bouts of sudden, vigorous contraction of the limbs and body into a twisted dystonic posture that may last for minutes or hours (Stevens 1966). There is no alteration of consciousness. The state is triggered in some individuals by a vigorous muscular effort and by a loud sound or startle in others. It is sometimes familial. No underlying pathology has been found. It is considered by some to be a form of epilepsy. It may be completely controlled by daily doses of diphenylhydantoin (Dilantin), carbamazepine (Tegretol), or primidone (Mysoline).

Gilles de la Tourette's Syndrome

This unusual syndrome consists of a sudden ticlike movement, usually of the face, head, or an upper extremity, accompanied by vocalization (Sweet et al 1973). The latter may be a grunt, a hissing sound, a few words, or a shouted profanity. There are no consistent neurologic or psychiatric abnormalities. Haloperidol (Haldol) usually will halt or reduce the intensity of the tics. A phenothiazine will occasionally help.

Postanoxic Action Myoclonus

This follows severe anoxia as may be caused by near-drowning, construction cave-ins, or narcotic drug overdoses. As the patient recovers consciousness, sudden jerks, or myoclonic movements, may be triggered by sound or a voluntarily initiated movement. There may be action or intention tremor as well. This particular kind of myoclonus is said to be helped by a combination of 5-hydroxytrytophan, the precursor to serotonin, and MK-486, an aromatic L-amino acid decarboxylase inhibitor that acts outside the nervous system (Van Woert and Sethy 1975) and which allows a very high level of serotonin to be achieved within the central nervous system. The last is still an experiment drug. No other therapy has helped for this condition, so this initial report is encouraging. While the mechanism of action of 5-hydroxytryptophan improving action myoclonus is unclear, it should be noted that this drug may aggravate the choreoathetosis in Huntington's chorea (Lee 1968).

Drug-Induced Motor Diseases

Some naturally occurring movement disorders can be mimicked by the action of certain drugs. For example, parkinsonian rigidity, akinesia, and tremor can be produced by some phenothiazines. Certain other movement disorders produced by drugs are quite unique. In both instances, it is important to recognize these drug-induced states (American College of Neuropsychopharmacology 1973).

Levodopa-Induced Dyskinesia

In the course of treatment of Parkinson's disease with large doses of levodopa, a new movement disorder was observed to develop. These movements are best described as choreoathetoid or dystonic. The head may be pulled back or to one side, or the arm extended and rotated. The hand may be flexed at the wrist, the forearm internally rotated, and the fingers extended. The trunk may be rotated. The jaws may be clenched or the eyelids held shut. While there are many manifestations, each patient has his own localized, individual dyskinesia.

The dystonic movements are usually seen in the first 3 to 12 months of treatment with levodopa, and usually occur at or near the dose necessary to benefit the parkinsonian symptoms, namely an average dose of about 4.5g per day (Markham et al 1974). These movements occur in as many as half of the cases. Usually a modest reduction in the dose of levodopa stops the dyskinesia. In a few cases such reduction has led to return of parkinsonian symptoms. One problem in regulating dosage in these patients is that a few would rather have a significant amount of choreoathetosis rather than parkinsonian symptoms.

The levodopa-induced dyskinesia is almost entirely confined to patients who also have parkinsonism. We have not seen it in those relatively few cases unresponsive to levodopa; possibly there were no nigral cells left in these. We did not see it in 6 normal persons who voluntarily took the medication (Ansel and Markham 1970). Nor have we seen it in patients with dystonia musculorum deformans or spasmodic torticollis who took large doses for many months. However, as noted above, levodopa can accentuate choreoathetosis in Huntington's chorea, a superficially similar dyskinesia but one which tends to involve all parts of the body, not one region. In both diseases one may speculate that parts of the striatum have become hypersensitive to dopamine. The role of aberrant sprouting of nigrostriatal terminations and of dopamine manufacture in nondopaminergic (serotoninergic) synaptic endings is presently unknown.

Dystonia

The phenothiazines, butyrophenones, and thioxanthenes, particularly those used in the treatment of psychosis, may produce a sudden and alarming dyskinesia. It is more likely to occur in children, and develops in the first few days of treatment, or when the dose is increased. The spasms affect head, face, and neck muscles especially. The face may be held in a fixed grimace, the tongue immobile. The eyes may be held fixed upward or to one side. The head may be pulled back or to one side and the back arched. There is no alteration of consciousness.

These dystonic movements abate when the offending drug is stopped or can be made to clear even more rapidly by parenteral administration of anticholinergic agents, antihistamines, and barbiturates.

The reaction is uncommon. While the offending drugs are considered to block receptors of dopamine (and serotonin and norepinephrine), there may be an initial excitatory effect produced by increasing synthesis and release of dopamine (Bedard and Larochelle 1973).

Parkinsonism

This state may be induced by reserpine and its analogs, by the phenothiazines, especially those with a piperazine side chain, eg, prochlorperazine (Compazine), trifluoperazine (Stelazine), and perphenazine (Trilafon), or with a substituted CF_3 group in the 2-position, eg, trifluopromazine (Vesprin); and by the butyrophenones, eg, haloperidol (Haldol) (Hornykiewicz et al 1970). It appears these drugs produce the parkinsonian state by either depleting dopamine from synaptic vesicles or by blocking the postsynaptic receptor site. The symptoms are quite similar to naturally occurring Parkinson's disease: akinesia, rigidity, tremor, and rarely oculogyric crises. Its occurrence is dose-related and does not continue if the offending medicine is decreased or stopped. Further, those individuals who have a relative with naturally occurring Parkinson's disease appear to have a greater susceptibility for this drug-induced state (Myrianthopolous et al 1969). It is well controlled by either reducing the drug or by giving levodopa or standard anticholinergic agents. The latter are simpler to use and usually quite effective.

Akathisia

This is another syndrome associated with the use of phenothiazines and butyrophenones. The patient acts in an extremely restless manner, getting up from a chair, sitting down, moving legs about, fiddling with a piece of paper. The patient is often intensely aware of this. The movements themselves are of the "normal" type rather than choreoathetoid. Akathisia is particularly likely to occur early in therapy and is usually precisely dose related. In our experience it is more common in adults. Its cause is unknown. Treatment involves reducing the dose or stopping the offending drug.

Tardive Dyskinesia

This is still another syndrome associated with the use of phenothiazines and butyrophenones. It usually appears after many months of therapy with large doses of one of the more potent compounds (see section above on Parkinson-producing drugs). Yet we have seen cases develop after treatment with moderate doses of thioridazine (Mellaril). It may be seen as the drug is being discontinued.

At its mildest, tardive dyskinesia may consist of pursing the lips. There may be tongue and face movements, torticollis, scoliosis or other choreoathetoid movements, or coarse tremors of almost any part of the body. These may be severe enough to prevent walking and they may continue for months or years, even after the offending drugs are stopped.

The similarity of these movements to those in Huntington's chorea and to levodopa-induced choreoathetosis in the treatment of Parkinson's disease has led to the speculation that tardive dyskinesia is due to dopamine receptor hypersensitivity (Klawans 1973). However, we have given 3 to 6 g of levodopa a day to such patients without worsening their tardive dyskinesia. While such a small trial does not rule out the above speculation, it does indicate some unexplained complications.

Treatment of this condition is unsatisfactory (Kazamatsuri et al 1972). If the movements are mild, perhaps no drug treatment is best. If severe, sometimes small doses of another antipsychotic drug may give benefit. Increasing the dose of the offending drug may also help, but this just aggravates the situation when the drug is finally withdrawn.

Ataxia and Incoordination

Diphenylhydantoin (Dilantin), a widely used anticonvulsant, can induce ataxia and a cerebellar type of incoordination in almost any individual. When used as an anticonvulsant at therapeutic dosages of 200 to 600 mg per day, possibly 15 percent of individuals have mild reversible ataxia. A blood level of 1 to 2 mg percent Dilantin is considered safe and effective, but we have had patients who were ataxic while receiving this dose range of the drug. In any case, most patients of the many who have taken Dilantin have no clinically discernible incoordination.

Patients who take an overdose of Dilantin in a suicide attempt or who receive a large amount in the course of treatment of status epilepticus may end up with permanent cerebellar symptoms and signs. On postmortem examination, such patients may have loss of cerebellar Purkinje cells, diffuse distribution of granule cells, and gliosis (Dam 1972). Chronic toxic doses of Dilantin given to rats also produce significant abnormalities of the membranes of Purkinje cells (Snider and del Cerro 1972).

A number of other drugs will produce ataxia and incoordination during acute overdosage. Alcohol is one. However, chronic use of alcohol in high amounts may produce degeneration of cellular elements in the anterior lobe of the cerebellum and be associated clinically with severe ataxia of gait (Victor et al 1959). Certain other drugs, such as the barbiturates and the benzodiazepines, may also produce ataxia in overdosage; the site of action for this effect is unclear.

References

American College of Neuropsychopharmacology—Food and Drug Administration Task Force: Neurological syndromes associated with antipsychotic drug use. Arch Gen Psychiatry 23:463, 1973

Ansel RD, Markham CH: Effects of L-Dopa in normal humans. In Barbeau A, McDowell F (eds): L-Dopa and Parkinsonism. Philadelphia, Davis, 1970, pp 69–72

Bak IJ, Hassler R, Kim JS, Kataoka K: Amantadine actions on acetycholine and GABA in striatum and substantia nigra of rat in relation to behavioral changes. J Neurol Trans 33:45, 1972

Bedard P, Larochelle L: Effect of section of strionigral fibers on dopamine turnover in the forebrain of the rat. Exp Neurol 41:314, 1973

Bernheimer H, Birkmeyer W, Hornykiewicz O: Verteilung des 5-Hydroxytryptamine (Serotonin) in Gehirn des Menschen und sein Verhalten bei Patienten mit Parkinson-Syndrom. Klin Wochenschr 39:1056, 1961

Chyatte SB, Birdsong JH, Roberson DL: Dantrolene sodium in athetoid cerebral palsy. Arch Phys Med Rehabil 54:365, 1973

Dam M: Diphenylhydantoin—neurological aspect of toxicity. In Woodbury DM, Penry JK, Schmidt RP (eds): Antiepileptic Drugs. New York, Raven, 1972, pp 227–235

Ehringer H, Hornykiewicz O: Verteilung von Noradrenalin und Dopamin (3-Hydroxytramin) im Gehirn des Menschen und ihr Verhalten bei Erkrankungen des extrapyramidalen Systems. Klin Wochenschr 38:1236, 1960

Gelenberg A, Poskanzer D: The effect of dantrolene sodium on spasticity in multiple sclerosis. Neurology 23:1313, 1973

Greenblatt DJ, Shader RI: Benzodiazepines (drug therapy). N Engl J Med 291:1011, 1974

Grelak RP, Clark R, Stump JM, Vernier VG: Amantadine-dopamine interaction: possible mode of action in parkinsonism. Science 169:203, 1970

Hillarp NA, Fuxe K, Dahlstrom A: Central monoamine neurons. In von Euler US, Rosell S, Urnas B (eds): Mechanisms of Release of Biogenic Amines. Oxford, Pergamon, 1966, pp 31–57

Hornykiewicz O, Markham CH, Clark WG, Fleming RM: Mechanisms of extrapyramidal side effects of therapeutic agents. In Clark WG, Del Guidice J (eds): Principles of Psychopharmacology. New York, Academic, 1970, pp 585–595

Kazamatsuri H, Chien CP, Cole JO: Therapeutic approaches to tardive dyskinesia. Arch Gen Psychiatry 27:491, 1972

Klawans HL Jr, Paulson GW, Ringel SP, Barbeau A: Use of L-Dopa in the detection of presymptomatic Huntington's chorea. N Engl J Med 286:1332, 1972

Klawans HL: The pharmacology of tardive dyskinesias. Am J Psychiatry 130:82, 1973

Lee DK, Markham CH, Clark WG: Serotonin (5-HT) metabolism in Huntington's chorea. In Life Sciences, Part I, Vol 7, No 13. New York, Pergamon, 1968, pp 704—712

Markham CH, Diamond SG, Treciokas LJ: Carbidopa in Parkinson disease and in nausea and vomiting of levodopa. Arch Neurol 31:128, 1974

————, Treciokas LJ, Diamond SG: Parkinson's disease and levodopa—a five-year follow-up and review. West J Med 121:188, 1974

Myrianthopolous NC, Waldrop FN, Vincent BL: A repeat study of hereditary predisposition in drug-induced parkinsonism. In Barbeau A, Brunette JR (eds): Progress in Neuro-Genetics. Amsterdam, Excerpta Medica Foundation, 1969, pp 486–491

Snider RS, del Cerro M: Diphenylhydantoin—proliferating membranes in cerebellum resulting from intoxication. In Woodbury DM, Penry JK, Schmidt RP (eds): Antiepileptic Drugs. New York, Raven, 1972, pp 237–245

Stevens H: Paroxysmal choreo-athetosis, a form of reflex epilepsy. Arch Neurol 14:415, 1966

Sweet RD, Solomon GE, Wayne H, Shapiro E, Shapiro AK: Neurological features of Gilles de la Tourette's syndrome. J Neurol Neurosurg Psychiatry 36:1, 1973

————, Blumberg J, Lee JE, McDowell FH: Propranolol treatment of essential tremor. Neurology 24:64, 1974

Treciokas LJ, Ansel RD, Markham CH: One to two year treatment of Parkinson's disease with levodopa. Calif Med 114:7, 1971

Van Woert MH, Sethy VH: Therapy of intention myoclonus with L-5-hydroxytryptophan and a peripheral decarboxylase inhibitor, MK-486 Neurology 25:135, 1975

Victor M, Adams RD, Mancall EL: Restricted form of cerebellar cortical degeneration occurring in alcoholic patients. Arch Neurol 1:579, 1959

the central mode of action of narcotic analgesic drugs

commentary

The search for an ideal pain-relieving medication is as old as mankind. Analgesic drugs are extremely important in the practice of medicine, for they enable the physician to relieve suffering, an achievement superior to that of prolonging life. To date, the most effective analgesics are opioids, the use of which dates from prehistoric times. However, this class of drugs has many disadvantages, including a strong addiction potential and the possibility of respiratory arrest. Physicians are sometimes fearful of using analgesic drugs in effective doses (see p 393). The more commonly used milder analgesics include aspirin, but these act on peripheral mechanisms, whereas the opioids act centrally. Pain is a phenomenon of great importance in medicine, but it is difficult to define and understand. Dr. Liebeskind and his colleagues have made important contributions to our understanding of the neural mechanisms underlying pain and how pharmacologic, surgical, and electrical approaches to control pain are best utilized.

During the past few years rapid progress has been made in elucidating the structure and locus of the morphine receptor. Also a number of endogenously occurring morphinelike substances have been isolated from the brain (Goldstein 1975, Hughes et al 1975, Simantov 1976). We can expect rapid progress in this field in the next few years.

References

Goldstein A: Isolation of the opiate receptor: a progress report. In Tower, DB (ed); The Nervous System, Vol. 1: The Basic Neurosciences. New York, Raven, 1975

Hughes J, Smith TW, Kosterlitz HW, et al: Identification of two related pentapeptides from the brain with potent opiate agonist activity. Nature 258:577–579, 1975

Simantov R, Snyder SH: Elevated levels of enkephalin in morphine-dependent rats. Nature 262:505–507, 1976

the central mode of action of narcotic analgesic drugs

Dell Lynn Rhodes, Ph.D.
John C. Liebeskind, Ph.D.

The task of relieving pain has always been of primary importance to the practice of medicine. Fortunately, two organic sources of analgesic compounds have been recognized since ancient times, the opium poppy from which the opiate alkaloids are derived and willow bark, which provides salicin, a chemical relative of the synthetic salicylates. These two classes of drugs—the narcotic analgesics, ie, the opiate alkaloids and their synthetic agonists, and the salicylates—are still the most effective and widely used pain-reducing agents available today.

It is generally accepted that the narcotics and the salicylates differ in their sites and mechanisms of analgesic action. In a classic experiment with the cross-perfused spleen of the dog, Lim et al (1964) demonstrated that the site of aspirin's analgesic action is the peripheral nervous system, whereas morphine produces analgesia by its activity on the central nervous system. More specifically, aspirin interacts with the process of pain reception at the site of injury, whereas morphine affects the processing of nociceptive signals after they have been initiated and sent to the central nervous system.

Recent studies have suggested a biochemical mechanism of action for aspirin. Using cell-free homogenates, Vane (1971) demonstrated that aspirin inhibits the synthesis of the prostaglandins PGE_2 and $PGF_{2\alpha}$ from arachidonic acid. Others have confirmed that aspirin has an effect on prostaglandins in physiologic systems by showing that it decreases the release of prostaglandins both from human blood platelets treated with thrombin (Smith and Willis 1971) and from dog spleen infused with adrenalin (Ferreira et al 1971). Finally, the prostaglandins have been implicated in pain production by the observation that slow infusion of concentrations of PGE_1, similar to those normally found in areas of inflammation, produced, over time, a sensitization of the infused area to mechanical and chemical stimuli (Ferreira 1972). It was concluded that aspirin may, by inhibiting the synthesis of the prostaglandins, prevent sensitization of pain receptors, which is necessary to the transduction of pain signals in inflamed tissue (Ferreira 1972).

The mechanism of analgesic action of narcotics has been much harder to pin down. Narcotic drugs affect a number of different functional systems within the organism, and it seems likely that pain perception is altered by these drugs in more than one way. Furthermore, the study of narcotic analgesia in man is complicated by the particularly strong contribution of psychologic factors to human pain perception. This chapter will focus on recent efforts to understand the basic mechanisms of narcotic analgesia. After briefly reviewing the clinical pharmacology of narcotic drugs, we will consider in more detail a group of very recent and exciting experimental findings that appear to be shedding important new light on the question of just how and where a narcotic drug, such as morphine, blocks the pain message.

The Clinical Pharmacology of Narcotic Drugs

The prototype narcotic analgesic drug is morphine. Effective doses of morphine for the relief of clinical pain of moderate to severe intensity average 10 mg per 70 kg, the usual routes of administration being intramuscular or intravenous (Jaffe 1970). Other effects that may be produced at these doses in man include respiratory depression (the most toxic), nausea and vomiting, sweating, pupillary constriction, constipation, drowsiness, mood changes (either euphoria or dysphoria), and mental clouding (Jaffe 1970). In addition, as has long been recognized, repeated use of morphine leads to the development of tolerance and physical dependence.

The dangers of tolerance and iatrogenic addiction limit the usefulness of morphine in the management of pain of more than brief duration (See p 419). Consequently, an extensive search has been conducted for a compound with the analgesic properties of morphine but relatively lacking in morphine's undesirable properties of respiratory depression, tolerance, and physical dependence (Eddy and May 1973). This search has led to a description of the necessary structural characteristics common to most morphine agonists (Schaumann 1940) as well as to the synthesis of several important morphine derivatives and synthetic compounds with morphinelike analgesic activity. Among the narcotics used clinically as analgesics are meperidine (Demerol), codeine, hydromorphone (Dilaudid), oxycodone (Percodan), levorphanol (Levo-Dromoran), methadone (Dolophine), pentazocine (Talwin), and dextrapropoxyphene (Darvon).

Unfortunately, none of the above drugs has proven to be the sought-after ideal. For most of them, there is a strong correlation between clinical antinociceptive effectiveness and the production of morphinelike physical dependence (Eddy and May 1973). An encouraging separation of these two actions has, however, been observed in the synthetic morphine agonist-antagonists which display the ability to mimic some actions of morphine while antagonizing others (Eddy and May 1973). The first of the agonist-antagonists to be discovered was nalorphine (Nalline), which, while antagonizing nearly all the effects of morphine, is itself almost equipotent with morphine in its analgesic properties (Lasagna 1964). Although repeated use of nalorphine leads to a type of physical dependence, it can be differentiated from the dependence produced by morphine and is particularly distinguished by a lack of drug-seeking behavior (Martin 1967). Nalorphine's clinical utility, however, is limited by its psychotropic effects, which resemble those of morphine at very low doses, but are identified as more psychotomimetic and barbituratelike at higher doses (Haertzen 1970).

More useful clinically is pentazocine (Talwin), which possesses a complex set of morphine-agonist, morphine-antagonist, and nalorphine-agonist properties (Jasinski 1973). At analgesic doses, pentazocine's subjective effects are usually morphinelike, although there is some evidence for a higher incidence of perceptual distortions and hallucinations with pentazocine than with pure morphine agonists (Wood et al 1974). Other side effects of pentazocine differ somewhat from those of morphine but do include significant respiratory depression. Most important, pentazocine's abuse potential is considerably lower than morphine's (Jasinski 1973). Although not controlled as a narcotic drug, pentazocine should be administered with the same caution as other opioids (Jaffe 1970), especially to dependency-prone persons (Dewey 1973).

Another important synthetic compound is naloxone (Narcan), which is distinguished by its ability to antagonize the effects of both morphine and nalorphine with little, if any, agonistic activity (Blumberg and Dayton 1973). It was hoped that, with proper doses, naloxone could be used to minimize the respiratory depressant and dependence-producing effects of morphine while sparing some analgesia. There seems to be little hope, however, that this separation of effects can be achieved by the combination of naloxone with morphine (Gupta and Dundee 1974).

In summary, the narcotic analgesics remain the drugs of choice for treating pain of moderate to severe intensity, especially over brief periods of time. Their utility is limited primarily by the development of tolerance and iatrogenic physical dependence. It may be cautioned on the one hand that the ready success these drugs enjoy in antinociception must never diminish the physician's zeal to discover and treat the condition causing pain. On the other hand, some physicians appear overly concerned with the dangers of drug dependence and, in refusing to prescribe narcotics, may permit needless suffering. We would not attempt here to deal further with this complex, medical-ethical issue. Suffice it to say that human suffering is as individual an experience as any can possibly be and hence cannot be approached with predetermined formulas.

Recent Evidence Concerning the Site and Mechanism of Action of Morphine

Excellent evidence is rapidly accumulating that morphine works by actively engaging a pain-inhibitory neural system in the brain and spinal cord rather than by passively blocking the afferent flow of the pain message. That is, instead of itself directly dulling "pain centers" in the nervous system (acting somehow centrally as a local anesthetic), morphine seems to ignite an endogenous mechanism of analgesia which has its own means of reducing or eliminating pain. In the remainder of this chapter we will review some of this evidence, much of which, admittedly, is so recent that it has not yet been subjected to the test of time.

As indicated above, Lim et al (1964) provided the most clearcut and elegant demonstration of the fact that morphine effects antinociception via its action on the central nervous system. Working with a vasoisolated but neurally innervated dog spleen cross-perfused by the blood supply of a donor dog, Lim and his associates recorded a reliable pain response to injections of the noxious substance, bradykinin, into the splenic artery of the recipient dog. This response was blocked by morphine injected into the recipient dog's circulation, where the drug had access to the animal's central nervous system, but not by morphine injected into the donor dog's circulation, which perfused only the recipient's spleen and its neural innervation. The opposite was true for aspirin.

The question of exactly where in the central nervous system morphine acts is still being investigated. There is reason to believe that morphine exerts its initial action on the brain and that its inhibitory effects on spinal nociceptive reflexes are mediated by the activation of descending pathways from the brain. A number of years ago, Irwin et al (1951) speculated on the existence of these descending pain-inhibitory paths. They found that a particular spinal nociceptive reflex in the rat was of greater amplitude after spinal transection, suggesting the presence of a tonically active descending inhibition in the intact animal. The transected rats were also much less sensitive to morphine than were unoperated animals. Similarly, in a more recent study it was shown that the suppressive effect of morphine on pain-evoked potentials in the spinal cord is blocked by a high spinal transection (Satoh and Takagi 1971). In fact, for morphine to be effective it was necessary to preserve the normal interconnections between the medulla and the cord. Interruption of the brain stem at higher than medullary levels did not diminish morphine's analgesic action (Satoh and Takagi 1971).

A number of recent studies appear to be pinpointing more precisely the site of morphine's analgesic action in the brain. By injecting minute quantities of morphine through fine cannulas stereotaxically placed in various brain structures, several investigators have found the periaqueductal gray matter in the caudal midbrain to be one of the most sensitive areas for eliciting analgesia in this fashion (Jacquet and Lajtha 1974, Sharpe et al 1974). From these and similar studies it may be concluded that there is a morphine-sensitive, medial, periventricular system extending from the periaqueductal gray matter rostrally into the caudal diencephalon and caudally into the pons and rostral medulla. Other workers have recently reported evidence of opiate receptors in the brain (Kuhar et al 1973, Lowney et al 1974, Pert and Snyder 1973). According to these studies, brain areas rich in opiate receptor sites include the medial diencephalon, the periaqueductal gray matter, and the caudal brain stem. Still another converging line of evidence derives from studies, including our own, which show that electrical stimulation of certain discrete brain regions through implanted electrodes can yield potent analgesia in laboratory animals (Liebeskind et al 1974, Mayer et al 1974, Rhodes 1975). Once again, it is these same medial, periaqueductal, and periventricular structures that provide the strongest and most reliable effects.

Many studies indicate that morphine's analgesic effectiveness depends upon the integrity of certain neurotransmitter systems in the central nervous system. These findings suggest that morphine works by activating neural pathways in which these transmitters are released. The cerebral monoamines (dopamine, noradrenaline, and serotonin) are almost certainly involved, since alterations in these transmitter systems cause important changes in morphine analgesia (Way and Shen 1971). Monoamine-containing neurons are also known to exist in the same core brain stem structures described above, some of their fibers extending upward into the forebrain and others descending and terminating in the spinal cord (Dahlström and Fuxe 1965, Lindvall and Björklund 1974). We were not surprised, therefore, to find that brain stimulation analgesia also depends upon these same transmitters (Akil and Liebeskind 1975).

It seems that the medial brain stem system concerned with pain inhibition can be activated *exogenously* either by direct electrical stimulation or by morphine administration and that synaptic transmission within at least some portions of this system occurs via the release of one or another of the monoamines. It may be assumed that this same system is also available to *endogenous* mechanisms of pain inhibition, perhaps accounting for some of the psychologic factors involved in pain control. A dramatic discovery by Hughes (1975) strongly supports this view. Hughes has succeeded in isolating from extracts of the brain stem of the rat an endogenous substance that has a specific morphinelike action in a bioassay. This action is blocked by the pure morphine antagonist, naloxone. It is tempting to speculate that morphine is effective because it structurally resembles this endogenous substance and hence occupies its receptor sites in the brain. Brain stimulation, on the other hand, may cause analgesia by releasing the endogenous substance.

The pathway from morphine's presumed initial site of action in the medial brain stem to the ultimate site or sites of pain inhibition is still almost completely a mystery. There is, however, growing evidence that at least one site of pain inhibition is located at the level of a particular class of sensory neuron found in the intermediate layers of the dorsal horn of the spinal cord. Wall (1967) and others have demonstrated the critical role in nociception played by these so-called lamina 5 cells. These cells respond most vigorously when a peripheral stimulus of cutaneous or visceral origin is noxious in quality. The pain-producing chemical, bradykinin, selectively activates these neurons (Besson et al 1972). It has recently been established that many of these cells project, via the spinothalamic tract, to the lower brain stem and the thalamus (Albe-Fessard et al 1974, Trevino et al 1973) and hence may inform the brain of the occurrence of a noxious stimulus. In fact, Melzack and Wall (1965) based a large portion of their now classic Gate Theory of pain on the actions of these cells and the interactions between large and small diameter fibers, which take place at this level. In view of this evidence relating lamina 5 cell activity to nociception, it is of considerable significance to note that morphine and related compounds exert a selective inhibition on spinal cord sensory cells of this type (Kitahata et al 1974, Maillard et al 1972). Similarly, we have shown that electrical stimulation of the medial brain stem selectively inhibits lamina 5 cells and may block completely their response to even intensely noxious stimuli (Oliveras et al 1974). Thus it is apparent that these spinal cord neurons are subject to descending inhibitory influences from the brain stem. At least one way in which morphine might induce analgesia is by reinforcing activity in such a descending path.

Another clue to the possible pathway underlying central mechanisms of morphine analgesia lies in the recent work of Vogt (1974) and of Anderson and his colleagues (Proudfit and Anderson 1974, Repkin et al 1974). These workers report that selective interference with the serotonin containing neurons of the medulla (whose axons are known to descend into the spinal cord) markedly reduces morphine's analgesic action. It has also been found that electrical stimulation of this brain region induces analgesia (Oleson and Liebeskind 1975, Oliveras et al 1975, Repkin et al 1974), and from preliminary evidence it seems that morphine may enhance the rates of spontaneous discharge of neurons in this area (Oleson and Liebeskind 1975). This region of the brain may, therefore, be a crucial link in the pathway between morphine's medial brain stem site of action and the spinal cord site of inhibitory interaction between the descending system and the afferent pain signal. Needless to say, many other essential links must be found and the suggestions of recent work must be confirmed and strengthened before the final chapter in this story will have been told.

In summary, it has been suggested that a pain-inhibitory system exists within the medial brain stem, and that this system is activated by morphine. One result of such activation is a powerful blockade of afferent transmission through spinal cord neurons thought to be involved in carrying the pain message. Although evidence for this particular mode of morphine action is strong, it in no way precludes the possibility that other central sites and mechanisms of narcotic analgesia exist in parallel.

References

Akil H, Liebeskind JC: Monoaminergic mechanisms of stimulation-produced analgesia. Brain Res 94:279, 1975

Albe-Fessard D, Levante A, Lamour Y: Origin of spino-thalamic tract in monkeys. Brain Res 65:503, 1974

Besson JM, Conseiller C, Hamann KF, Maillard MC: Modifications of dorsal horn cell activities in the spinal cord after intra-arterial injection of bradykinin. J Physiol (Lond) 221:189, 1972

Blumberg H, Dayton HB: Naloxone and related compounds. In Kosterlitz HW, Collier HOJ, Villareal JE (eds): Agonist and Antagonist Actions of Narcotic Analgesic Drugs. Baltimore, University Park Press, 1973, p 110

Cox BM, Goldstein A, Li CH: Opioid activity of a peptide, β-lipotropin (61-91) derived from β-lipotropin. Proceedings NAS USA 73:1821–1832, 1976

Dahlström A, Fuxe K: Evidence for the existence of monoamine neurons in the central nervous system. II. Experimentally induced changes in the intraneuronal amine levels of bulbospinal neuron systems. Acta Physiol Scand 64: (Suppl 247) 5, 1965

Dewey WL: The pharmacology of pentazocine. Int Anesthesiol Clin 11:139, 1973

Eddy NB, May EL: The search for a better analgesic. Science 181:407, 1973

Ferreira SH: Prostaglandins, aspirin-like drugs and analgesia. Nature New Biol 240:200, 1972

———, Moncada S, Vane JR: Indomethacin and aspirin abolish prostaglandin release from the spleen. Nature New Biol 231:237, 1971

Gupta PK, Dundee JW: Morphine combined with doxapram or naloxone: A study of post-operative pain relief. Anaesthesia 29:33, 1974

Haertzen DA: Subjective effects of narcotic antagonists cyclazocine and nalorphine on the Addiction Research Center Inventory (ARCI). Psychopharmacologia 18:366, 1970

Hughes J: Isolation of an endogenous compound from the brain with pharmacological properties similar to morphine. Brain Res 88:295, 1975

———, Smith TW, Kosterlitz HW et al: Identification of two related pentapeptides from the brain with potent opiate agonist activity. Nature 258:577–597, 1975

Irwin S, Houde RW, Bennett DR, Hendershot LC, Seevers, MH: The effects of morphine, methadone and meperidine on some reflex responses of spinal animals to nociceptive stimulation. J Pharmacol Exp Ther 101:132, 1951

Jacquet YF, Lajtha A: Paradoxical effects after microinjection of morphine in the periaqueductal gray matter in the rat. Science 185:1055, 1974

Jaffe JH: Narcotic analgesics. In Goodman LS, Gilman A (eds): The Pharmacological Basis of Therapeutics. New York, Macmillan, 1970, p 237

Jasinski DR: Effects in man of partial morphine agonists. In Kosterlitz HW, Collier HOJ, Villareal JE (eds): Agonist and Antagonist Actions of Narcotic Analgesic Drugs. Baltimore, University Park Press, 1973, p 94

Kitahata LM, Kosaka Y, Taub A, Bonikos K, Hoffert M: Lamina-specific suppression of dorsal-horn unit activity by morphine sulfate. Anesthesiology 41:39, 1974

Kuhar MJ, Pert CB, Snyder SH: Regional distribution of opiate receptor binding in monkey and human brain. Nature (Lond) 245:447, 1973

Lasagna L: The clinical evaluation of morphine and its substitutes as analgesics. Pharmacol Rev 16:47, 1964

Liebeskind JC, Mayer DJ, Akil H: Central mechanisms of pain inhibition: studies of analgesia from focal brain stimulation. In Bonica JJ (ed): Advances in Neurology, Vol 4, Pain. New York, Raven, 1974, p 261

Lim RKS, Guzman F, Rodgers DW, Goto K, Braun C, Dickerson GD, Engle RJ: Site of action of narcotic and nonnarcotic analgesics determined by blocking bradykinin-evoked visceral pain. Arch Int Pharmacodyn 152:25, 1964

Lindvall O, Björklund A: The organization of the ascending catecholamine neuron systems in the rat brain as revealed by the glyoxylic acid fluorescence method. Acta Physiol Scand 412 (Suppl):1, 1974

Lowney LI, Schulz K, Lowery PJ, Goldstein A: Partial purification of an opiate receptor from mouse brain. Science 183:749, 1974

Maillard M-C, Benoist J-M, Conseiller C, Hamann K-F, Besson J-M: Effets de la phénopéridine sur l'activité des interneurones de la corne dorsale de la moelle chez le Chat spinal. C R Acad Sci (Paris) 274:726, 1972

Martin WR: Opioid antagonists. Pharmacol Rev 19:463, 1967

Mayer DJ, Liebeskind JC: Pain reduction by focal electrical stimulation of the brain: an anatomical and behavioral analysis. Brain Res 68:73, 1974

Melzack R, Wall PD: Pain mechanisms: A new theory. Science 150:971, 1965

Oleson TD, Liebeskind JC: Relationship of neural activity in the raphe nuclei of the rat to brain stimulation-produced analgesia. Physiologist 18:338, 1975

Oliveras JL, Besson J-M, Guilbaud G, Liebeskind JC: Behavioral and electrophysiological evidence of pain inhibition from mid-brain stimulation in the cat. Exp Brain Res 20:32, 1974

———, Redjemi F, Guilbaud G, Besson JM: Analgesia induced by electrical stimulation of the inferior centralis nucleus of the raphe in the cat. Pain 1:139, 1975

Pert CB, Snyder SH: Opiate receptor: demonstration in nervous tissue. Science 179:1011, 1973

Proudfit HK, Anderson EG: Blockade of morphine analgesia by destruction of a bulbospinal serotonergic pathway. Pharmacologist 16:203, 1974

Repkin AH, Proudfit HK, Anderson EG: Primary afferent depolarization as a mechanism of morphine analgesia. Pharmacologist 16:203, 1974

Rhodes DL: A behavior investigation of pain responsiveness following electrical stimulation of the rostral brain stem of the rat. Unpublished Doctoral Dissertation, UCLA, 1975

Satoh M, Takagi H: Enhancement by morphine of the central descending inhibitory influence on spinal sensory transmission. Eur J Pharmacol 14:60, 1971

Schaumann O: Über eine neue Klasse von Verbindungen mit spasmolytischer und zentral analgetischer WirksamKeit unter besonderer Berücksichtigung des 1-Methyl-4-phenyl-piperidin-4-carbonsäure-äthylesters (Dolantin). Arch Exp Pathol Pharmakol Naunyn-Schmiedebergs 196:109, 1940

Sharpe LG, Garnett JE, Cicero TJ: Analgesia and hyperreactivity produced by intracranial microinjections of morphine into the periaqueductal gray matter of the rat. Behav Biol 11:303, 1974

Simantov R, Snowman AM, Snyder SH: A morphine-like factor enkephalin in rat brain: subcellular localization. Brain Res 107:650–657, 1976

Smith JB, Willis AL: Aspirin selectively inhibits prostaglandin production in human platelets. Nature New Biol 231:235, 1971

Trevino DL, Coulter JD, Willis WD: Location of cells of origin of spinothalamic tract in lumbar enlargement of the monkey. J. Neurophysiol 36:750, 1973

Vane JR: Inhibition of prostaglandin synthesis as a mechanism of action for aspirin-like drugs. Nature New Biol 231:232, 1971

Vogt M: The effect of lowering the 5-hydroxytryptamine content of the rat spinal cord on analgesia produced by morphine. J Physiol (Lond) 236:483, 1974

Wall PD: The laminar organization of dorsal horn and effects of descending impulses. J Physiol (Lond) 188:403, 1967

Way EL, Shen F: Catecholamines and 5-hydroxytryptamine. In Clouet DH (ed): Narcotic Drugs: Biochemical Pharmacology. New York, Plenum, 1971, p. 229

Wood AJJ, Moir DC, Campbell C, et al: Medicines evaluation and monitoring group: Central nervous system effects of pentazocine. Br Med J 1:305, 1974

drugs and brain lesions

commentary

Although a certain number of patients in every practice will have brain damage, the reserve capacity of the brain is so great that it is frequently difficult to make a diagnosis. Dead brain tissue cannot be replaced, but there have been some studies which indicate that the homeostatic repair of brain damage could be facilitated by stimulant drugs (Mishkin et al 1953). Changes in brain function due to congenital brain damage, trauma during lifetime, or brain damage induced by diseases, such as pituitary disorders or senility, may or may not yield to drug treatment, but there is every reason to believe that pharmacologic treatment should be useful in such cases. Although this is largely a research-oriented chapter, there are points of extreme interest to practicing physicians. In years to come, the diagnosis of brain damage will become easier with the advent of computerized brain scans and other advanced neurodiagnostic procedures.

A common form of brain damage treated with drugs is parkinsonism, in which levodopa seems to be distinctly helpful (see p 127). However, another common cause of brain damage, the cerebrovascular accident, has not yet yielded to any particular drug treatment. It is clear that more research, such as that of Dr. Glick, is highly necessary in this important area.

Reference

Mishkin M, Rosvold HE, Pribram KH: Effects of nembutal in baboons with frontal lesions. J Neurophysiol 15:155–159, 1953

drugs and
brain
lesions

Stanley Glick, M.D., Ph.D.

The administration of drugs to brain-damaged patients is common practice in clinical medicine. The rationale for using a particular drug in the treatment of a particular disorder is sometimes quite specific, but in other cases it is quite nebulous. For example, the use of levodopa in parkinsonism is founded on the theoretical restoration of dopaminergic function in the corpus striatum. In contrast, the use of amphetamines in the treatment of minimal brain dysfunction is based entirely upon empirical findings rather than on any generally accepted principle or theory. This chapter will be concerned primarily with the discussion of experimental studies, in animals, involving drugs and brain lesions. It is hoped that by furthering an understanding of the interactions of drugs and brain damage, fundamental principles will emerge which eventually will be applicable to many clinical settings.

Experimental studies involving drugs and brain lesions usually stem from three approaches. Most commonly, an investigator wishes to determine the neuroanatomic site of action of the drug. The underlying assumption in some of these studies is that if one removes that part of the brain at which the drug normally acts, the drug will then have little or no effect. In other site of action studies, emphasis is placed on comparing the effects of drugs and brain lesions. If similar behavioral effects are produced by a particular drug and a specific brain lesion, then it may be surmised that the drug normally inhibits that specific area of the brain. Finally, other investigators studied changes in drug sensitivity as a function of time after brain damage in order to provide inferences as to what kinds of neuronal changes may be involved in the recovery of function, which often occurs after brain damage. Based on such inferences, an attempt can be made to understand rational ways of using drugs to facilitate recovery. By necessity, most of the experimental work in this area is done in animals. In the sections to follow, examples of each of these three drug lesion approaches will be considered in more detail.

Ablating the Site of Drug Action

If the behavioral effects of a drug are mediated by synaptic activating effects (eg, stimulating postsynaptic receptors or releasing a neurotransmitter from presynaptic terminals) in a particular brain region, then a lesion that includes some or all of those synapses upon which the drug acts should decrease or abolish the behavioral potency of the drug. In most cases, however, it is likely that a drug has multiple sites of action, contributing to each of possibly many behavioral effects. In some instances, though, it has been possible to implicate a major site of action for one or more specific behavioral effects of a drug. One such example is a syndrome of abnormal behavior elicited by high doses of amphetamines (ie, D-amphetamine, L-amphetamine, DL-amphetamine, or methamphetamine). In most species of mammals, including man, high doses of amphetamines induce stereotypic compulsive movements. In man, the syndrome, which may appear as aimless and repetitive searching activity, often precedes or occurs concomitantly with other manifestations of an amphetamine-induced paranoid psychosis. In the rat, stereotypic movements include rearing, gnawing, crouching, and sniffing (see p 467). Much evidence indicates that the stereotypic effects of amphetamines in rats, as well as in humans, are mediated by a presynaptic action of amphetamines on dopaminergic neurons projecting from the substantia nigra to the corpus striatum. In several studies with rats, it has been found that lesions of the substantia nigra or corpus striatum diminish or abolish amphetamine-induced stereotypy (Neil et al 1974). Complementing the data on lesions are other neurochemical results in which the effects of amphetamines on striatal dopamine metabolism have been correlated with the intensity of stereotypic behavior (Taylor and Synder 1970). Although there is some uncertainty as to whether or not an action of amphetamine on other structures also contributes to their stereotypic effects, it seems clear that the corpus striatum is the major site of action involved (Creese and Iverson 1974).

If a drug produces its effects by synaptic blocking actions (eg, blocking postsynaptic receptors or inhibiting release of a neurotransmitter from presynaptic terminals) in a particular brain region, then a lesion that includes some of those synapses upon which the drug acts would not necessarily be expected to lessen the behavioral potency of the drug. In fact, it might be expected that the drug would produce a larger behavioral effect than in a normal animal since, following the lesion, there would be fewer neurons for the drug to block. If the lesion were total, in the sense that all synapses at which the drug acts were destroyed, animals with such lesions might exhibit, without any drug, behavioral effects similar to those induced by the drug in normal animals. In these lesioned animals, the drug should then produce no further effect beyond that of the lesion. The lesion would thus have resulted in decreased drug sensitivity but only because the lesion had already produced a maximal or "ceiling" effect in the same system affected by the drug. The case involving a subtotal lesion and increased drug sensitivity would appear to be the more common occurrence in view of the fact that drugs usually act in many regions of the brain. For example, although its precise mechanism of action is still controversial, LSD is generally thought to induce many of its behavioral and hallucinogenic effects by inhibiting serotonin turnover in the brain (Aghajanian et al 1968). Serotoninergic neurons in the brain originate from the raphe nuclei in the midbrain. In support of the serotonin hypothesis of the action of LSD, it has been found that partial lesions of the midbrain raphe lower the threshold for an LSD-induced depression of bar pressing in rats (Appel et al 1970). Presumably, the effect of the lesion and the effect of LSD are additive with respect to a decrease in function of serotoninergic pathways.

Mimicking the Effects of Lesions with Drugs

Because of the limited conclusions that can be made on the basis of correlations alone, studies specifically concerned with comparing the behavioral effects of drugs and brain lesions are relatively few. One example of this approach is the similarity between the effects of anticholinergic drugs (eg, scopolamine and atropine) and lesions of the septum or hippocampus. In several behavioral situations (eg, active and passive avoidance behavior), scopolamine and atropine have been found to produce effects that partly, at least, mimic those produced by lesions of the septum or hippocampus in rats (Leaton 1971). These include diminished habituation to stimuli and vicious attack behavior. Injections of scopolamine or atropine into the septum or hippocampus also mimic the effects of septal or hippocampal lesions (eg, Hamilton and Grossman 1969). These results have suggested that the behavioral effects of anticholinergic drugs are mediated, at least in part, by blockade of cholinergic pathways between the septum and hippocampus.

Time-Dependent Changes in Drug Sensitivity and Recovery of Function

Several years ago it was reported that rats with bilateral ablations of the frontal cortex became increasingly sensitive to the activity stimulant effect of amphetamine with increasing time following surgery (Adler 1961). This time-dependent development of drug hypersensitivity was attributed to the occurrence of denervation supersensitivity in the central nervous system. Denervation supersensitivity generally refers to the observation that when a postsynaptic membrane is deprived of input, usually by destruction of presynaptic neurons (ie, denervation), postsynaptic sensitivity to chemical stimulation, either by the neurochemical normally mediating synaptic transmission or by others, increases (ie, supersensitivity) as a function of time after denervation. Although this phenomenon has been directly demonstrated in the peripheral nervous system (Trendelenburg 1963), it has only been indirectly inferred in the central nervous system (Sharpless and Jaffe 1968). Adler's data (1961), were presented as evidence for this inference. Frontal cortical lesions were envisioned as partially denervating subcortical structures; amphetamine presumably released catecholamines from remaining input to such structures, thus activating supersensitive postsynaptic receptors. Subsequent studies confirmed Adler's findings (Glick 1972). Inasmuch as recovery of function after brain damage depends on temporal factors, it has been proposed that denervation supersensitivity would be a likely compensatory mechanism to mediate recovery phenomena (Glick 1974).

Other studies with different lesions have supported both theories—that denervation supersensitivity occurs in the central nervous system and that denervation supersensitivity may be, at least in part, responsible for recovery of function. There have been several studies concerned with lesions of the dopaminergic nigrostriatal system. Following a unilateral lesion in any part of the nigrostriatal system (eg, in either the substantia nigra, nigrostriatal bundle, or corpus striatum), rats will rotate or turn in circles toward the side of the lesion (Crow 1971). When, after a few days, such rats recover from the tendency to rotate spontaneously, administration of amphetamine will reelicit this ipsilateral rotational behavior (eg, Ungerstedt 1971a). The cause of such rotation is an imbalance in nigrostriatal function on the two sides of the brain; rats rotate contralateral to the more active side. Amphetamine, by releasing dopamine from nigral input, apparently stimulates the intact nigrostriatal system and enhances the imbalance. In contrast, apomorphine, a drug which directly stimulates dopaminergic receptors, has very different effects, depending upon the location of the lesion within the nigrostriatal system. Following a unilateral lesion of the corpus striatum, apomorphine, like amphetamine, will potentiate or induce ipsilateral rotation; this would be expected to occur because apomorphine should predominantly activate receptors in the intact striatum. Following a unilateral lesion of either the substantia nigra or the nigrostriatal bundle, the effects of apomorphine will vary with the duration of the time interval after the lesion (Ungerstedt 1971b). Immediately after such a lesion, apomorphine produces very little effect. With increasing time after surgery, however, apomorphine increasingly induces contralateral rotation (ie, circling toward the side opposite the lesion). The nigral lesion denervates dopaminergic receptors in the striatum, which appear to become progressively supersensitive as a function of time following the denervation. As supersensitivity occurs, therefore, apomorphine has a greater effect on the denervated striatum than on the intact striatum. Since amphetamine's action depends upon intact presynaptic terminals containing dopamine, its ipsilateral rotation effect varies very little with time after surgery.

It is well known that bilateral lesions of the lateral hypothalamus in the rat produce a syndrome of aphagia and adipsia terminating in death, unless rats are kept alive by intragastric tube feedings. If initially maintained alive with force feedings, recovery of spontaneous feeding may eventually occur (Teitelbaum and Epstein 1962). Several kinds of data have implicated an important role of catecholamines in both normal feeding behavior and in the aphagic adipsic syndrome following lateral hypothalamic lesions (eg, Berger et al 1971). (There is presently some controversy as to which catecholamine, norepinephrine or dopamine, is primarily involved in feeding and to what extent the lateral hypothalamic syndrome is attributable to damage of nigrostriatal fibers adjacent to the hypothalamus [eg, Marshall et al 1974]). Following lateral hypothalamic lesions, denervation supersensitivity of remaining neurons to remaining catecholaminergic inputs might be responsible for recovery of feeding. If functional recovery involves denervation supersensitivity, it should be possible to facilitate recovery by administering treatments that induce supersensitivity in the pathways mediating recovery. Data consistent with this idea were reported in a study with alpha-methyl-p-tyrosine (α-MpT). a drug that interferes with the synthesis of catecholamines. Alpha-methyl-p-tyrosine was administered to rats for 3 days before lateral hypothalamic lesions were made; drug administration was discontinued 1 day prior to surgery. Doses of α-MpT, which were effective in partially depleting the brain of catecholamines, facilitated the recovery of feeding (Glick et al 1972). By administering α-MpT prior to surgery, the neurons subserving recovery should have been functionally denervated before surgery and sufficiently supersensitive sooner after surgery for recovery to occur. Termination of drug treatment before surgery should have allowed intact inputs that remained after surgery to become functional again.

Clinical Implications

Consideration of the ways in which drugs may interact with brain damage suggests a basis for some current as well as potential therapeutic practices. For example, although levodopa is thought to restore dopaminergic function in parkinsonism, the question arises as to how such restoration is possible if, as a result of the disease process, many fewer presynaptic terminals are left in the corpus striatum to synthesize dopamine. Several explanations have been proposed to account for this (eg, Hornykiewicz 1974). One very plausible reason for the efficacy of levodopa is denervation supersensitivity. Supersensitivity of dopamine receptors, resulting from the loss of many nigrostriatal neurons, would partially compensate for the greatly reduced input; further compensation would occur if, by the administration of levodopa, remaining nigrostriatal neurons could synthesize and release moderately increased amounts of dopamine to activate the supersensitive receptors.

Using special regimens of administration, drugs may eventually be of benefit in some specific cases of stroke or tumor surgery. As a precondition for such drug administration, extensive knowledge of the damaged brain area would be required to the extent that functional roles of particular neurotransmitters could be evaluated. If damage to such a brain area was anticipated (eg, in tumor surgery), then a drug or drugs interfering with the actions of the most relevant neurotransmitters might be administered before the damage occurred in order to promote the development of supersensitivity in the system to be affected by the damage. Faster recovery following the damage might then be expected. If the damage occurs serendipitously (eg, stroke), the drug might be administered for a short period of time after the damage. Clinical symptomatology might temporarily be worse than if the drug were not administered, inasmuch as the drug would produce a functional, but reversible lesion, summating with the actual lesion. However, when drug treatment is terminated, recovery should occur faster than if the drug were not administered because, as a result of the initially greater denervation induced by the drug, the compensatory mechanism (ie, denervation supersensitivity) mediating recovery would develop faster (Glick and Greenstein 1974).

In recent years there has been a great deal of publicity about hyperactive children with learning difficulties. The publicity has been related most often to treatment of these children with stimulant drugs such as amphetamines. Such children have frequently been found to have a "paradoxic" response to these drugs; instead of being stimulated as a normal child would be, the hyperactive child is sedated. As a result, the drug-treated hyperactive child is now able to concentrate better and hence his learning ability improves. Much of the publicity is probably attributable to difficulties in correctly diagnosing the condition, which is usually referred to as minimal brain dysfunction. That is, hyperactivity and retarded learning may result from many causes, environmental (eg, poor teaching conditions, home-related problems) as well as organic (eg, brain damage, endocrine disorders). It appears, however, that drug treatment will help those children in whom neurologic evidence of minimal but real brain damage is demonstrable (eg, Satterfield et al 1973, Millichap 1973). The basic diagnostic difficulty, therefore, lies in readily being able to discriminate different reasons for the same kinds of abnormal behaviors.

Recent research has begun to elucidate the reasons for the "paradoxic" benefit of drug treatment in minimal brain damage. It appears that the paradoxic nature of the drug effect may not, indeed, be truly paradoxic but reflect instead, drug hypersensitivity, ie, a quantitative rather than a qualitative effect. In both normal animals and humans, low doses of stimulant drugs "stimulate" or increase activity, whereas high doses "depress" or decrease activity (eg, Kelleher and Morse 1968, Glick and Milloy 1973). Drug hypersensitivity would result in an apparent paradoxic response to a low dose—a hypersensitive individual would react to a low dose as if it were a high dose. In rats it has been shown that particular kinds of brain damage (eg, Glick 1975) will produce such hypersensitivity to amphetamine-type drugs; such research may eventually tell us which parts of the brain are the source of dysfunction in minimal brain damage. Furthermore, we may have a potential diagnostic tool. For example, using small doses of amphetamines, one might determine the sensitiviyy of an individual to the drug's effect in some laboratory test of attentiveness. It could then be predicted that only those children showing a hypersensitive drug response would benefit from drug treatment.

References

Adler MW: Changes in sensitivity to amphetamine in rats with chronic brain damage. J Pharmacol Exp Ther 134:214–221, 1961

Aghajanian GK, Foote WE, Sheard MH: Lysergic acid diethylamide: sensitive neuronal units in the midbrain raphe. Science 161:706–708, 1968

Appel, JB, Lovell RA, Freedman DX: Alterations in the behavioral effects of LSD by pretreatment with p-chlorophenylalanine and α-methyl-p-tyrosine. Psychopharmacologia 18:387–406, 1970

Berger BD, Wise CD, Stein L: Norepinephrine: reversal of anorexia in rats with lateral hypothalamic damage. Science 172:281–284, 1971

Creese I, Iversen SD: The role of forebrain dopamine systems in amphetamine induced stereotyped behavior in the rat. Psychopharmacologia 39:345–357, 1974

Crow TJ: The relationship between lesion site, dopamine neurones and turning behaviour in the rat. Exp Neurol 32:247–255, 1971

Glick SD: Changes in amphetamine sensitivity following frontal cortical damage in rats and mice. Eur J Pharmacol 20:351–356, 1972

———. Changes in drug sensitivity and mechanisms of functional recovery after brain damage. In Stein DG, Rosen JJ, Butters N (eds): Plasticity and Recovery of Function is the Central Nervous System. New York, Academic, 1974, 339–372

———: Recovery of function and changes in sensitivity to amphetamine after caudate lesions in rats. Behav Biol 13:239–244, 1975

———, Greenstein S: Facilitation of lateral hypothalamic recovery by postoperative administration of α-methyl-p-tyrosine. Brain Res 73:180–183, 1974

———, Greenstein S, Zimmerberg B: Facilitation of recovery by α-methyl-p-tyrosine after lateral hypothalamic damage. Science 177:534–535, 1972

———, Milloy S: Rate-dependent effects of d-amphetamine on locomotor activity in mice: possible relationship to paradoxical amphetamine sedation in minimal brain dysfunction. Eur J Pharmacol 24:266–268, 1973

Hamilton LW, Grossman SP: Behavioral changes following disruption of central cholinergic pathways. J Comp Physiol Psychol 69:76–82, 1969

Hornykiewicz O: The mechanisms of action of L-dopa Parkinson's disease. Life Sci 15:1249–1259, 1974

Kelleher RT, Morse WH: Determinants of the specificity of behavioral effects of drugs. Ergeb Physiol 60:1–56, 1968

Leaton R: The limbic system and its pharmacologic aspects. In Rech RH, Moore KE (eds): An Introduction to Psychopharmacology. New York, Raven, 1971, p 137–174

Marshall JF, Richardson JS, Teitelbaum P: Nigrostriatal bundle damage and the lateral hypothalamic syndrome. J Comp Physiol Psychol 87:808–830, 1974

Millichap GL: Drugs in management of minimal brain dysfunction. Ann NY Acad Sci 205:321–334, 1973

Neil DB, Boggen WMO, Grossman SP: Behavioral effects of amphetamine in rats with lesions in the corpus striatum. J Comp Physiol Psychol 86:1019–1030, 1974

Satterfield JH, Lesser LL, Saul RE, Cantwell DP: EEG aspects in the diagnosis and treatment of minimal brain dysfunction. Ann NY Acad Sci 205:274–282, 1973

Sharpless SK, Jaffe JH: Pharmacological denervation supersensitivity in the CNS: a theory of physical dependence. In Wiker A (ed): The Addictive States. Baltimore, Williams & Wilkins, 1968

Taylor KM, Snyder SH: Amphetamine: differentiation by D and L isomers of behavior involving brain norepinephrine or dopamine. Science 168:1487–1489, 1970

Teitelbaum P, Epstein AN: The lateral hypothalamic syndrome: recovery of feeding and drinking after lateral hypothalamic lesions. Psychol Rev 69:74–90, 1962

Trendelenburg U: Supersensitivity and subsensitivity to sympathomimetic amines. Pharmacol Rev 15:225–227, 1963

Ungerstedt U: Striatal dopamine release after amphetamine or nerve degeneration revealed by rotational behaviour. Acta Physiol Scand Suppl 367:49–68, 1971a

————: Postsynaptic supersensitivity after 6-hydroxy-dopamine induced degeneration of the nigro-striatal dopamine system in the rat brain. Acta Physiol Scand Suppl 367:69–93, 1971b

distribution of drugs to the brain

commentary

Clinical pharmacology is concerned with the absorption, fate, and distribution of drugs. One factor that plays a most important role in the pharmacokinetics of psychiatric drugs is the blood-brain barrier. A molecular modification can influence the readiness with which drugs pass into the brain, and consequently their central effects. Thus, the brain uptake index of heroin is more than 20 times as great as that of morphine and may explain its greater addiction liability. It is fortunate that certain substances, like colchicine and catecholamines, penetrate the blood-brain barrier with difficulty while others, such as imipramine and caffeine, get through easily.

Dr. Oldendorf provides a concise, readable account of the blood-brain barrier, with a list of various drugs and their relative ability to reach the brain.

distribution of drugs to the brain

William H. Oldendorf, M.D.

Following its introduction into the body, a drug must be distributed to the fluid environment of brain nerve cells if it is to directly affect their function. If the drug is swallowed, it must resist degradation by stomach acid and other intestinal contents, penetrate the wall of the gut, survive passage through the microcirculation of the liver, remain in free solution in blood plasma, and penetrate capillary walls in the brain (the blood-brain barrier) to enter the brain extracellular fluid. When injected parenterally, the drug enters the general extracellular fluid directly, thereby circumventing the actions of the intestines and liver. Many drugs, given orally or parenterally, have little of no effect on the central nervous system because they never enter the brain.

We shall largely be concerned here with the mechanisms governing distribution to the brain once a drug has appeared in blood plasma.

Capillary Characteristics

Capillaries in tissues other than the brain are freely permeable to all molecules that have a molecular weight less than 20,000 to 40,000. This nonspecific permeability is based upon several characteristics of endothelial cells, which are joined together in such a way that there is a slit between the cells just large enough to permit passage of molecules smaller than about 20,000 to 40,000 molecular weight.

Many capillaries also have fenestrae, which are covered by an ill-defined membrane that probably also restricts large molecules.

As a result of this permeability, more than 80 percent of small molecules are lost by diffusion from plasma within the first minute after intravenous injection. Blood plasma constitutes about 20 percent of the total extracellular fluid. When an injected tracer is distributed from plasma to this larger compartment, most of it will have left the blood. There are also many pinocytotic vesicles that probably

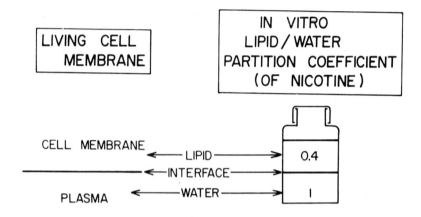

Fig. 1. Left. The brain capillary wall is the blood-brain barrier. It is composed of a continuous layer of flat endothelial cells joined tightly in such a way that there is no possibility even small molecules can leak between them. A drug molecule entering the brain must be able to move through the capillary cell. It must be able to enter the lipid of the plasma membrane, pass through the cytoplasm, and enter and penetrate to the lipid of the outer membrane. Although some enzymatic degradation may take place in the cell cytoplasm, the major obstacle to blood-brain barrier penetration is the cell membrane lipid. Whether or not a drug will enter the membrane depends upon specific molecular structural characteristics other than molecular size. The small rectangle indicates the domain shown on the right. **Right.** Entry into the endothelial cell membrane is determined by the drug's relative affinities for four major molecular species present at the plasma-membrane interface. These are: plasma water, plasma protein, membrane lipid, and membrane carrier proteins. Plasma and membrane carrier proteins give these compartments special affinities not easily predicted on the basis of drug structure. An ionized drug is anchored in water and perhaps to plasma proteins. Even though un-ionized, drugs may form hydrogen bonds to water molecules (such as shown here for -OH and /NH$_2$ groups) and this will reduce their likelihood of entering membrane lipid. By forcing them to pass through capillary cells to enter the brain, drugs are exposed to possible degradation by cytoplasmic enzymes before they can reach brain cells.

carry small packets of plasma (containing molecules of all sizes) across the endothelial cell. These vesicles probably cause the capillary wall to be slightly permeable to even large molecules.

The brain capillary is quite different in structural and permeability characteristics (Fig. 1); nonspecific routes of exchange are missing in nonneural capillaries. The intercellular clefts are sealed shut and there are tight continuous junctions between adjacent cells. There are no fenestrae and almost no pinocytotic vesicles.

Since substances in plasma cannot penetrate the capillary wall between cells, as in nonneural tissues, they must pass directly through the endothelial cell to penetrate the blood-brain barrier, which behaves like a single, very large thin cell because brain capillary cells are fused together. The rate at which the two cell membranes and the interposed thin layer of cytoplasm are penetrated by a drug is determined by its specific molecular characteristics.

The blood-brain barrier is best thought of as a selectively permeable capillary bed. This selectivity is based upon the ability of a drug to leave plasma water, enter the capillary cell membrane lipid, and, thereafter, pass completely through the capillary cell. All molecules in blood plasma are distributed to the brain to a measurable degree, but the range of relative rates of penetration is very large. Some appear as freely in the brain as in any other tissue, whereas others enter the brain to a barely measurable degree. The chemical structural difference between two drugs exhibiting such widely different characteristics may be very slight.

In plasma a portion of the drug molecules is bound to plasma protein and the remainder is in free solution in water. Since the protein-drug complex probably cannot enter membrane lipid, it is generally considered that only that portion in free solution has a possibility of penetrating the blood-brain barrier. Whereas the protein-bound fraction does not penetrate, the blood-brain barrier may be freely permeable to the unbound-fraction, the concentration of which in brain extracellular fluid may be the same as that of the unbound fraction in plasma.

Molecular Characteristics

The most crucial molecular characteristics governing the permeability of the blood-brain barrier to a drug is the relative affinity of the drug for water and for cell membrane lipid. This *relative* affinity, not the absolute solubility of the drug in membrane lipid or in water, is important.

The membrane-plasma water interface can be simulated in vitro

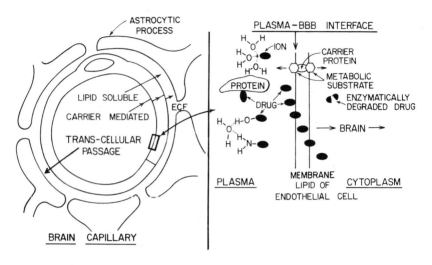

Fig. 2.   The plasma water-capillary cell membrane interface can be approximated in vitro by a simple two-phase system. Some olive oil (or octanol)
and some buffered water are placed in a bottle with some of the drug: in this
illustration nicotine. After thorough shaking and allowing the oil and water
to separate, the concentration of drug in oil divided by its concentration in
water equals the partition coefficient of the drug. The interface between the
oil and water in the bottle represents the interface between endothelial cell
membrane lipid and plasma water in the living organism. Such a simple
system can only approximate the blood-brain barrier because the lipid is not
the same; there are no plasma proteins and there are no carrier proteins in
the lipid which could cause these compartments to show unpredictable
affinities.

by a two-phase lipid-water system (Fig. 2). Olive oil or octanol
commonly are used as lipid phases and buffered saline as the water
phase. A few milliliters of olive oil can be placed in a bottle with a
similar volume of water buffered to pH 7.4. Some of the drug can be
added, the bottle capped and shaken violently, and the mixture allowed to settle back to two distinct phases. The concentration in oil
divided by the concentration in water is the oil-water partition
coefficient of the drug. As indicated in Figure 13-2, the partition
coefficient for nicotine (olive oil-water) is about 0.4. This value suggests that nicotine in plasma water will distribute readily into the
adjacent endothelial cell membrane lipid and freely penetrates the
blood-brain barrier.

The molecular characteristics determining the partition coefficient
can be predicted from the amount of drug ionized at body pH and the
hydrogen bonding capability of the nonionized drug. An ionized

drug molecule strongly attracts adjacent water molecules and becomes firmly anchored in the water. As a result, ions have very low partition coefficients and do not readily penetrate biologic membranes unless there is some mechanism strong enough to overcome this charge-dipole attraction to water. Since the fraction of drug ionized is often strongly influenced by pH, the degree of ionization present at pH 7.4, the pH at the plasma-blood-brain barrier interface, must be known. If the drug has a dissociation constant near this pH, the fraction of ionized drug may change considerably with even the moderate pH shifts that occur in vivo in acid-base disturbances. This could alter the permeability of the blood-brain barrier to the drug. Even though ions penetrate this barrier slowly, it is important to realize that it is not completely impermeable to any substance. Because of the great range of pH encountered during passage through the gut, considerable shifts in ionization may occur there.

The affinity of nonionized drugs for water is established largely by the number and total strength of the hydrogen bond-forming sites on each molecule. The strongest hydrogen bonds in common drugs are formed by -OH and $-NH_2$ groups, which are of about equal strength. Other groups form weaker hydrogen bonds. As groups forming hydrogen bonds are added to a molecule, the affinity of the molecule for water rises and its affinity for lipid falls. Such increasing polarity correspondingly reduces the molecule's ability to penetrate the blood-brain barrier.

Drugs with high partition coefficients often are described simply as *lipid soluble*, and it is generally recognized that such drugs readily penetrate the blood-brain barrier. The same characteristics that facilitate penetration of the blood-brain barrier also facilitate penetration of intestinal epithelial cells. For this reason, drugs that have prominant affects on the central nervous system usually are effective when taken orally. On this same basis drugs that penetrate the blood-brain barrier also can penetrate brain cell membranes and enter brain cells.

Ethanol, for example, penetrates all of the epithelial surfaces it contacts in the mouth, esophagus, stomach, and small intestine. Its partition coefficient is about 0.05, indicating that its concentration in an oil-water system is about 20 times greater than that in the water phase. Some of the ethanol in the portal venous blood is entrapped by liver and, if sufficient ethanol is ingested, some escapes into the systemic circulation. It readily penetrates the capillary walls of all tissues, including the blood-brain barrier, and distributes throughout all extracellular fluid. Since ethanol can penetrate lipid cell membranes, it also distributes itself throughout the intracellular fluid of all cells.

When thiopental is injected intravenously into adult humans, it emerges from the left heart within 10 seconds, and, in the resting patient, about 20 percent is delivered to the brain. Being quite lipid soluble (partition coefficient equals 3) it readily penetrates the blood-brain barrier and enters brain cells, where it results in an immediate loss of consciousness. The partition coefficient of thiopental is so high and the blood-brain barrier so permeable to it, essentially all of the drug delivered to brain leaves the blood, since

TABLE 1
PARTITION COEFFICIENTS AND BRAIN UPTAKE OF VARIOUS RADIOLABELED DRUGS FOLLOWING CAROTID INJECTION.*

Test substances	Brain uptake index† (BUI) (% of ^{3}HOH)	Partition coefficients (Olive oil/water)
^{3}HOH reference	100	—
Nicotine	131	0.39
Imipramine	128	86
BCNU	114	2.87
Procaine	113	0.34
Isopropanol	110	—
Ethanol	104	0.046
Caffeine	90	0.084
Antipyrine	68	0.040
Heroin	68	0.2
Levomethadone	42	14.0
Cyanide	41	0.15
5,5-Diphenylhydantoin	31	6.83
Codeine	26	0.16
Phenobarbital	22	0.57
L-Ascorbic acid	3.0	0.0046
Morphine‡	2.6	0.016
Methotrexate‡	2.3	0.00024
Acetylsalicylic acid‡	1.8	0.0037
Benzylpenicillin‡	1.7	0.0051
Cytosine arabinoside‡	1.6	0.00010
5-Iodo-2-deoxyuridine‡	1.5	0.0047

*Modified from Oldendorf WH, Ketano M: Proc Soc Exp Biol Med 141:940, 1972.

†Signifies percentage of drug remaining in the brain 15 seconds after abrupt carotid arterial injection in the rat, expressed relative to a labeled diffusable reference, tritiated water, injected simultaneously 90 percent of which is known to be cleared by the brain during a single brain passage.

‡Uptake of these drugs cannot be measured accurately because very little is retained in the brain and the background of the method used is about 2 percent.

the volume of brain tissue to which it can freely distribute is very much larger than the volume of capillary plasma. Such distribution, in which essentially all of the drug is cleared by a tissue during a single circulatory passage, is referred to as flow-limited distribution. The amount of drug delivered to a tissue is proportional to the fraction of cardiac output to that tissue. In the case of thiopental an initially large concentration appears immediately in the brain (thus its rapid onset of action). The drug washes quickly out of brain as it redistributes to other tissues in proportion to the partition coefficients of the various tissues. This rapid redistribution out of the brain largely explains thiopental's very short duration of action.

Various analogs of morphine demonstrate the effects of hydrogen bonding on blood-brain barrier penetration. Morphine has two hydroxyl groups, which cause it to have a low partition coefficient; accordingly very little morphine penetrates the blood-brain barrier. Methylating one hydroxyl forms codeine, a less polar drug that enters the brain much more readily. Acetylating both hydroxyls further reduces polarity, and thus heroin penetrates the blood-brain barrier more rapidly. This can be determined experimentally by measuring the percentage of a drug injected intra-arterially and lost to rat brain during a single circulatory passage (Table 1).

Derivative of β-phenethylamine also show the influence of polarity due to hydrogen bonding. The unsubstituted parent compound readily penetrates the blood-brain barrier. Adding polar groups, creating various sympathomimetic amines, increases polarity, and most of these derivatives have correspondingly little affect on the central nervous system. The least polar of these drugs, amphetamine and methampethamine, have strong central nervous system actions, probably based largely on their free penetration of the blood-brain barrier. Norepinephrine and epinephrine are much more polar because of their extra hydroxyl group and, accordingly, penetrate slowly.

Lipid Affinity

A drug with an extremely high affinity for lipid accumulates in body fat depots from which it is slowly washed out by blood. Therefore, it remains in the blood for long periods of time. This probably is a factor in the prolonged after-effects of cannabis smoking, since the partition coefficient of tetrahydrocannabinol exceeds 5000. Very little ethanol accumulates in lipid because, as indicated earlier, its partition coefficient is quite low and correspondingly little of the alcohol is distributed to fat depots.

174 Experimental Psychopharmacology: Drugs as Tools

Drugs commonly taken for their mental effects, such as ethanol, caffeine, amphetamine, nicotine, cocaine, tetrahydrocannabinol, heroin, and barbiturates are at least moderately soluble in lipid and their partition coefficients are large enough to allow them to penetrate the blood–brain barrier rapidly (Table 1). The mental effects of most of these drugs were discovered empirically in nontechnical cultural settings. The early onset of their effects probably fostered their recognition. Had these effects been delayed, the association between administration and effect might never have been formed.

The olive oil-water partition coefficient of most of these common drugs is between about 0.04 and 1.0. This range is desirable because it allows the drug to penetrate the blood-brain barrier rapidly but does not result in depot fat storage. As a result the effects are largely limited to the first few hours after administration. Such brief duration of action usually is desirable, if the resulting altered mentation is not to seriously disrupt the user's life pattern.

Rapid penetration of the blood-brain barrier does not always result in a rapid onset of central nervous system effects. Even though therapeutic brain concentrations are achieved immediately, the mechanism of drug action may require some time to evolve. Imipramine, for example, appears immediately in the brain, but several days are usually required before this drug becomes therapeutically effective. Similarly the affects of LSD, which presumably also appears immediately in brain, are delayed several hours.

In addition to the predictable lipid-mediated penetration of the blood-brain barrier by nonpolar drugs, it is also possible that some of the selective transport mechanisms for metabolic substrates, such as glucose, will be shown to have an affinity for some drugs. Such an affinity would be much less predictable.

References

Goldstein A, Aronow L: The durations of action of thiopental and pentobarbital. J Pharmacol Exp Ther 128:1, 1960

Kreuz DS, Axelrod J: Delta-9-tetrahydrocannabinol: localization in body fat. Science 179:391, 1973

Landis EM, Pappenheimer JR: Exchange of substances through capillary walls. In Dow P, Hamilton WF (eds): Handbook of Physiology, Sect 2, Circulation, Vol 2. Washington, DC, American Physiological Soc, 1963, p 961

Oldendorf WH: Brain uptake of radiolabeled amino acids, amines, and hexoses after arterial injection. Am J Physiol 221:1629, 1971

———, Kitano M: The early disappearance of extracellular tracers from plasma after intravenous injection. Proc Soc Exp Biol Med 141:940, 1972

————, Hyman S, Braun L, Oldendorf SZ: Blood brain barrier: penetration of morphine, codeine, heroin, and methadone after carotid injection. Science 178:984, 1972

————: Blood brain barrier permeability to drugs. Annu Rev Pharmacol 14:239, 1974

Stein WD: The Movement of Molecules Across Cell Membranes. New York, Academic, 1967

drugs and electroencephalographic effects
commentary

Our indices of what psychotropic drugs are doing to the brain are necessarily indirect. Neither the radiologist nor the pathologist can detect function in the brain. It is still difficult to see into the brain, and one must rely on peripheral manifestations of brain action of drugs as revealed in behavior and peripheral physiologic changes. The one exception is the electroencephalogram, which is a mirror of brain function. The electroencephalogram reflects the average activity of millions of neuronal and possibly glial units. These can be studied individually in animals and on occasion in man. Sophisticated electronic and computerized equipment is needed to reveal changes in amplitude and frequency of electrical activity, which can be recorded from various parts of the scalp. The full potentialities of these techniques are still in their infancy. The major characteristics of electroencephalographic changes induced by psychotherapeutic drugs are briefly described.

drugs and electroencephalographic effects

Keith F. Killam, Jr., Ph.D.

Remarkable strides in the chemotherapeutic control of abnormal behavior have been made in the past 25 years. Neurochemical, neuropsychopharmacologic and electrophysiologic studies have been carried out in parallel, in part in an attempt to provide a scientific foundation for the use of psychotherapeutic compounds. Other studies have examined the proposed sites of action of drugs as functional units in systems that elaborate or control behavior. Obviously the details of all studies must be worked out in animals so that brain biopsies and depth electrical recordings are made possible.

The search continues for bridges between the patient and the experimental animal. One such bridge is the bioelectric activity generated as a result of biochemical events associated with the firing patterns of neurons in the brain. In man bioelectric activity is recorded noninvasively from the scalp by means of the electroencephalogram.

The electroencephalogram was first described by Berger (1929) as a phenomenon that might be useful in monitoring brain function and behavior. Subsequently normal characteristics of the electroencephalogram have been described with respect to characteristic frequencies, to site specificity for the localization of those frequencies across the skull and thence the underlying brain, to the responsiveness of patterns to changes in external stimuli and to variations in behavioral attention and sleep.

Until recently the electroencephalogram has been used clinically primarily in the diagnosis of seizure states and to localize sites of space-occupying lesions, such as brain tumors. The development of

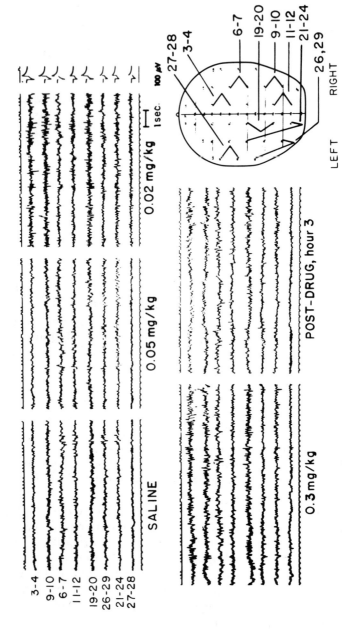

Fig. 1. Bipolar EEG recordings illustrating the effects of chlorpromazine. (From Gehrmann, Killam: unpublished data.)

digital computers has made possible more precise estimates of the frequency and power content of the electroencephalogram. Extensive studies have been conducted to evaluate nonparoxysmal abnormalities of the electroencephalogram from the states of sleeping and waking. The sleep-wakefulness continuum was found to have characteristic cyclicity (p 105); norms have been established for latencies and durations of the infradian and ultradian cycles; circadian rhythms recur approximately every 24 hours.

Drugs may shift the sleep-wakefulness cycle or restrict variability of the electroencephalogram in given behavioral states. Drugs may uncouple the relationship between behavior and the electroencephalogram. Drugs may alter the anatomic site specificity of the electrical parameters. And drugs may induce characteristics not usually found in the electroencephalogram.

Among many others, Bente (1961), Brazier (1964), Fink (1959 and 1968), and most recently Florio et al (1976) have attempted to correlate therapeutic responses to changes in the electroencephalogram. The more salient features occurring at therapeutic dose ranges will be summarized here:

Phenothiazines. In general there is a shift of the frequency content of the electroencephalogram to slower frequencies. The more sedative the drug, the more pronounced the shift, eg, chlorpromazine versus fluphenazine. The drugs with less sedative properties also increase the incidence of frequencies in the so-called alpha band (10 per second), eg, trifluoperazine (Fig. 1).

Butyrophenones. The butyrophenones exhibit changes similar to those seen with chlorpromazine, ie, a shift in the frequency content of the electroencephalogram to slower frequencies without an increase of power in the alpha band.

Lithium salts. The pattern of the electroencephalogram after chronic treatment with lithium salts closely resembles that characteristic of chlorpromazine. However, stabilization of the electroencephalogram into a particular state is less obvious.

Antidepressant drugs. These agents, (impramine or amitriptyline) exhibit increases in both high and low frequencies in the electroencephalogram without significant changes in amplitude. In contrast, psychomotor stimulants such as D-amphetamines are characterized by an increase in fast frequency components but with a significant decrease in the overall amplitude of the electroencephalogram.

Antianxiety (anxiolytic) drugs. Fink (1968) reports few distinguishing features between patterns seen after benzodiazepines (diazepam), barbiturates (pentobarbital), and sedatives

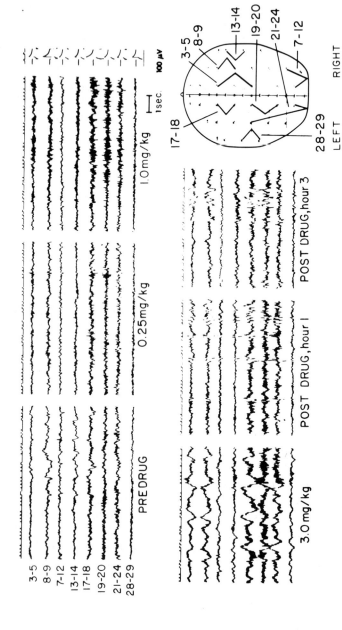

Fig. 2. Bipolar EEG recordings illustrating the effects of diazepam. (From Gehrmann, Killam: unpublished data.)

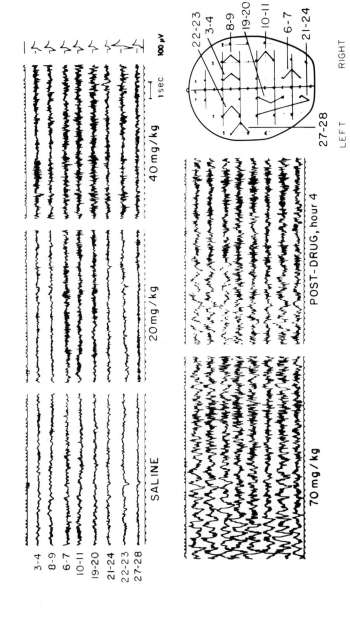

Fig. 3. Bipolar EEG recordings illustrating the effects of amobarbital. (From Gehrmann, Killam: unpublished data.)

183

(glutethimide and meprobamate). The pattern includes an increase in the high-frequency components of the electroencephalogram, particularly in the so-called beta 1 band, with a decrease in variability and an increase in overall amplitudes. However, using different analytic techniques, Joy et al (1971) report distinguishing features between benzodiazepines and barbiturates in the electroencephalograms from subhuman primates, and Gehrmann and Killam (1975) report recognizable differences in the spectral changes induced (Figs. 2,3).

With the advent of objective analytic techniques to characterize the electroencephalogram, classification schemes are in the process of development. Although the limitations are obvious, they are noted: For a given patient the quality of the electroencephalographic record obtained will influence the validity of the characteristics established; usefulness in prognosis would require longitudinal studies on a particular subject. More critically, little is known as yet about the influence of drug interactions. The summary of these descriptors was from subjects exposed to one drug at a time, but such a drug regimen is rare or practically nonexistent in therapeutic situations. Hopefully, using the electroencephalogram as an intellectual bridge, animal studies with controlled interactions, supported with measurements of blood levels of the drugs, would aid in the evaluation of electroencephalographic changes in man induced by mixtures. The potential of the electroencephalogram as a noninvasive method of assessing drug efficacy or simply as a quantitative determinant is still unresolved. Indeed, the values of limitations of the measurement of brain bioelectrical activity in drugged subjects has yet to be fully explored.

References

Berger H: Uber das Elektrenkephalogramm des Menschen. Arch Psychiatr Nervenkr 87:527–570, 1929

Bente D: Elektroencephalographische Gesichtspunkte zur Klassifikation neuro- und thymoleptischer Pharmaka. Med Exp (Basel) 5:337–346, 1961

Brazier MAB: The effects of drugs on the electroencephalogram of man. Clin Pharmacol Ther 5:102–112, 1964

Fink M: EEG classification of psychoactive compounds in man: A review and theory of behavioral associations. In Efron DH, Cole JO, Levine J, Wittenborn JR (Eds): Psychopharmacology: A review of Progress 1957–1967. Public Health Service Publication 1836, 1968, pp 497–507

————: EEG and behavioral effects of psychopharmacologic agents. In Bradley PB, Deniker P, Radouco-Thomas C (Eds): Neuropsychopharmacology, Vol 1. Amsterdam, Elsevier, 1959, pp 441–446

Florio V, Longo VG, Verdeaux G: Antipsychotics, tranquilizers and antidepressants. In Remond A (ed): Handbook of Electroencephalography. Amdam, Elsevier, 1976

Gehrmann JE, Killam KF: In Kagan F, Harwood T, Rickels K, Rudzik, Sour H (Eds): Hypnotics. New York, Spectrum, 1975, pp 241–282

Itil T: Elektroencephalographische Befunde zur Klassifikation neuro und thymoleptischer Medikamente. Med Exp (Basel) 5:347–363, 1961

Joy RM, Hance AJ, Killam KF: A quantitative electroencephalographic comparison of some benzodiazepines in the primate. Neuropharmacology 10:483–497, 1971

hormones
and
behavior

commentary

There is increasing interest in the role of endocrine glands in behavior, particularly in rhythmic activities, such as sleep, in which the endocrine organs seem to play a major role. Many of the drugs used in the treatment of mental disorders have pronounced endocrine influences, and these are discussed.

Of the seven anterior pituitary hormones, four (ACTH, LH, FSH, TSH) have feedback from peripheral glands (adrenal cortex, gonads, thyroid), and three (growth hormone, prolactin, and MSH) are inhibited by the hypothalamus. All seven have hypothalamic releasing factors. The CNS control of several metabolically important hormones is more subtle (insulin, parathormone, aldosterone, gastrin, and glucagon). Antipsychotic drugs, by blocking dopamine receptors, prevent release of prolactin-inhibiting factors in the brain and thereby cause enhanced release of prolactin.

Some interesting, newer developments involve the use of polypeptide hormones or derivatives for the control of mood and learning.

hormones
and
behavior

Robert Rubin, M.D.
Jon F. Sassin, M.D.

General Concepts of Neuroendocrine Function

Since the mid-1960s, there has been a virtual explosion of research on the central nervous system control of endocrine glands and, conversely, the influence of hormones on brain function. Based on hundreds of studies within this new field of research, neuroendocrinology, it is now well established that a major controlling factor in endocrine regulation is the central nervous system. In the human, correlative studies of the neuroendocrinology of both sleep and wakefulness have contributed to this concept. Sleep studies are useful because sleep is a well-defined period during which there are major shifts in the activity of the central nervous system, such as the regular transition between slow-wave sleep and rapid eye movement or dreaming sleep. The importance of the central nervous system in endocrine functioning is gaining recognition in the classic endocrinology literature, as evidenced by the following quote from the new edition of Williams' *Textbook of Endocrinology* (Reichlin 1974):

> An important practical consequence of sleep related endocrine rhythms is the recognition that adequate evaluation of endocrine function requires study over the full twenty four hours of one day. An important theoretical consequence of this new information is that the bulk of anterior pituitary secretion is under open loop nonhomeostatic control.

Thus, it is now appreciated that the secretion rates of the anterior pituitary hormones depend on the balance between central nervous system activity, driving the hypothalamus (open loop mechanisms) and negative feedback to the pituitary and brain by the seven anterior pituitary hormones and their target organ hormones (closed loop mechanisms; Fig. 1). As a representative example the secretion of ACTH from the anterior pituitary depends on a balance between the central nervous system secretory "program" and the negative feedback by glucocorticoids from the adrenal cortex.

The importance of open loop or central nervous system driving mechanisms in the regulation of ACTH may be inferred from several lines of recently developed evidence. (a) Both ACTH and cortisol are released in a pulsatile, episodic pattern (Gallagher et al 1973), rather than being secreted in a smooth fashion as would be found with closed loop, negative feedback regulation. (b) ACTH normally has a prominent circadian (24-hour) rhythm (DeLacerda et al 1973), with plasma concentrations increasing between 3 and 8 AM, and then declining throughout the rest of the day and the first part of the night. The increasing plasma concentrations of ACTH and cortisol between 3 and 8 AM are caused by a greater number of secretory episodes, with higher amplitude during these hours. This normal circadian rhythm is abolished in animals by severing the nerve inputs to the medial basal hypothalamus, indicating that this rhythm

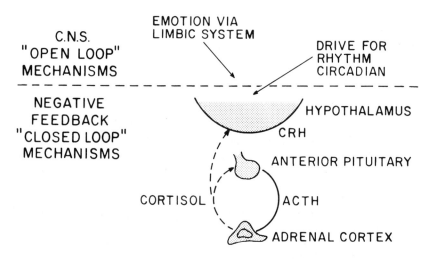

Fig. 1.   Schematic representation of central nervous system open loop and negative feedback closed loop control of the hypothalamo-anterior pituitary-adrenal cortical axis. ACTH—adrenocorticotropic hormone; CRF—corticotropin releasing factor.

is under the control of the central nervous system. Other areas of the brain, in addition to the hypothalamus, have been shown to influence the regulation of ACTH release. Stimulation of the amygdala and hippocampus, two parts of the limbic system, has been shown to increase and decrease corticosteroids, respectively, in depth electrode studies of the central nervous system in humans (Rubin et al 1966). (d) Beginning with Selye's description of the general adaptation syndrome almost 40 years ago (Selye 1973), a plethora of studies have revealed that ACTH release is exquisitely sensitive to many different kinds of psychologic stress, both naturally occurring and experimentally contrived (Rubin and Mandell 1966, Mason 1971).

Central Nervous System Neurotransmitters and Neurohormones

Since the mid-1960s, many neurochemical investigations have elucidated the roles of a number of compounds as central nervous system neurotransmitters; ie, substances that convey nerve impulses across the synapses between neurons (Baldessarini and Karobath 1973). The putative central nervous system neurotransmitters that have been most extensively investigated are the catecholamines, dopamine and norepinephrine; the indoleamine, serotonin (5-HT); and acetylcholine (see pp 35, 231, 467). Other postulated neurotransmitters also are receiving attention, including γ aminobutyric acid, histamine, and glycine. On the basis of considerable evidence, dopamine, norepinephrine, and serotonin have been implicated in the affective disorders of mania and depression; in the transition from wakefulness to sleep and the orderly progression through various sleep stages; in aggressive behavior, along with influential hormones such as testosterone; in temperature regulation; in the hypothalamic mechanisms of hunger and satiety; and in the secretion of the hypothalamic-hypophysiotropic hormones (pituitary hormone releasing and inhibiting factors, Rubin 1975). Many neuropharmacologic studies have involved manipulating the levels of these neurotransmitters by the use of compounds that release them from their stores in presynaptic endings, that are precursors for their formation, that block the enzymes participating in their synthesis, that block their inactivation, that act as false neurotransmitters, or that block the postsynaptic receptors for these neurotransmitters. By the alteration of various neurotransmitter activities in the central nervous system, effects can be produced on affective states, sleep cycling, aggressive behavior, body temperature, feeding behavior, and the secretion patterns of the anterior and posterior pituitary hormones.

Another major area of research has been the investigation of the "hypothalamic-hypophysiotropic hormones" (Schally et al 1973). These neurohormones (releasing and inhibiting factors) are small polypeptides produced in the neurosecretory cells of the hypothalamus. They are secreted into the portal blood vessels of the pituitary stalk and carried to the cells of the anterior pituitary (hypophysis), where they exert their trophic effects. The pituitary hormones that have negative feeback mechanisms from target organ hormones (ACTH, LH, FSH, TSH) appear to have only a hypothalamic releasing factor. On the other hand, pituitary hormones that do not have a distinct negative feedback relationship with a target organ hormone (growth hormone, prolactin, MSH) appear to have both a hypothalamic releasing factor and an inhibiting factor. Several of these hypothalamic-hypophysiotropic hormones have been characterized and synthesized. Thyrotropin releasing factor (TRF) is a tripeptide; LH-FSH releasing factor (LRF) is a decapeptide, growth hormone inhibiting factor (somatostatin) is a tetradecapeptide, and MSH inhibiting factor (MIF) may be a tripeptide or a pentapeptide. Synthetic analogs of these hypothalamic hormones have been prepared and some are commercially available; they are employed in clinical endocrinology for provocative tests of pituitary integrity. Also, some of them, notably TRF, have been claimed to exert antidepressant and other effects when given in pharmacologic doses (Kastin et al 1972, Prange et al 1972). The behavioral effects of these hypothalamic hormones will be considered later.

Hormone Biorhythms

The study of changes in endocrine secretion both during sleep and during the daytime hours is an important tool for the investigation of the regulation of endocrine functioning by the central nervous system. During the time of sleep there are large qualitative shifts in the activity of the central nervous system, eg, slow-wave (Stage 3–4) or "deep" sleep versus rapid eye movement (REM) or "dreaming" sleep. These shifts are regular, being part of a basic rest-activity cycle detectable throughout the entire 24-hour period (Kleitman 1969). This basic rest-activity cycle has a length of approximately 90 to 110 minutes in normal individuals. Thus, this ultradian (less than 24 hours) rhythm provides another pattern of changing central nervous system activity, in addition to the circadian sleep-wake cycle.

The various pituitary hormones have unique secretion patterns, some of which are closely linked to these central nervous system rhythms and others of which are not (Rubin et al 1974); (Fig. 2). For example, the aforementioned ACTH-cortisol circadian rhythm is not closely linked to the sleep-wake cycle, in that sleep-wake reversal studies have indicated that the cortisol rhythm takes approximately 2 weeks to shift around to the new sleep-wake pattern. On the other hand, prolactin is closely linked to the sleep-wake cycle, with in-

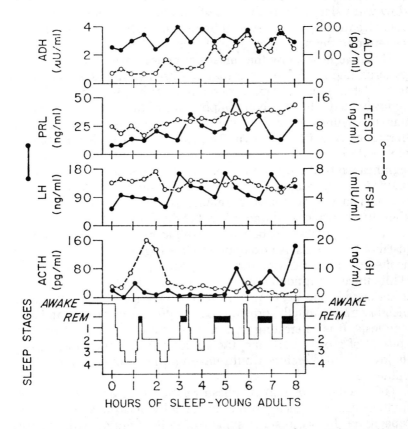

Fig. 2. Composite representation of the typical secretion patterns (plasma levels) of 8 hormones during a normal 8-hr sleep period in a young adult man. REM—rapid eye movement sleep; ACTH—adrenocorticotropic hormone; GH—growth hormone; LH—luteinizing hormone; FSH—follicle-stimulating hormone; PRL—prolactin; TESTO—testosterone; ADH —antidiuretic hormone; ALDO—aldosterone. Hormones named on left side of figure depicted by dots and solid line; those named on right side depicted by open circles and dashed line.

creasing blood levels at the time of sleep onset and peak levels approximately 5 hours into the sleep period (Sassin et al 1973). Sleep-wake reversal immediately shifts the prolactin rhythm (Sassin et al 1973), and daytime naps result in the release of prolactin (Parker et al 1974).

Another pituitary hormone, growth hormone, appears to be linked specifically to slow-wave sleep, in that the major secretion of growth hormone in the normal adult during the entire 24-hour period occurs in conjunction with the first entry into slow-wave (Stage 3–4) sleep within the first hour or two of the sleep period. Deprivation of slow-wave sleep blunts this growth hormone release (Sassin et al 1969a), and sleep-wake reversal immediately shifts growth hormone secretion to the new sleep time (Sassin et al 1969b).

Thus, we now know that most hormones have unique secretion patterns, and many have circadian or ultradian rhythms that appear to be determined by central nervous system driving mechanisms. Unfortunately, the metabolic importance of these circadian and ultradian rhythms as well as the episodic release patterns of these hormones is quite unknown. The influence of each hormone on metabolic processes has been studied thoroughly, but the special significance of the dynamic aspects of these secretion patterns remains to be elucidated. Curtis (1972) has pointed out that circadian rhythms suggest that most hormones are secreted either during or slightly in advance of the active part of the daily cycle, during which most energy intake (anabolism) as well as most energy expenditure (catabolism) occurs. An exception to this is growth hormone which, as mentioned, is released during the early part of the sleep period. While the exact function of this major secretion of growth hormone is unknown, one possibility is that it serves to help consolidate memory traces from the previous day by promoting protein and RNA synthesis. It is interesting that, at the time of this major secretory episode of growth hormone, the glucocorticoid concentration is at its lowest and therefore would have minimum opposing catabolic influence.

The alteration of normal phase relationships among endocrine rhythms can occur as a result of unusual living schedules; impaired capacity of the organism to synchronize its rhythms with environmental cues, such as probably occurs in patients with severe depressive disorders; or as a result of sudden overwhelming environmental stress, such as stress-induced anovulatory cycles in women (Kiritz and Moos 1974, Lund 1974). The alteration of these normal phase relationships could have a major impact on overall hormone balance and, consequently, on many metabolic processes. It is well known in clinical medicine that a number of illnesses frequently are preceded by psychologic stress (Rubin 1975), but the neurophysiologic mechanisms that transduce perceived psychologic stress and anxiety into pathophysiologic consequences are still generally unknown.

Psychopharmacologic Influences on Hormone Release

As mentioned, the biogenic amines—dopamine, norepinephrine and serotonin—as well as acetylcholine, appear to be neurotransmitters in hypothalamic neural circuits that influence the hypothalamic hormones. In turn, the latter hormones influence secretion of anterior pituitary hormones (Ganong 1972, deWied and deJong 1974). Many of the drugs used in clinical psychiatry have a primary effect on these neurotransmitters by a number of mechanisms, such as depleting neurotransmitter stores in the presynaptic nerve endings (eg, reserpine), blocking the enzymes that metabolize neurotransmitters (eg, tranylcypromine or Parnate), blocking or enhancing their inactivation (reuptake) from the synapse (eg, imipramine or Tofranil), acting as false neurotransmitters (eg, LSD or lysergic acid diethylamide), or blocking the postsynaptic receptors (eg, chlorpromazine or Thorazine).

The antipsychotic agents, predominantly the butyrophenones and phenothiazines, have a strong dopamine blocking effect at the postsynaptic receptor, and this currently is believed to be the neurochemical basis for their antipsychotic properties (Snyder et al 1974). Not only do they block dopamine receptors in certain areas of the limbic system that may influence the schizophrenia thought disorder, but they also block dopamine receptors elsewhere. Thus, they have regular extrapyramidal side effects, including Parkinson-like syndromes, dystonias, and so forth. Also, they strongly influence the dopamine system in the median eminence of the hypothalamus, thereby altering pituitary hormone release. The clinical side effects of amenorrhea (based on the blocking of the ovulatory surge of the gonadotropins) and galactorrhea (based on the reduction of prolactin inhibiting factor) are well-known neuroendocrine side effects of these drugs (Beumont et al 1974). Indeed, the antipsychotic potency of the individual drugs correlates well with their ability to induce prolactin release in the rat (Clemens et al 1974).

These antipsychotic drugs also have norepinephrine blocking properties as well as certain anticholinergic properties. Thus, it is an oversimplification to attribute their neuroendocrine effects entirely to their dopamine blockade. The determining factor for the secretion of hypothalamic hormones appears to be the balance between a number of competing neural systems, utilizing different neurotransmitters, rather than the isolated effect of a single neurotransmitter system.

Other psychopharmacologic agents also have been shown to influence pituitary hormone release. The tricyclic antidepressant imipramine abolished the slow-wave, sleep-related growth hormone secretion in 2 of 4 subjects; the phenothiazine chlorpromazine did not abolish growth hormone release during sleep (Takahashi 1974). Whereas chlorpromazine has noradrenergic and dopaminergic blocking effects, the tricyclic antidepressants enhance neurotransmitter activity by blocking their inactivation, via reuptake, after they are released into the synaptic cleft. The dopamine precursor levodopa has been shown to enhance growth hormone release during the day (Boyd et al 1970). Thus, it can be seen that the regulatory mechanism for even a single pituitary hormone becomes rather complex when approached by various psychopharmacologic manipulations.

Hormones as Psychopharmacologic Agents

Up to this point, we have been considering the influence of the central nervous system on endocrine functioning and the ways in which pharmacologic manipulation of this system alters patterns of hormone release via drug effects on neurotransmitter systems. Because the brain is a tissue embodying the same principles of metabolic activity that govern all other tissues of the body, it is quite susceptible to the influence of various hormones. Thus, there is a reciprocal relationship between the functions of the central nervous system on the one hand and patterns of hormone release on the other. These endocrine effects cover the spectrum from very general systemic influences to specific central nervous system effects (see p 3). An example of the former, a general effect, would be the disturbance in consciousness produced by the hypoglycemia resulting from increased insulin levels. An example of the latter, a very specific central nervous system effect, would be the euphoria frequently produced by exogenous glucocorticoid administration or the rather stereotyped myxedema psychosis seen in patients with profound hypothyroidism. Indeed, practically any endocrine imbalance will have concomitant disturbances in central nervous system functioning and behavior (Smith et al 1972).

An interesting area of recent research is the male-female

dichotomy in the organization of brain mechanisms and behavior. The male versus female pattern of hypothalamic functioning, ie, the tonic release of gonadotropins versus their cyclic ovulatory release, is determined very early in the life of the organism via exposure of the brain to androgenic steroids at a critical time in its development. Depending on the species, this time may be prenatal or postnatal. If the animal is exposed to androgen at the proper time, the hypothalamus becomes "masculine," ie, tonic, and the animal is "defeminized" in behavior. If the animal is not exposed to androgen, then the hypothalamus remains cyclic and a feminine-behaving animal results. While this has been demonstrated most clearly in the laboratory rat, the same principles appear to hold for primates as well as for humans. Money and Ehrhardt (1972) give many clinical examples of altered hormone balance in infants in whom the expected male-female behavior patterns were altered in later years. Thus, hormones have long-lasting organizational effects on the central nervous system as well as immediate ongoing effects on the metabolic processes of central nervous system tissue.

In this regard other clinical psychopharmacologic effects of hormones should be mentioned. The advent of synthetic progestational contraceptive agents has resulted in changing the balance of female gonadal steroids in millions of women. A number of psychiatric disturbances have been reported with the use of these hormones, including both depression and euphoria, with some relationship between symptoms and the prior personality status of the individual (Weissman and Slaby 1973). It is difficult to predict how any particular woman will respond psychologically to oral contraceptives, and many contraceptive agents are available with varying amounts of hormones in them. Careful research on the psychiatric effects of contraceptive agents therefore must consider these diverse factors (Cullberg 1972).

Finally, as mentioned earlier, some of the hypothalamic hormones have been synthesized and are available for clinical use. Thyrotopin releasing factor (TRF), in particular, has been claimed to have important antidepressant properties in depressed patients (Kastin et al 1972, Prange et al 1972). This effect is considered to be specific for TRF, and not secondary to its influence on TSH release and the consequent release of thyroid hormones. Studies on depressed patients who responded to TRF with relief of their depression revealed that, if anything, the TSH response was blunted compared to normal patients. Other investigators, however, have failed to replicate these findings (Coppen et al 1974) so that the ultimate clinical usefulness of TRF as an antidepressant remains in serious doubt.

Summary

The field of neuroendocrinology is one of the most exciting areas of current research. It appears that the central nervous system exerts a major influence on the release patterns of many different hormones throughout the body. In particular, the anterior and posterior pituitary hormones appear to be intimately governed by central nervous system mechanisms. Psychologic stress, sleep versus waking, sleep-stage cycling within the sleep period, and the pharmacologic manipulation of central nervous system neurotransmitters all influence the release patterns of pituitary hormones. The ultimate metabolic effects of these changes in hormone release patterns remain as the next major area for research investigation.

Conversely, hormones themselves have manifold influences on central nervous system functioning. The lifelong organization of the central nervous system, in terms of the male-female dichotomy, both with respect to hypothalamic control of gonadotropin release and with respect to certain patterns of behavior, appears to be under the influence of androgenic steroid hormones at a critical time in early life. Also, hormones influence many aspects of behavior in an ongoing way, such as the mood changes seen with the menstrual cycle and the use of contraceptive agents. Many clinical endocrinopathies have concomitant disturbances of brain function. The hypothalamic hormones (releasing and inhibiting factors) themselves may have pharmacologic effects on the central nervous system, such as TRF possibly possessing certain antidepressant properties. Clearly this field of research, neuroendocrinology, has yielded much exciting information in the past 10 years, but this represents only the beginning of our understanding of the interplay between brain and body.

References

Baldessarini RJ, Karobath M: Biochemical physiology of central synapses. Ann Rev Physiol 35:273–304, 1973

Beumont PJV, Corker CS, Friesen HG, Gelder MG, Harris GW, Kolakowska T, MacKinnon PCB, Mandelbrote BM, Marshall J, Murray MAF, Wiles DH: The effects of phenothiazines on endocrine function: I and II. Br J Psychiatry 124:413–430, 1974

Boyd AE, Lebovitz HE, Pfeiffer JB: Stimulation of human-growth-hormone secretion by L-DOPA. N Engl J Med 283:1425–1429, 1970

Clemens JA, Smalstig EB, Sawyer BD: Antipsychotic drugs stimulate prolactin release. Psychopharmacologia 40:123–127, 1974

Coppen A, Peet M, Montgomery S, Bailey J, Marks V, Woods P:

Thyrotrophin-releasing hormone in the treatment of depression. Lancet 2:433–435, 1974

Cullberg J: Mood changes and menstrual symptoms with different gestogen/estrogen combinations: a double-blind comparison with a placebo. Acta Psychiat Scand Suppl 236:9–86, 1972

Curtis GC: Psychosomatics and chronobiology: possible implications of neuroendocrine rhythms: a review. Psychosom Med 34:235–256, 1972

De Lacerda L, Kowarski A, Migeon CJ: Integrated concentration and diurnal variation of plasma cortisol. J Clin Endocrinol Metab 36:227–238, 1973

deWied D, deJong W: Drug effects and hypothalamic-anterior pituitary function. Ann Rev Pharmacol 14:389–412, 1974

Gallagher TF, Yoshida K, Roffwarg HD, Fukushima DK, Weitzman ED, Hellman L: ACTH and cortisol secretory patterns in man. J Clin Endocrinol Metab 36:1058–1068, 1973

Ganong WF: Pharmacological aspects of neuroendocrine integration. Prog Brain Res 38:41–57, 1972

Kastin AJ, Schalch DS, Ehrensing RH, Anderson MS: Improvement in mental depression with decreased thyrotropin response after administration of thyrotropin-releasing hormone. Lancet 2:740–742, 1972

Kiritz S, Moos RH: Physiological effects of social environments. Psychosom Med 36:96–114, 1974

Kleitman N: Basic rest-activity cycle in relation to sleep and wakefulness. In Kales A (ed): Sleep: Physiology and Pathology. Philadelphia, Lippincott, 1969, pp 33–38

Lund R: Personality factors and desynchronization of circadian rhythms. Psychosom Med 36:224–228, 1974

Mason JW: A re-evaluation of the concept of "non-specificity" in stress theory. J Psychiatr Res 8:323–333, 1971

Money J, Ehrhardt AA: Man and Woman: Boy and Girl. Baltimore, Johns Hopkins University Press, 1972

Parker DC, Rossman LG, VanderLaan EF: Relation of sleep-entrained human prolactin release to REM-nonREM cycles. J Clin Endocrinol Metab 38:646–651, 1974

Prange AJ, Lara PP, Wilson IC, Alltop LB, Breese GR: Effects of thyrotropin-releasing hormone in depression. Lancet 2:999–1002, 1972

Reichlin S: Neuroendocrinology. In Williams RH (ed): Textbook of Endocrinology, 5th ed. Philadelphia, Saunders, 1974, p 805

Rubin RT: Mind-brain-body interaction: elucidation of psychosomatic intervening variables. In Pasnau R (ed): Consultation-Liason Psychiatry. New York, Grune & Stratton, 1975, pp 73–85

————, Mandell AJ: Adrenal cortical activity in pathological emotional states: a review. Am J Psychiatry 123:387–400, 1966

————, Mandell AJ, Crandall PH: Corticosteroid responses to limbic stimulation in man, localization of stimulus sites. Science 153:767–768, 1966

————, Poland RE, Rubin LE, Gouin PR: The neuroendocrinology of human sleep. Life Sci 14:1041–1052, 1974

Sassin JF, Parker DC, Johnson LC, et al: Effects of slow wave sleep deprivation on human growth hormone release in sleep: preliminary study. Life Sci 8:1299–1307, 1969a

————, Parker DC, Mace JW, Gotlin RW, Johnson LC, Rossman LG: Human growth hormone release: relation to slow wave sleep and sleep-waking cycles. Science 165:513–515, 1969b

————, Frantz A, Weitzman E, Kapen S: Human prolactin: 24-hour pattern with increased release during sleep. Science 177:1205–1207, 1972

————, Frantz A, Kapen S, Weitzman E: The nocturnal rise of human prolactin is dependent on sleep. J Clin Endocrinol Metab 37:436–440, 1973

Schally AV, Arimura A, Kastin AJ: Hypothalamic regulatory hormones. Science 179:341–350, 1973

Selye H: The evolution of the stress concept. Am Scientist 61:692–699, 1973

Smith CK, Barish J, Correa J, Williams RH: Psychiatric disturbance in endocrinologic disease. Psychosom Med 34:69–86, 1972

Snyder SH, Banerjee SP, Yamamura HI, Greenberg D: Drugs, neurotransmitters and schizophrenia. Science 184:1243–1253, 1974

Takahashi Y: Growth hormone secretion during sleep: a review. In Kawakami M (ed): Biological Rhythms in Neuroendocrine Activity. Tokyo, Igaku-Shoin, 1974, pp 316–325

Weissman MM, Slaby AE: Oral contraceptives and psychiatric disturbance: evidence from research. Br J Psychiatry 123:513–518, 1973

part III
clinical psychopharmacology
rationale of drug treatment

Introduction

Until the mid-1950s, pharmacotherapy was considered only symptomatic treatment in psychiatry. At the turn of the century, the main drugs for this purpose were morphine, alcohol, bromides, and the newly discovered barbiturates. In the 1930s amphetamine was synthesized by Alles (1933) and used as an appetite depressant and a stimulant. Its use in hyperactive children was suggested only shortly after its discovery in the 1930s. Anxiety was and continues to be treated with phenobarbital, but better drugs are available today. During the 1950s, the antipsychotic, antidepressant, and antimanic drugs were introduced or became popular. They will be discussed below. Children and the aged have some special problems because certain psychiatric disorders are especially common at these times of life. The practicing physician should find suggestions in chapters on nonprescription drugs and on the use of narcotic drugs especially thought provoking.

The primary practice physician is involved with clinical psychopharmacology every day and is apt to encounter all of the problems discussed in this part. The advice given by these experts is based on many years of experience and much knowledge. The reader may even disagree with some of the conclusions of certain authors, but he should scrutinize these chapters even more carefully if he does. None of the drugs mentioned can be considered truly curative in that none eliminates the disease. But sometimes the disease remits spontaneously, and the drug will allow the patient to lead a more comfortable and productive life in the interim.

Reference

Alles GA: The comparative physiological actions of DL-β-phenylisopropylamines. 1. Pressor effect and toxicity. J Pharmacol Exp Ther 47:399–354, 1933

pharmacotherapy of psychosis

commentary

Since their discovery 20 years ago, much has been learned about the efficacy and toxicity of antipsychotic drugs. The most commonly used drugs are the phenothiazines and butyrophenones, but the thioxanthines and one indole derivative are also used. All agents that are significantly more effective than a placebo are dopamine antagonists and all produce extrapyramidal effects. Antiparkinsonian drugs are frequently administered with antipsychotic drugs. Repository preparations are useful when patient compliance is a problem. No differences in the efficacy of any of these agents has been demonstrated, but their side effects are significantly different.

Tardive dyskinesia, the most perplexing of the many side effects of the phenothiazines, sometimes responds to either a reduction or an increase in dose, but frequently is refractory to any type of treatment at all. If any of the newer antipsychotic agents can convincingly be shown not to produce this dreaded disorder, they will certainly supplant the phenothiazines. In the meantime, the antipsychotic drugs discussed in this chapter are the only demonstrably useful treatment for major psychoses, and it is questionable whether traditional psychotherapy has a beneficial effect (May 1968, Grinspoon 1972). Obviously, psychotic individuals require support and advice in addition to drug treatment.

References

Grinspoon L: Schizophrenia: Pharmacotherapy and Psychotherapy. Baltimore, Williams & Wilkins, 1972

May PRA: Treatment of Schizophrenia. New York, Science House, 1968

pharmacotherapy of psychosis

Jonathan O. Cole, M.D.

Antipsychotic Drugs

History of Development

The chance discovery of the antipsychotic drug, chlorpromazine, by Laborit, a surgeon, and its verification as an antipsychotic agent by the French psychiatrists, Delay and Deniker (Swazey 1974), in 1952 heralded a new era of treatment for the seriously mentally ill. Chlorpromazine and a growing number of pharmacologically similar antipsychotic agents have made a major contribution to the recent emptying of mental hospitals in the United States. To be sure, the drugs have been aided by a variety of community mental health philosophies and procedures; it may well be that neither the drugs nor the community mental health practices alone would have resulted in a major reshaping of American psychiatric care, but the combination has certainly had a massive effect. As an example, Boston State Hospital, the hospital with which this author is most familiar, had an inpatient population of over 3000 in the late 1950s and was kept to this size only by its practice of transferring chronic patients to other state hospitals in Massachusetts. Currently the inpatient population at Boston State Hospital is under 400 and is shrinking. The availability of antipsychotic drugs has enabled acutely psychotic schizophrenic patients to be handled in emergency rooms without hospitalization and has allowed many chronically psychotic individuals to be stabilized in the community with their families or in a variety of sheltered environments, such as

TABLE 1
ANTIPSYCHOTIC AGENTS

Antipsychotic agent	Daily dosage range* (mg)	Dose ratio equivalent to 300 mg chlorpromazine†
Phenothiazine		
Aliphatics		
Chlorpromazine (Thorazine)	100–1000	300
Triflupromazine (Vesprin)	20–150	100
Piperidines		
Thioridazine (Mellaril)	30–800‡	300
Mesoridazine (Serentil)	50–400	150
Piperacetazine (Quide)	20–160	30
Piperazines		
Trifluoperazine (Stealzine)	2–30	25
Perphenazine (Trilafon)	2–64	28
Carphenazine (Proketazine)	25–400	75
Acetophenazine (Tindal)	40–80	50
Butaperazine (Repoise)	30–50	30
Prochlorperazine (Compazine)	15–125	60
Thiopropazate (Dartal)	6–30	30
Fluphenazine (Prolixin)	0.5–20	6
Thioxanthene		
Chlorprothixene (Taractan)	10–600	300
Thiothixene (Navane)	6–60	25

206

TABLE 1 (cont.)

Antipsychotic agent	Daily dosage range* (mg)	Dose ratio equivalent to 300 mg chlorpromazine†
Butyrophenones		
Haloperidol (Haldol)	1–100	15
Indoles		
Molindone (Moban)	15–225	60

*Dosage ranges derived from package inserts published in 1974 Physicians Desk Reference. Upper limits are "recommended."
†Dosage equivalents prepared by George Gardos, M.D., Boston State Hospital, on basis of other available estimates and clinical experience.
‡Mandatory upper limit because of retinitis pigmentosa.

nursing homes, halfway houses, or boarding houses. Although one can argue with passion as to whether or not chronically psychotic individuals are really better off in nursing homes or in some of the other community settings chosen for them by mental health administrators, it is nevertheless very clear that antipsychotic drugs plus current mental health practices have successfully prevented the severe chronic institutionalization and deterioration in behavior so often seen on the back wards of mental hospitals 20 years ago.

There are currently 16 antipsychotic drugs approved for general prescription use in the United States (Table 1). Most of these are phenothiazines, meaning that they are chemically related to chlorpromazine, differing in the chemical attached at two points to the characteristic tricyclic structure. Two of the other compounds are thioxanthines (thiothixine and chlorprothixine) and are chemically very similar to the phenothiazines, differing slightly in the composition of the tricyclic ring. The other two, haloperidol, a butyrophenone, and molindone, an indole compound, are radically different structurally from each other and from the tricyclic antipsychotics. However, all of these drugs are really very similar to each other in their animal pharmacology and in their actions in man. Although the dose at which various antipsychotic drugs are effective varies widely, as can also be seen in Table 1, their overall effectiveness in the treatment of acute or chronic schizophrenia is probably roughly comparable. Attempts to find clear differential indications for the use of one drug over another in a particular kind of psychotic patient have generally not met with success. The drugs appear to differ from each other more markedly in their side effects than in their therapeutic effects.

Mechanism of Action

Persuasive evidence implicates dopamine (a brain biogenic amine believed to play a role not only in the etiology of Parkinson's disease but in the transmission of nerve impulses within the brain) in the etiology of schizophrenia and in the mechanism of action of antipsychotic drugs. D-amphetamine and related drugs can produce, in high doses in human subjects, a psychotic state almost indistinguishable from paranoid schizophrenia (Bell 1973). All of the potent antipsychotic drugs effectively block D-amphetamine-induced bizarre behaviors in animals and are effective in the treatment of amphetamine psychosis in man. The neurologic side effects so commonly produced by the antipsychotic drugs resemble naturally occurring Parkinson's disease. Both phenomena appear to be related to a lack of dopaminergic neuronal activity in the central nervous system. The antipsychotic drugs act by blocking transmission at dopaminergic (dopamine-run) synapses (Snyder et al 1974). At a more behavioral level, Irwin (1974) has noted that the antipsychotic drugs reduce activity in animals, reduce the animal's response to environmental stimuli, and reduce anxiety. In contrast the antianxiety drugs reduce anxiety while increasing activity and while increasing the animal's response to environmental stimuli. Antipsychotic drugs may therefore be thought of as protecting the psychotic patient by decreasing his responsiveness to his environment and decreasing the likelihood that he will exhibit psychotic behaviors. Calloway (1970) has advanced a similar theory in which he envisions the schizophrenic's brain as a malfunctioning computer and the antipsychotic drugs as agents that delay response to environmental or internal stimuli, thereby leading the schizophrenic patient to process his information more thoroughly and arrive at a more accurate and less psychotic behavior or verbal response.

Efficacy and Clinical Use

There is reasonable evidence that all of the antipsychotic drugs listed in Table 1 are reasonably effective in the treatment of both acute and chronic schizophrenia and, on the basis of less firm evidence, in the treatment of manic excitement (Davis and Cole 1976). These drugs are also widely used at necessarily far lower doses in the treatment of agitated or disturbed geriatric patients. They are also occasionally used in the treatment of behavior disorders of childhood, where they are less clearly effective and, also at lower doses, in the treatment of anxious outpatients. There is even reasonable evidence that two of the antipsychotic agents, chlorpromazine and thioridazine, are useful in the treatment of depression (Hollister 1973). Because of the problem posed by tardive dyskinesia, a condition to be discussed below, these drugs cannot be recommended for routine or regular use in conditions other than schizophrenia or acute mania, since better antianxiety or antidepressant drugs exist for use in other conditions. The antipsychotic drugs should only be used in anxious or depressed patients or in patients with behavior disorders or agitated senile states if the benzodiazepines and the tricyclic antidepressants have failed to provide symptomatic relief.

Schizophrenia. When the antipsychotic drugs are used in the treatment of schizophrenic patients, the dose at which symptomatic improvement begins to occur is highly variable. Some patients improve greatly on as little as 150 mg of chlorpromazine a day, while others require 3000 mg a day. Often, intramuscular medication is found to be substantially more effective on a milligram-per-kilogram basis than oral medication, and this is certainly true for chlorpromazine. There is beginning evidence that in crisis situations intramuscular medication can bring about a rapid reduction in psychotic ideation if heroic doses are used. For example, haloperidol, in doses of 10 mg intramuscularly every hour, has been reported to bring disturbed schizophrenic patients under good behavioral control within a few hours (Anderson and Kuehnle 1974). It should be noted that for many years, chlorpromazine has been considered the drug of choice for use in emergency rooms and emergency situations in psychiatry. Evidence is beginning to show that other drugs, at least mesoridazine (Hamid and Wertz 1973) and haloperidol (Anderson and Kuehnle 1974), may be more useful in such situations if the aim is to improve psychotic behavior. The probable reason for this is that chlorpromazine is more likely than some of the more potent drugs to cause a drop in blood pressure and to cause marked initial sedation when it is first administered. For this reason patients given chlorpromazine intramuscularly in large amounts tend to have a marked drop in blood pressure and to be profoundly sedated and almost unarousable. Comparable doses of haloperidol will leave a patient slightly drowsy but in good contact and able to function free from troublesome hypotension.

It is common practice to raise the dose of antipsychotic drugs fairly rapidly, early in the first few days of treatment, and then to lower the dose as patients improve or side effects become manifest. After patients are cognitively reconstituting and significantly improved, it is often desirable to give all of the antipsychotic medication at bedtime. These drugs are quite long acting and are even about as effective when given three times a week as they are when given daily. For many, but not all patients, a single bedtime dose improves the reliability with which the drug is taken and permits sedative or other mild short-term side effects to pass during the night while the patient is asleep. It should also be noted that the cost of these medications is not a direct function of dose. A 200 mg chlorpromazine tablet, at least in public mental hospitals in Massachusetts, costs only three times as much as a 25 mg tablet. In the interests of cost, it is therefore wise to prescribe the smallest number of tablets of the highest unit dosage whenever possible. Liquid medication forms are generally more expensive than tablets, but have the advantage in that it is harder for a patient to avoid taking the medication.

Clinical Response.   The clinical response in schizophrenia patients is usually pervasive and broad. Essentially all symptoms commonly found in schizophrenics have been shown to improve to a significantly greater extent on antipsychotic drug treatment than on placebo. The greatest improvement is usually seen during the first week of treatment, with significant further improvement continuing, on the average, for at least 13 weeks (Davis 1965). The "fly" in the therapeutic ointment is the fact that some patients hospitalized or treated for schizophrenia as outpatients had an unsatisfactory level of social functioning and mental health before the onset of an overt psychotic breakdown. Even if the drug relieves major psychotic symptoms, such as delusions, hallucinations, or thought disorder, the patient's level of social and vocational functioning may still be distinctly impaired. In other patients antipsychotic drugs serve to suppress many symptoms of psychosis, but the patient may be left with decreased initiative, vague thinking, and residual paranoid ideation. The patient may be improved but is by no means well. Therefore, although the drugs are a great improvement over available social therapies and are probably more benign than biologic treatments (electroconvulsive therapy, insulin coma treatment, and lobotomy) available prior to 1952, there are still far too many patients who are inadequately helped. For manic excitement, recent evidence from a controlled study supports the belief that lithium carbonate is a more effective treatment for manic excitement than either haloperidol and chlorpromazine (Shopsin et al 1975). However an earlier and larger VA-NIMH study showed chlorpromazine to be more effective than lithium in the treatment of severely manic patients (Prien et al 1972).

Long Acting Injectables. The major innovation in antipsychotic drug therapy during the past 10 years is the development of long-acting injectable forms. Currently, fluphenazine enanthate and decanoate are the only such medications available in the United States (Groves and Mandel 1976). A single injection of either drug tends to last between 2 and 4 weeks. They appear to be generally far safer than was initially suspected. Since there is excellent evidence that ambulatory chronic schizophrenic patients tend to relapse with high frequency if they do not take their medication, this long-acting injectable preparation can be used to ensure that patients actually are receiving active medication. The injection can be given in a clinic or in a doctor's office, but it can also be given in the home by a visiting nurse. Although many patients tolerate the injectable medication well, some show a tendency toward neurologic side effects after almost every injection, despite the prophylactic use of antiparkinsonian drugs.

Side Effects

Anticholinergic and Antidopaminergic. The antipsychotic drugs can be conceived as of varying significantly in their degree of antidopaminergic effect and also in their degree of anticholinergic (atropinelike) effect (Snyder et al 1974). The antidopaminergic effects produce a variety of neurologic symptoms. The anticholinergic effects tend to counteract the antidopaminergic effects. Anticholinergic drugs (eg, benztropine) have long been used in the treatment of parkinsonism. The anticholinergic effects include dry mouth, blurred vision, drop in blood pressure, increase in heart rate, and sometimes difficulty urinating. One may conceive of the antipsychotic drugs as a continuum. At one end is thioridazine, which produces a relatively low incidence of neurologic side effects but tends to cause a drop in blood pressure, blurred vision, dry mouth, and other autonomic symptoms. It is also the drug most likely to cause mild changes in the electrocardiogram, of currently unknown significance. At the other extreme would be drugs like haloperidol or fluphenazine which have very strong antidopaminergic effects and very weak anticholinergic effects. Generally, the lower the dose at which a drug is effective as an antipsychotic, the more potent its antidopaminergic actions are and the less marked its anticholinergic actions are.

Neurologic. The neurologic side effect which usually occurs earliest in treatment is dystonia. This consists of spasms of muscle systems, usually in the neck and face, of acute onset lasting a few minutes to hours. It is harmless but often frightening to the patient and to observers. It can be rapidly relieved by intravenous or intramuscular injection of antiparkinsonian drugs such as benztropine or diphenhydramine. Somewhat later in treatment, after 2 days to several weeks, patients may develop two other symptoms. One of these, pseudoparkinsonism, is characterized by muscular stiffness, stooped posture, shuffling gait, masklike facies, and drooling. The syndrome resembles naturally occurring parkinsonism very closely, although tremor is less common in drug-induced parkinsonism. Pseudoparkinsonism is generally relieved by antiparkinsonian drugs.

The third acute neurologic side effect, akathisia, is characterized by an inner feeling of restlessness and discomfort in the muscles (Van Putten 1974). Some patients may just complain of feeling badly while others may find it impossible to sit still and may pace up and down or move about constantly when sitting. This subjective somatic discomfort is usually not incorporated into the patient's psychiatric complaints and symptoms, but must of course be distinguished from psychotic agitation. It again is relieved by antiparkinsonian agents.

In choosing antiparkinsonian agents, there is little firm evidence on which to base a choice. However, it seems reasonable that diphenhydramine, a relatively sedative and somewhat less anticholinergic agent, might be preferable in patients who need additional sedation, while a drug like benztropine or biperiden might be more useful in patients who are already substantially drowsy.

Other reported side effects of antipsychotic drugs (Shader and DiMascio 1970), such as agranulocytosis or jaundice, are quite rare and cannot be picked up by routine laboratory testing. Staff in contact with patients on antipsychotic drugs should, however, be watchful for sore throat and fever and obtain a blood count on patients showing such signs during the first few months of treatment. Similarly, patients with abdominal distress or who appear jaundiced should have liver function studies. Agranulocytosis is a serious complication; the effects of these drugs on the liver appear to be a minor inconvenience. Occasionally, in susceptible patients, these drugs, which tend to lower the convulsive threshold, will precipitate a seizure. However, patients with preexisting epilepsy have often been treated safely without showing any increase in the frequency of convulsions. Chlorpromazine produces photosensitivity. Patients on this drug will often experience very severe sunburns after a relatively brief exposure to sun. Other phenothiazines do not appear to share this property. Thioridazine tends initially to cause delayed ejaculation, and after more prolonged use it can cause impotence. Other drugs may share this action to a lesser extent. Antipsychotic drugs also stimulate the secretion of prolactin and, in some patients, this produces breast engorgement or even slight lactation.

Problems of Long-Term Administration

For the first 10 to 15 years during which antipsychotic drugs were used, no long-term side effects were recognized and the drugs appeared to be quite safe. At present, however, there is clear evidence that some phenothiazines, certainly chlorpromazine and possibly others, produce pigmentary deposits in the skin, causing exposed areas to turn a brownish, grayish, purplish shade (Greiner and Barry 1964). Similar deposits have been observed in the cornea and lens of the eye. These eye changes are almost invariably found only on slit-lamp examination and almost never interfere with vision (Prien et al 1970).

Two other concerns associated with long-term antipsychotic drug therapy are (a) the possibility that sudden death occurs more often than it should in chronic psychiatric patients receiving antipsychotics. However, sudden unexplained death in psychiatric patients was considered a problem long before the antipsychotic drugs were discovered, and there is no clear evidence that the frequency of such deaths has in fact increased (Moore and Book 1970). (b) There is also the possibility that chronic drug therapy of any sort may affect the fetus during its development. To date, there is no evidence that the incidence of fetal abnormalities in patients treated with antipsychotic drugs is any greater than that in pregnant women not receiving such drugs. It is still well to remember that pregnant women, particularly during the first trimester, should receive drugs only if absolutely necessary.

Tardive Dyskinesia.   The serious concern in the long-term use of antipsychotic drugs is the appearance of tardive dyskinesia, a chronic, often persistent movement disorder (ACNP-FDA Task Force 1973). About 10 years ago, it was noticed, for the first time, that chronic mental patients showed a variety of abnormal movements. The most characteristic were chewing, smacking movements of the lips with writhing, and, occasionally, protrusion of the tongue. Such patients also showed body twisting, rocking, and pelvic thrusting movements as well as athetoid twisting movements of the arms and legs. The late recognition that this disorder was drug related is undoubtedly due to the fact that such movement disorders have occurred with a considerably lower incidence in psychiatric

patients for centuries (Marsden et al 1976). The disturbing fact is
that the proportion of patients, on chronic psychiatric wards, showing such movements (generally to a minimal or mild extent) is generally climbing, and at Boston State Hospital, at present, the prevalence ranges between 25 and 50 percent, depending on the criteria
used to assess their presence or absence. Also, the disorder is appearing in patients who have received antipsychotic medications for
nonpsychiatric conditions; this author has personally seen four such
patients in the past year with clear tardive dyskinesia. In all four
cases, the patients developed abnormal movements of the mouth
and tongue and, in some cases, of the extremities after only a year's
treatment. The drugs involved were respectively, thioridazine,
chlorpromazine, fluphenazine, and thiothixene. The patients ranged
in age from late 30 to early 70. All had been originally treated for
either depressive reactions or severe anxiety states. The range of
drugs involved in my small series and in the general literature is so
great as to leave one convinced that any antipsychotic drug can
produce the syndrome in a predisposed individual. Dose or duration
of treatment do not seem to correlate highly with the occurrence of
the disorder.

In conclusion, the antipsychotic drugs provide a very valuable
tool in the treatment of acute schizophrenia and are generally effective in preventing severe psychotic manifestations in more chronic
schizophrenic patients. They are also of significant use in the treatment of acute mania. Despite their occasional usefulness in nonpsychotic disorders, such as anxiety states and depressive syndromes, their use in such conditions should be generally avoided and
other treatment possibilities exhausted first, because tardive dyskinesia is a risk.

References

ACNP-FDA Task Force: Neurologic syndromes associated with antipsychotic drug. N Engl J Med 290:427–428, 1973

Anderson WH, Kuehnle JC: Strategies for the treatment of acute psychosis.
JAMA 229:1884–1889, 1974

Bell DS: The experimental reproduction of amphetamine psychosis. Arch
Gen Psychiatry 29:35–40, 1973

Calloway E: Schizophrenia and interference. Arch Gen Psychiatry
22:193–208, 1970

Davis JM: The efficacy of the tranquilizing and anti-depressant drugs. Arch Gen Psychiatry 13:552–572, 1965

————, Cole, JO: Antipsychotic Drugs. In Freedman DX (ed): Handbook of Psychiatry. New York, Basic Books, 1976

Greiner AC, Berry K: Skin pigmentation and corneal and lens opacities with prolonged chlorpromazine therapy. Can Med Assoc J 90:663–665, 1964

Groves JE, Mandel MR: The long acting phenothiazines. Arch Gen Psychiatry 33, 1976

Hamid T, Wertz W: Mesoridazine versus chlorpromazine in acute schizophrenia. Am J Psychiatry 130:689–692, 1973

Hollister L: Clinical Use of Psychotherapeutic Drugs. Springfield, Ill, Thomas, 1973

Irwin S: The use and potential hazards of psychoactive drugs. Bull Menninger Clinic 38:14–48, 1974

Marsden CD, Tarsy D, Baldessarini RJ: Spontaneous and drug-induced movement disorders in psychotic patients. In Benson H, Blumer D (eds): Psychiatric Complications of Neurological Diseases. New York, Grune, 1976

Moore MT, Book MH: Sudden death in phenothiazine therapy. Psychiatr Q 44:389–395, 1970

Prien, RF, Caffey EM, Klett CJ: Comparison of lithium and chlorpromazine in the treatment of mania. Arch Gen Psychiatry 26:146–153, 1972

————, Delong SL, Cole JO, Levine J: Ocular changes occurring with prolonged high dose chlorpromazine therapy. Arch Gen Psychiatry 23:464–467, 1970

Shader RI, DiMascio A: Psychotropic drug side effects. Baltimore, Williams & Wilkins, 1970

Shopsin B, Gershon S, Thompson H, Collins P: Psychoactive drugs in mania. Arch Gen Psychiatry 32:34–42, 1975

Snyder S, Greenberg D, Yamamura H: Antischizophrenic drugs and brain cholinergic receptors. Arch Gen Psychiatry 31:58–67, 1974

Swazey J: Chlorpromazine: the history of a psychiatric discovery. Cambridge, MIT Press, 1974

Van Putten T: Why do schizophrenic patients refuse to take their drugs? Arch Gen Psychiatry 31:67–71, 1974

diagnosis of affective disorders

commentary

There are estimates that up to 15 percent of the population may at some time suffer from depression or mania sufficiently severe to be called an illness. In this chapter a distinction is made between major depressive illness and minor depressive disorder. The temporal patterns in affective disorders have diagnostic, therapeutic, and prognostic implications. Delusions, hallucinations, and thought disorder help differentiate between affective illness, schizophrenic disorder, and schizophrenia. Particularly in older patients, organic brain syndrome may mimic or overlap an affective disorder.

diagnosis of affective disorders

Frederick K. Goodwin, M.D.

Syndrome Versus Symptom

What does the term *affective illness* or, more specifically, *depression* or *mania* mean to the psychopharmacologist? This question is most subtle in relation to depression, since as a *symptom* it is part of everyday life, one of the hosts of normal responses to the great variety of stresses, losses, and reversals that are part of the human condition. However, as physicians we have all come to recognize individuals in whom symptoms of depression or sadness are only a part of a larger whole, that is, the *syndrome* of depression. For years psychiatrists have speculated that the depressive syndrome, especially in its more severe forms, reflected a biologic dysfunction for a number of reasons. (a) There is good evidence that the depressive syndrome tends to run in families, a tendency that suggests a genetic predisposition (Winokur et al 1969, Gershon et al 1971). (b) A major depression has the characteristics of an illness, in that it has a relatively clear onset, course, and prognosis with a reasonably consistent and definable group of symptoms.

Criteria For Identifying Depression Syndrome

I will attempt to define the syndrome of depression in a way that tells us whether drug treatment is necessary or appropriate in a given patient. In so doing I am aware that there are many other purposes for which depression is defined (eg, biologic research, genetic studies, psychotherapy studies) and that the definitional criteria largely depend on the use to which the definition is to be put. For our purposes, then, three general criteria should be met before one can properly identify the syndrome of depression. These criteria involve (a) a *cluster* of symptoms, (b) sufficient *duration*, and (c) *functional* incapacity. Thus, (a) the primary symptom of a depressed or dysphoric mood (which often has a distinct quality different from grief) must occur as part of a *cluster* of varied symptoms. These varied symptoms should include at least several of the following: sleep disturbance (especially difficulty staying asleep); loss of appetite, often with weight loss; psychomotor retardation (and /or agitation); anxiety; loss of energy and excessive tiredness; vague aches and pains; decreased capacity to feel pleasure; loss of interest; suicidal thoughts (and acts); decreased ability to think, concentrate, or remember; and thought patterns dominated by helplessness, hopelessness, self-depreciation, and excessive guilt, any of which can reach psychotic proportions. The symptoms often show a distinct diurnal variation (worse in the morning) and a relative lack of reactivity to the environment. (b) The problem should have been evident for at least 2 to 3 weeks. (c) The symptoms should have been of sufficient severity to have objectively interfered with the individual's occupational and interpersonal functioning. Additional features of the history often include a prior depressive episode and a family history of affective illness.

Research Diagnostic Criteria. Recent efforts to improve classification in psychiatry (Feighner et al 1972) have led to the development of the research diagnostic criteria (RDC) (Spitzer et al 1975). The RDC, which will become the basis for the revised diagnostic manual of the American Psychiatric Association (DMS III), represents a significant advance in the rational classification of affective disorders. Briefly, the RDC defines criteria for major depressive illness as distinguished from minor dysphoric illness; these criteria are essentially those listed above for the syndrome of depression. Table 1 lists the RDC for major primary depressive illness.

In the RDC system, major depressive illness is further described by the application of specific groups of criteria which can overlap. For example, a given major depressive episode may be *primary* (rather than secondary to another diagnosable psychiatric or medical condition), *endogenous* (having a specific cluster of symptoms such as diurnal variation, lack of reactivity to the environment, early-morning awakening, and so forth), *recurrent, psychotic* (based on the presence of delusions, not on severity), *situational* (apparent close relationship to significant life events), and *incapacitating* (reflecting major functional impairment, often requiring hospitali-

TABLE 1
RESEARCH DIAGNOSTIC CRITERIA FOR MAJOR, PRIMARY DEPRESSIVE ILLNESS*

A. DYSPHORIC MOOD: Prominent and persistent with feelings of depression, hopelessness, emptiness, and so forth.

B. CLUSTERS OF SYMPTOMS, including at least *five* of the following:
appetite disturbance (decrease or increase)
sleep disturbance (decrease or increase)
loss of energy
psychomotor retardation (or agitation)
loss of interest in usually pleasurable activities
slowed thinking, decreased ability to concentrate or remember
self-blame and inappropriate guilt
recurrent thoughts of death or suicide

C. DURATION of the above, at least *two weeks*

D. *IMPAIRED FUNCTIONING, requiring hospitalization*†

E. PRIMARY, ie, no prior evidence of schizophrenia, anxiety state, phobic disorder, obsessive—compulsive disorder, antisocial personality, drug dependence, serious physical illness, or other diagnosable psychiatric disorders.

*(From Spitzer et al: Am J Psychiatry 32:1187, 1976.)
†Hospitalization required in National Institute of Mental Health criteria

zation). Each of the descriptive categories addresses itself to a different aspect of the depression. These categories are especially useful because they are *not mutually exclusive* and do not require forced choices. In the traditional, less empirically based system for the classification of depression it was implicit that the terms *psychotic, incapacitating, nonsituational, severe,* and *endogenous* were more or less synonymous. It remains to be seen to what extent these various independent descriptive categories interrelate and overlap in clinical application. In regard to the question of drug treatment addressed in this chapter, data on the relationship between specific RDC categories and drug response are not yet available.

The Depressive Spectrum

In making a decision about an individual patient it is useful to conceptualize depression as a spectrum, as illustrated in Figure 1. As a general rule, the closer the individual is to the right end of the spectrum, the more suitable he is for drug therapy. Note that in this model there is no definite cutoff point for defining drug-treatable

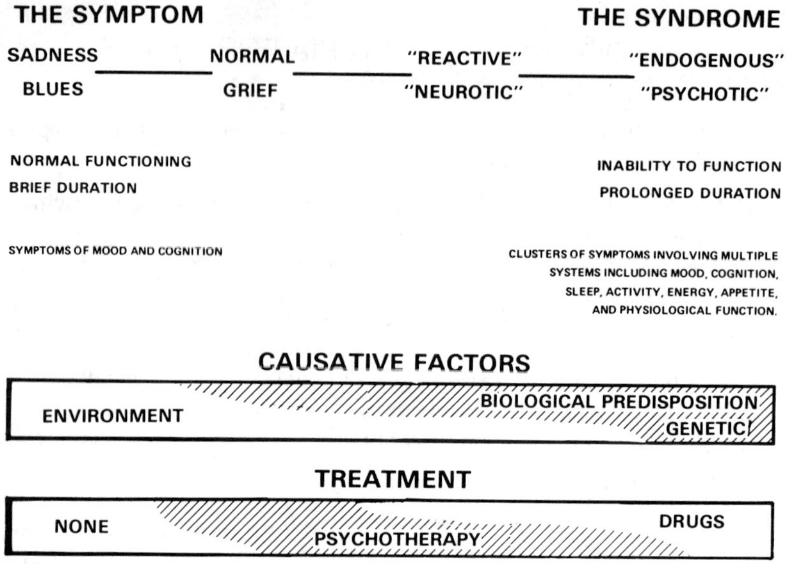

THE SYMPTOM   **THE SYNDROME**

SADNESS	NORMAL	"REACTIVE"	"ENDOGENOUS"
BLUES	GRIEF	"NEUROTIC"	"PSYCHOTIC"

NORMAL FUNCTIONING   INABILITY TO FUNCTION

BRIEF DURATION   PROLONGED DURATION

SYMPTOMS OF MOOD AND COGNITION   CLUSTERS OF SYMPTOMS INVOLVING MULTIPLE
                                                   SYSTEMS INCLUDING MOOD, COGNITION,
                                                   SLEEP, ACTIVITY, ENERGY, APPETITE,
                                                   AND PHYSIOLOGICAL FUNCTION.

CAUSATIVE FACTORS

ENVIRONMENT   BIOLOGICAL PREDISPOSITION

                                                   GENETIC

TREATMENT

NONE   PSYCHOTHERAPY   DRUGS

Fig. 1.   Depression—a spectrum.

depression, and note also that there is a large intermediate area of the spectrum in which drugs and psychotherapy may both be indicated.

As noted above in the discussion of the RDC, by employing a spectrum model, I do not wish to imply that the features at either end of the spectrum are necessarily mutually exclusive (Kendell 1968). Factor analytic studies make it clear that the validity of the distinction between *reactive* (or neurotic) and *endogenous* depression rests on the presence or absence of endogenous features, not on the presence or absence of neurotic symptoms or reactive features (Kiloh et al 1972, Paykel 1971). In other words, some patients with the endogenous syndrome may have neurotic or reactive features (including clear precipitating events, Leff et al 1970, Paykel et al 1969), while some may not. On the other hand, the diagnosis of neurotic or reactive depression depends on the relative absence of endogenous features. Confusion in the use of these dichotomous terms (particularly reactive versus endogenous and neurotic versus psychotic) is probably responsible for apparent discrepancies in the earlier literature on the types of depression most appropriately treated with drugs. The issue of severity also needs some clarification; while it is obvious that overall severity of the problem generally increases as you go toward the endogenous end of the spectrum, it is nevertheless possible for an individual with a severe neurotic depression (absence of endogenous features) to be in more distress than another patient with a mild or moderate depression with endogenous features. Later I will outline more specifically the clinical information needed to make a decision about drug therapy and to choose between a variety of available agents if drug therapy is deemed appropriate.

Episode Duration

The expected duration of a depressive episode should also influence treatment decisions. Large-scale, recently completed long-term studies are of help here (Grof et al 1973). For most untreated major depressive episodes, the duration is 4 to 6 months or less; substantially longer episodes are encountered among individuals with *involutional* depressions (a relatively severe depressive syndrome usually occurring in association with the menopause and in which prominent agitation and paranoid features are exhibited; there may or may not be a prior history of depression). Episodes substantially shorter than 4 months are more often seen in cyclic manic-depressive illness. Where there has been a previous episode, its duration often may be used to estimate the expected duration of the current episode since longitudinal studies indicate that the duration of the episodes tends to be relatively constant in a given patient in whom the illness is recurrent (Grof et al 1973).

Patterns of Recurrence in Affective Illness—The Unipolar-Bipolar Distinction

One of the most important and yet most often overlooked aspect of major affective illness is that it is almost always a recurrent illness (Winokur et al 1969, Grof et al 1973). Although it has long been generally assumed that roughly one-half to two-thirds of depressed patients will experience only a single episode in their lifetime, careful long-term follow-up studies of a large number of patients who had been hospitalized at least once for an affective episode indicate that *virtually every one of these seriously depressed patients experienced more than one episode* (Grof et al 1973).

There are basically two patterns of recurrence in the major affective disorders—the *unipolar* and the *bipolar*. The unipolar pattern involves depressions alone, while in the bipolar pattern a history of both depression and mania (or hypomania) is noted. The unipolar

TABLE 2
DIFFERENTIAL CLINICAL CHARACTERISTICS OF
UNIPOLAR AND BIPOLAR DEPRESSED PATIENTS

UNIPOLAR	BIPOLAR
Low incidence of mania in family history	Higher incidence of mania in family history
Late age of onset (40s)	Early age of onset (20s)
Moderate to high levels of measured activity during depression	Low levels of measured activity during depression
Psychomotor agitation and /or retardation	Psychomotor retardation
Higher ratings of anxiety and physical complaints	Lower ratings of anxiety and physical complaints
Abnormal MMPI during depression	Normal MMPI during depression
Lower frequency of postpartum depression	Higher frequency of postpartum depression

and bipolar patterns appear to reflect two different illnesses which can be differentiated clinically, genetically, biologically, and pharmacologically. Clinical features that differentiate unipolar and bipolar depressed patients are listed in Table 2. Instances of unipolar mania have been reported (Winokur et al 1969, Perris 1966), although this phenomenon is extremely rare; some reports of unipolar mania (Abrams and Taylor 1974) can be questioned in regard to the method used to ascertain a prior history of depression.

The Syndrome of Mania

The typical manic episode may start with a sudden "switch" from a depressive phase or it may develop gradually out of a depression or a normal period. The initial phase of the episode is characterized by increased psychomotor activity. At this point the accompanying mood is usually labile, with a predominance of euphoria, although irritability may become apparent when the individual's many demands are not met. The cognitive state during this phase is characterized by expansiveness, grandiosity, and overconfidence. Thoughts are coherent although often tangential. An individual is often aware of the mood change at this point, frequently describing it as "going high" or as having racing thoughts. In many instances the "high" does not go beyond this level of severity and is designated as hypomania. In some instances, however, the episode progresses with further increases in psychometer activity, including increased initiation in rate of speech, while the mood state becomes more of a mixture of euphoria and dysphoria. The irritability observed initially progresses to open hostility and anger, and the accompanying behavior is frequently explosive and assaultive. Racing thoughts progress to a definite flight of ideas, with increasing disorganization of the cognitive state. Preoccupations present earlier and become more intense, with grandiose and paranoid trends now apparent as frank delusions. In some patients the manic episode can progress to an undifferentiated psychotic state, experienced by the patient as clearly dysphoric and accompanied by frenzied psychomotor activity. Thought processes that earlier had been only difficult to follow now become incoherent; definite loosening of associations is often seen (Kraepelin 1921, Rennie 1942, Carlson and Goodwin 1973). Delusions are often bizarre and idiosyncratic, and some patients in this phase even experience ideas of reference and disorientation. This phase of the syndrome is difficult to distinguish from an acute schizophrenic psychosis (Carlson and Goodwin 1973, Abrams et al 1974). Obviously, in the severe phase of mania, patients require hospitalization. The borderline between mild hypomanic excitement and normal mood elevation is sometimes difficult to distinguish, but, in general, if the patient and /or his family has experienced the mood state as abnormal, and it has resulted in any interruption in normal role functioning, it should be considered hypomanic.

Differentiating Affective Disorder, Schizoaffective Disorder, and Schizophrenia

The complex topic of schizophrenia is discussed elsewhere in this volume (see p 205). As a cardinal rule, a diagnosis of affective illness is not considered unless the affective state of depression (or mania) is a prominent part of the clinical picture and unless the patient has at least several of the specific symptoms noted above as part of the depressive (or manic) syndrome.

What about those patients who fulfill the criteria for the syndrome of depression or mania but in addition have "schizophreniclike" symptoms, such as delusions, hallucinations, or formal thought disorder? In other words are there guidelines that can be used to differentiate "pure" affective illness from schizoaffective disorder? Delusions per se neither rule out a diagnosis of affective disorder nor require a diagnosis of schizoaffective disorder. Delusions that represent psychotic extensions of excessively lowered or elevated self-esteem can be especially characteristic of affective illness; examples of affect-laden delusions are: "I am so awful my body is rotting," (depressive) or, "The President came to see me today" (manic). Paranoid or persecutory delusions can accompany major depressions, particularly menopausal or postmenopausal (involutional) depression; paranoid delusions are commonplace in mania.

Schizoaffective disorder should be considered if the content of the delusions is especially bizarre, if they are multiple, or if the delusions are elaborated into a formal system. Prominent examples here are delusions of one's own feelings, thoughts, and actions being controlled from outside; of one's thoughts being broadcast; and of others' thoughts being inserted into one's mind.

The presence of persistent hallucinations is generally not consistent with a diagnosis of affective disorder. Exceptions to this are hallucinations which are clearly related to the disordered moods, such as the depressed patient who hears accusing voices.

The existence of formal thought disorder, in the presence of the depressive (or manic) syndrome, requires a diagnosis of schizoaffective disorder. The diagnosis of a formal thought disorder (incoherence, loosening of associations, grossly illogical thinking, poverty of content) involves very subtle judgments and should not be based on material included in delusions. Psychiatric consultation is often necessary here. The usefulness of the distinction between affective and schizoaffective disorder, as it relates to drug therapy, will be discussed in the following chapter.

Differentiating Affective Illness from Organic Brain Syndrome

Major affective illness is often accompanied by some of the symptoms prominently associated with organic brain disease, and, at times, this differential diagnosis can be difficult. The extent to which a major depression can interfere with cognitive functions is often not fully appreciated. The depressed patient can present with serious impairment of recent memory, confusion, and even the appearance of disorientation—all symptoms classically associated with chronic organic brain disease—ie, the dementias.

The problem is additionally complicated by the fact that many patients undergoing an organic brain syndrome will experience depressive symptoms in response to their awareness of decreased functional capacity (the so-called catastrophic reaction). Also, the age range at which many patients experience depression overlaps with the age range for organic brain disease.

In making the differential diagnosis it is important to know first of any past history of depression, and second, the nature of the *initial symptoms* in the present episode. Thus, if the patient's difficulties started with memory loss or with episodes of confusion one should pursue evidence that might corroborate a diagnosis of organic brain disease; further evaluation would include a more rigorous and detailed clinical examination of the sensorium, psychologic testing, and full neurologic work-up. If, on the other hand, the initial symptoms of the episode were affective (such as depressed mood, sleep loss, and so forth) rather than primarily organic, one could make a presumptive diagnosis of affective illness, taking care to follow the evolution of organic symptoms.

Similarly, a manic patient in the most severe phase of the illness can show many of the symptoms of an acute delirium (Kraepelin 1921, Carlson and Goodwin 1973). If one encounters this without knowledge of the history or the initial symptoms of the episode, it is advisable to rule out obvious causes of acute brain syndrome, such as drug ingestion, head injury, or other neurologic problems.

References

Abrams R, Taylor MA: Unipolar mania: a preliminary report. Arch Gen Psychiatry 30:441–443, 1974

———, Taylor MA, Gartanopa P: Manic depressive illness and paranoid schizophrenia: A phenomenologic, family, history, and treatment and response study. Arch Gen Psychiatry 31:640–642, 1974

Carlson GA, Goodwin FK: The stages of mania: a longitudinal analysis of the manic episodes. Arch Gen Psychiatry 28:221–228, 1973

Feighner JP, Robins E, Guze SB, et al: Diagnostic criteria for use in psychiatric research. Arch Gen Psychiatry 26:57–63, 1972

Gershon ES, Dunner DL, Goodwin FK: Toward a biology of affective illness: genetic contributions. Arch Gen Psychiatry 25:1–15, 1971

Grof P, Angst J, Haines T: The clinical course of depression: practical issues. Symposia Medica Hoechst 8:141–148, 1973

Kendell RE: The Classification of Depressive Illness. London, Oxford, 1968

Kiloh LH, Andrews G, Neilson M, Bianchi GN: The relationship of the syndromes called endogenous and neurotic depression. Br J Psychiatry 121:183–196, 1972

Kraepelin E: Manic-depressive Insanity and Paranoia. Edinburgh, Livingston, 1921

Leff MJ, Roatch JF, Bunney WE Jr: Environmental factors preceding the onset of severe depressions. Psychiatry 33:293–311, 1970

Paykel ES: Classification of depressed patients: a cluster analysis derived grouping. Br J Psychiatry 118:275–288, 1971

―――, Myers JK, Dieuelt MN, et al: Life events and depression. Arch Gen Psychiatry 21:753–760, 1969

Perris C: A study of bipolar (manic-depressive) and unipolar recurrent depressive psychoses. Acta Psychiatr Scand 42: Suppl 194:9–189, 1966

Rennie TAC: Prognosis in manic-depressive psychosis. Am J Psychiatry 98:801–814, 1942

Spitzer RL, Endicott J, Robins E: Clinical criteria for psychiatric diagnosis and DSM III. Am J Psychiatry 32:1187–1192, 1975

Winokur C, Clayton PJ, Reich T: Manic-Depressive Illness. St. Louis, Mosby, 1969

biologic basis of drug action in the affective disorders

commentary

The regular cyclicity of affective disorders, the demonstration of a genetic component, the usefulness of drug therapy, and the availability of modern analytic chemical technology has made theorizing about the biologic basis of this disorder very profitable. The implication of neurotransmitter in the genesis of depression and mania has paralleled the development of an understanding of the role of these transmitters in the central nervous system. The simplest statement of the catecholamine theory associated depression, with a deficit of brain norepinephrine and mania with an excess of this substance. Dr. Goodwin discusses the variations of this theme and its vicissitudes. As with many theories of mental illness, it now appears that the facts are not as simple as the original formulation, but that a number of brain transmitters are involved in the neuropathology of affective illness and in the action of antidepressant and antimanic drugs.

biologic basis of drug action in the affective disorders

Frederick K. Goodwin, M.D.

The major hypotheses concerning biochemical factors in affective illness center on the possibility that these disorders are related to disturbances in central neuronal systems involving one or more of the neurotransmitter catecholamines (norepinephrine, NE; or dopamine, DA) or indoleamines (serotonin, 5HT). A great variety of basic work over the past 15 years has identified and categorized these neuronal systems as the primary regulatory circuits in those areas of the brain which subserve functions broadly related to appetitive behaviors, drives, arousal, and "emotions" (including their neuroendocrine and psychophysiologic concomitants), and to the integration of these functions with a wide range of other brain components. As in all neuronal circuits, the flow of impulses is primarily regulated at the synaptic junction. The complex nature of the processes responsible for synthesis, storage, release, reuptake, and metabolism of the amine neurotransmitters provides many possibilities for drug effects as well as for internal regulatory processes.

The amine neurotransmitter systems have enormous functional significance in spite of the relatively modest number of neurons, a situation which can be appreciated when their neuroanatomic distribution is considered. Briefly, these systems are made up of neurons with very long axonal processes and a very large number of terminal branchings such that a single nerve cell receiving input from multiple sources can synapse with as many as 75,000 other neurons. These amine systems are heavily concentrated in midline brain stem structures and have their cell bodies primarily in the upper brain stem and midbrain, with projections throughout the

limbic system, cerebral cortex, neocortex, hypothalamus, and lower
brain stem, in effect interacting with virtually every major functional
area of the brain (Kety 1967, Cooper et al 1974). Given the complexity of the syndrome of affective illness with its interrelated cognitive, emotional, psychomotor, appetitive, and autonomic manifestations one can understand that these very widely distributed systems
have become the focus of neurobiologic investigations.

Figure 1 illustrates schematically the function of norepinephrine
at the nerve ending. First, tyrosine, a dietary amino acid, is taken up
into the neuron by an active transport process where it undergoes a
ring hydroxylation (the rate-limiting step in norepinephrine synthesis), a subsequent decarboxylation to dopamine, and then a process
of uptake into a storage vesicle with an associated side chain hydroxylation to form norepinephrine. With the arrival of a nerve impulse, a complex process is set in motion involving calcium and
other ionic shifts, as a result of which the vesicle migrates to the
inner wall of the neuronal membrane, fuses with it, and releases its

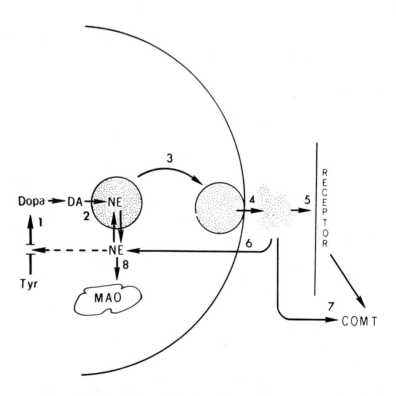

Fig. 1.   Schema of a noradrenergic synapse.

contents into the synaptic junction, where the neurotransmitter can interact with the postsynaptic receptor, ultimately setting in motion another neuronal event. Some of the released neurotransmitter is taken back into the neuron by an active transport process following which it can again be stored or metabolized by monoamine oxidase. The synaptic mechanisms for serotonin and dopamine are basically similar to those for norepinephrine.

The initial suggestion that there may be a relationship between the functional state of one or more of these neurotransmitters and the clinical state of depression was the result of a chance observation concerning the effects of the drug reserpine. Associated with its widespread use in the early 1950s as an antihypertensive agent, it was discovered that a significant percentage of patients on the drug experienced symptoms of depression (Lemieux et al 1956, Ayd 1956, Quetsch et al 1959). At about the same time it was found in animal experiments that reserpine was capable of depleting nerve endings of their stores of serotonin, dopamine, and norepinephrine (Shore and Brodie 1957, Carlsson et al 1957). These two sets of observations, one from the clinic, the other from the biochemical laboratory, came to be associated because of the alertness of individuals trained both clinically and biochemically; as a result of this association, the amine hypothesis of affective disorders was formulated (Prange 1973, Bunney and Davis 1965, Schildkraut 1965). In its simplest form, the amine hypothesis states that depression is associated with a functional deficit of one or more brain neurotransmitter amines at specific central synapses, and that conversely mania is associated with a functional excess of one or more of these amines.

Shortly after the observations concerning reserpine, there was another serendipitous observation concerning the drug iproniazid, which was being used in the treatment of tuberculosis. Some patients on this drug were noted to have mood elevation with reversal of the depression often associated with chronic illness (Kline 1958). At about the same time, it was independently discovered that this drug was capable of elevating brain amine levels by inhibiting the metabolizing enzyme, monoamine oxidase (MAO) (Davidson 1958). It was shown in animals that a series of monoamine oxidase inhibitors could prevent or reverse the syndrome of sedation and depression produced by reserpine (Brodie et al 1959). At this point, therefore, one had the observation of a mood elevating drug (monoamine oxidase inhibitor) that also elevated brain amines and a mood depressing drug (reserpine) that decreased brain amines. Furthermore, amphetamine and cocaine, both stimulants in man, were found to increase amine function at the synapse through a variety of mechanisms.

Another important piece of evidence was provided by the discovery of the tricyclic antidepressants (Kuhn 1957), drugs that were originally developed as derivatives of the major tranquilizers. Because these drugs did not alter the levels of brain amines in animals, their relevance to the amine hypothesis of affective disorder was initially unclear. However, it was subsequently found that tricyclics could inhibit the uptake process by which the amines in the synaptic cleft were taken back into the neuron (Glowinski and Axelrod 1964). This inhibition of reuptake had the effect of increasing the amount of amine available to interact with the receptor. Thus, the role of the tricyclic antidepressants seemed also to fit neatly into the amine hypothesis of affective illness.

Lithium, a drug with dramatic antimanic properties (Schou 1968), also seemed to fit the hypothesis since animal data suggested that its action on amines at the synapse was to enhance reuptake (Colburn et al 1968) and inhibit release (Katz et al 1968)—an effect "opposite" to the tricyclic antidepressants. Thus the presumed lithium-induced reduction in the amount of amine in the synaptic cleft was consistent with the hypothesis associating mania with elevated amines.

Although the foregoing pharmacologic data have provided a major impetus to the development of hypotheses concerning affective illness, there are a number of difficulties in fitting all of the data into any straightforward amine hypothesis; these observations are summarized in Table 1. First, drugs that are stimulants in normal individuals (eg, cocaine, amphetamine) are not generally found to be therapeutic in patients suffering from major depressive illness (Klein and Davis 1969, Post et al 1974). Conversely those drugs that do have antidepressant activity are not stimulants in normal individuals (Oswald et al 1972). These data on differential responses to drugs support the concept that depression may not simply represent a quantitative extension of a normal mood state but probably reflect a qualitatively different psychobiologic substrate (Goodwin and Sack 1973). A second inconsistency relates to the clinical efficacy of the MAO inhibitors, which apparently have a spectrum of effectiveness different from that of the tricyclic antidepressants. This is difficult to reconcile with a conclusion implicit in the amine hypothesis, namely, that both drugs work by increasing brain amine function.

In addition there are some problems in the interpretations of the clinical effects of the drugs that made up the foundations of the catecholamine hypothesis. In relation to the original observations on reserpine it should be noted that the incidence of patients who experienced major depressive symptoms (those analogous to endogenous depressions) was almost identical to the percent incidence of individuals with prior histories of depression (Goodwin et al 1971).

TABLE 1
DRUG-CATECHLOAMINE RELATIONSHIPS

Drug	Effect on Catecholamines at Receptor	Behavioral Effects in Man			
		Normals	Predisposed to Affective Illness	Depressed Patients	Manic Patients
MAOI	↑	No Effect or Mild sedation	Can precipitate mania	Some antidepressant Activity	?
Tricyclics	↑	No effect or mild sedation	Can precipitate mania Prevent recurrences of depression(?)	Antidepressant	Antimanic (?)
Amphetamine	↑	Stimulation	Can precipitate mania (?)	Poor antidepressant	?
Cocaine	↑	Stimulation	Can precipitate mania (?)	Poor antidepressant	?
L-Dopa	↑	No effect	Can precipiiate hypomania	Activation without antidepressant effect	?
Reserpine	→	Sedation	Can precipitate depression	?	Sedation and/or tranquilization
Lithium	→	No effect or mild sedation	Prevent recurrences of mania and depression	Moderate antidepressant effect in some	Antimanic
AMPT	→	Sedation	?	Sedation	Antimanic (?)
Fusaric acid (DBH inhibitor)	↓ (NE)	No effect	?	No effect	Not antimanic; psychosis increased

Thus it appears more likely that reserpine is capable of precipitating depression in susceptible individuals rather than inducing it *de novo*, an important distinction. Additionally, as will be discussed later, lithium does have antidepressant effects in some patients, both acutely and prophylactically, and this finding is difficult to reconcile with its ability to decrease amines, which of course is consistent with its antimanic effects. Thus the relevance of lithium to the amine hypothesis is important, since the amine hypothesis in effect implies that depression and mania represent opposite poles of a single biochemical continuum, whereas lithium, a single agent, has therapeutic effects in both depression and mania, suggesting interactions with some underlying processes similar in the two conditions.

Another problem in the interpretation of drug-amine relationships in affective illness is that our concepts concerning the neurochemical action of a drug have been largely derived from acute (short-term) studies in animals, whereas the clinical effects of these drugs may require weeks to become evident. This issue is all the more important recently because of new evidence that the chronic effects of drugs on amine systems may be different from (even opposite to) the acute effects (Mandell 1975, Goodwin et al 1975).

In spite of these inconsistencies an overall examination of the drug-amine relationships in Table 1 reinforces the sense that brain amines are in some way involved in the action of these mood related drugs, although the more simplified versions of the "too much–too little" concepts will need continuing revision.

TABLE 2
DIFFERENTIAL BIOLOGIC CHARACTERISTICS OF UNIPOLAR AND BIPOLAR DEPRESSED PATIENTS

Unipolar	Bipolar
Normal or elevated 17-OHCS excretion	Low 17-OHCS Excretion
Plasma magnesium unchanged on lithium	Increased plasma magnesium on lithium
Red cell COMT markedly reduced	Red cell COMT slightly reduced
Normal platelet MAO activity	Low platelet MAO activity
Higher urinary MHPG	Lower urinary MHPG
"Reducer" on AER	"Augmenter" on AER

A final issue to be considered is that of biologic heterogeneity in the affective disorders. Recently a number of studies have reported differential biologic findings among hospitalized depressed patients subdivided according to the absence (unipolar) or presence (bipolar) of a prior history of mania. The breadth of these findings (Table 2), taken together with the clinical and genetic differences between these two subgroups, strongly suggest that two separable illnesses exist. This has important implications for drug treatment.

References

Ayd FJ: Thorazine and serpasil treatment of private neuropsychiatric patients. Am J Psychiatry 113:16, 1956

Brodie BB, Spector S, Shore PA: Interaction of drugs with norepinephrine in the brain. Pharmacol Rev 11:548–564, 1959

Bunney WE Jr, Davis JM: Norepinephrine in depressive reactions. Arch Gen Psychiatry 13:483, 1965

Carlsson A, Rosengren E, Bertler A, Nilsson J: Effect of reserpine on the metabolism of catecholamines. In Garattini S, Ghetti V (eds): Psychotropic Drugs. Amsterdam, Elsevier, 1957

Colburn RW, Goodwin FK, Murphy DL, Bunney WE Jr, Davis JM: Quantitative studies of norepinephrine uptake by synaptosomes. Biochem Pharmacol 17:957, 1968

Cooper JR, Bloom FE, Roth RH: The Biochemical Basis of Neuropharmacology, 2nd ed. New York, Oxford, 1974

Davidson AN: Physiological role of monoamine oxidase. Physiol Rev 38:729–747, 1958

Glowinski J, Axelrod J: Inhibition of uptake of tritiated noradrenaline in the intact rat brain by imipramine and structurally related compounds. Nature 204:1318–1319, 1964

Goodwin FK, Ebert M, Bunney WE Jr: Mental effects of reserpine in man. In Shader RI (ed): Psychiatric Complications of Medical Drugs. New York, Raven, 1971

———, Sack RL: Affective disorders: the catecholamine hypothesis revisited. In Usdin E, Snyder S (eds): Frontiers in Catecholamine Research. New York, Pergamon, pp 1157–1164, 1973

———, Post RM, Sack RL: Clinical evidence for neurochemical adaptation to psychotropic drugs. In Mandell AJ (ed): Neurobiological Mechanisms of Adaptation and Behavior. New York, Raven, 1975, pp 33–45

Katz RJ, Chase TN, Kopin IJ: Evoked release of norepinephrine and serotonin from brain slices: inhibition by lithium. Science 162:466–467, 1968

Kety SS: The central physiological and pharmacological effects of biogenic amines and their correlations with behavior. In Quarton GC, Melnechuck T, Schmitt FO (eds): The Neurosciences: A Study Program. New York, Rockefeller, 1967

Klein DF, Davis JM: Diagnosis and Drug Treatment of Psychiatric Disorders. Baltimore, Williams & Wilkins, 1969

Kline NS: Clinical experience with iproniazid (Marsilid). J Clin Exp Psychopathol 19:72–78, 1958

Kuhn R: Uber die Behandlung depressiver zustaende mit einem Iminodibenzylderivat (G22355). Schweiz Med Wochenschr 87:1135–1140, 1957

Lemieux G, Davignon A, Genest J: Depressive states during Rauwolfia therapy for arterial hypertension: a report of 30 cases. Can Med Assoc J 74:522, 1956

Mandell AJ: Neurobiological mechanisms of presynaptic metabolic adaptation and their organization: implications for a pathophysiology of affective disorders. In Mandell AJ (ed): Neurobiological Mechanisms of Adaptation and Behavior. New York, Raven, 1975, pp 1–33

Oswald I, Brezinova V, Dunleavy DLF: On the slowness of action of tricyclic antidepressant drugs. Br J Psychiatry 120:673–677, 1972

Post RM, Kotin J, Goodwin FK: Effects of cocaine in depressed patients. Am J Psychiatry 131:511–517, 1974

Prange AJ Jr: The use of drugs in depression: its theoretical and practical basis. Psychiatr Ann 3:56–75, 1973

Quetsch RM, Achor RWP, Litin EM, Faucett RL: Depressive reactions in hypertensive patients. A comparison of those treated with Rauwolfia and those receiving no specific antihypertensive treatment. Circulation 19:366, 1959

Schildkraut JJ: The catecholamine hypothesis of affective disorders: a review of supporting evidence. Am J Psychiatry 122:509, 1965

Schou M: Special review: lithium in psychiatric therapy and prophylaxis. J Psychiat Res 6:67–95, 1968

Shore PA, Brodie BB: Influence of various drugs on serotonin and norepinephrine in the brain. In Garattini S, Ghetti V (eds): Psychotropic Drugs. Amsterdam, Elsevier, 1957

drug treatment of affective disorders: general principles

commentary

The drugs used in the treatment of depression are the tricyclic antidepressants, the monoamine oxidase inhibitors and lithium. Mania is treated with librium, phenothiazines, or butyrophenones. Electroconvulsive shock is still a useful treatment that should be considered.

Dr. Goodwin discusses a variety of diagnostic considerations that will aid the physician in making a decision about what kind of treatment to institute and how long to continue it. Affective disorders yield to drug treatment, perhaps better than most forms of mental illness, and when suicide is a risk, they may be lifesaving.

drug treatment of affective disorders: general principles

Frederick K. Goodwin, M.D.

Pretreatment Evaluation of Depression

In dealing with the acutely depressed (and perhaps suicidal) patient, the physician faces an urgent and, at times, even an emergency situation. There is thus great pressure to begin treatment immediately, perhaps before adequate information has been obtained. Adding to this difficulty is the fact that depressed patients may be too preoccupied by their symptoms or too confused or retarded to give a comprehensive history in the all too short time that many busy practioners give them.

It cannot be overemphasized that the time and care invested in the pretreatment evaluation is vital to the success of the therapeutic effort. Whenever possible, the patient's spouse or other close family member should also be seen; often at this stage, only they can provide detailed and reliable information about the functional and symptomatic state of the patient and about key aspects of the past history, particularly any past history of affective disorder. In the special case of evaluating mania or hypomania, it is absolutely essential that corroborating data be obtained from family members, since the patient will characteristically deny and distort the extent of the symptoms. Interviewing the spouse can of course also provide a quick overview of the patient's marital and family relationships —factors which may be important in understanding a given depression and its treatment. Furthermore, with many seriously depressed (or manic) patients, the active collaboration of the spouse may be essential to any drug treatment program, particularly if the patient is to be kept out of the hospital.

The general kinds of information needed can be described under several headings:

1. The nature of the present episode: Each of the symptoms of the depressive syndrome should be investigated. With *each* symptom it is important to know how long it has been present: was its onset sudden or gradual, has it been constant or fluctuant, and has the patient experienced any similar symptoms before in his life? It is very important to determine whether one is dealing with a relatively acute problem, or simply an exacerbation of a chronic depression. In this regard it is often helpful to ask when the patient has last felt himself, or felt really well. It is also important to ascertain to what extent the depressive syndrome (or any of its individual symptoms) changes for better or worse in relation to alterations in the environmental situation.

2. Past history of affective episode: In exploring past history, it is important to know the age of onset of the first definable depressive (or manic) episode, and the general characteristics of each episode, including severity, duration, and nature of symptoms. For purposes of visualizing overall patterns, it is often helpful to chart the episodes on a graph so that patterns in the duration, frequency, and regularity of cycles can readily be seen.

3. Past treatment history: The single most important piece of information bearing on a treatment decision in psychopharmacology is what drug that individual may have responded to (or failed to respond to) in the past. Often it requires careful and persistent detective work to obtain accurate information; it is particularly important to determine whether a past trial was optimal—that is, was the dose and duration of treatment adequate and was patient cooperation sufficient to ensure that the drug was actually taken as prescribed. Obviously a false negative conclusion about a previous drug trial is worse than having no information at all, since it could result in the appropriate drug being passed over.

4. Family history of response to drug treatment: In the presence of a positive history of depression (or mania) in a first-degree relative, the physician should attempt to determine the nature of the response to drug treatment. This is important since there is evidence suggesting that response characteristics to tricyclic antidepressants, monoamine oxidase inhibitors, and/or lithium tend to have a familial component and therefore have predictive utility.

5. General medical status of the patient, past and present: This constitutes an extremely important part of the pretreatment evaluation and may require the collaboration of a specialist. The evalua-

tion is focused around several important questions: First, is there anything about this patient's medical condition which may constitute a contraindication to any of the drugs being considered? Here one is primarily interested in cardiovascular, hepatic, and renal function. Second, has the patient been on any drug which may have contributed to the depression (or mania), such as cortisone, reserpine preparation, or antimetabolites? Third, are there any medical conditions which may be contributing to the depression or which could affect the response to drug treatment? Of special importance here is the functional status of the endocrine systems, particularly the thyroid, parathyroid, adrenal, and gonadal systems. This information is important since it is possible that primary correction of the medical dysfunction or removal of an offending drug can be enough to reverse the depressive process without the requirement of specific antidepressant drug treatment. It is important to inquire not only about present symptoms, but also about any past history suggestive of endocrine dysfunction. For example, many females with depression on careful investigation reveal a history of having been evaluated for thyroid dysfunction earlier in life, but report no current symptoms. We will discuss the evidence that some depressed patients may have borderline low function in other endocrine systems as well, and that antidepressant response can be potentiated by the simultaneous administration of small doses of the appropriate endocrine substance.

General Indications for the Drug Treatment of Depression

There are rough clinical criteria which can be used to estimate which type of antidepressant might be the most suitable for a given patient. In general, the indications for an antidepressant drug trial are outlined in Table 1.

It is often said that drug treatment should be reserved for depressions of at least moderate severity. Although this assertion is difficult to contest, it is equally difficult to apply it in the absence of precise criteria for judging severity. More useful as a clinical guideline is the following: *The more completely the clinical picture fits the description of the depressive syndrome the more certainly are drugs indicated.* In evaluating this "fit" one notes the degree and duration of functional impairment and then looks for the so-called *endogenous* cluster of symptoms, especially the characteristic pattern of sleep disturbance (middle and late insomnia), psychomotor

TABLE 1
GENERAL INDICATIONS FOR DRUG THERAPY
IN DEPRESSION*

Clinical Features Likely to be Associated with Good Drug Response
Presence of clear "endogenous" symptoms (see)
Pervasiveness of the depressive syndrome
Clear onset of the depressive syndrome
Decrease in functional capacity
Prior history of drug response
Family history of affective illness
Family history of drug response

Clinical Features Likely to be Associated with Poor Drug Response
Depressive symptoms integral to another psychiatric diagnosis
Depressive symptoms of long-standing duration (chronic)
Prominent features of hysteria, complaining, blaming others
History of multiple previous drug failures
History of exaggerated sensitivity to drug side effects
Multiple somatic symptoms with history of somatic preoccupation
Presence of schizo-affective features

*It should be appreciated that these criteria are for the most part overlapping, and no single pathognomonic sign can determine the suitability for drug treatment.

retardation (or agitation), diurnal variation (worse in the morning), relative lack of reactivity to the environment, and depressive thoughts and feelings. If some endogenous features are present and have been so for two weeks or more, one then looks for a clear-cut onset starting from a reasonably "well" state. If the depressive symptoms have arisen as one part of a larger psychiatric problem, such as a well-defined anxiety neurosis or schizophrenia, then drug approaches are likely to be complicated by poor response, intensification of the primary illness, or both. Similarly, if the depressive symptoms represent simply an exaggerated manifestation of a long-standing personality disturbance (characterologic depression), drug approaches are less successful.

The age of the patient has been identified as an important variable in large studies of drug response in mixed depressive populations, with the older patients tending to show more drug responsiveness (Klerman and Cole 1965, Raskin et al 1970). However, we should not attempt to use age by itself to predict drug response or nonresponse in an individual patient. It is the presence or absence of the identifying feature of the *syndrome* which is important. The age relationship holds essentially because the *syndrome* of depression is more likely to occur in older individuals for a variety of reasons. Thus age appears to have little or no *direct* relationship to drug response (Angst 1961).

It has sometimes been thought that neurotic or reactive features of the depression weigh against drug response. This can be misleading. The presence or absence of presumed precipitating events should not by itself influence the decision about drug therapy; on the other hand, if a depression once established shows a high degree of ongoing reactivity to the environment, then drug approaches are less likely to succeed.

Often the clinician may be faced with difficult drug treatment decisions when dealing with a patient who has depressive symptoms that have arisen as part of a normal grief reaction. In general, drug treatment is not indicated if the symptoms are not severely debilitating and if the grieving process has not evolved into a true clinical depression, such as might be evidenced by a qualitative shift of symptoms toward severe guilt, suicidal ideation, and despair. In normal grief reactions, after a few weeks the individual will have begun to partially mobilize some of his own resources to deal with the loss, although some overt depressive symptoms can persist for months (Fig. 1).

In some situations, in spite of clinical features or preexisting factors, which in general might weigh against drug responsiveness, the clinician may elect a drug trial because of the unavailability of psychotherapy, on the basis of a prior history of inadequate response to psychotherapy or as a diagnostic test, for example to distinguish characterologic depressive symptoms from drug responsive depressive illness.

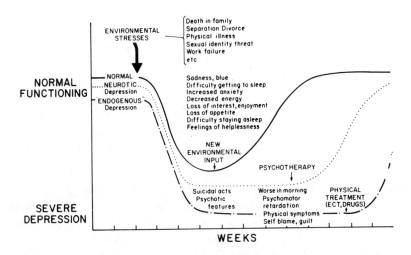

Fig. 1.   Course of normal and depressive pathologic reactions.

Special Issues: Hospitalization and Electroconvulsive Therapy

The great majority of drug treatable depressions can be managed on an outpatient basis. When is hospitalization advisable? There are no universal guidelines here, but in considering each patient's individual situation it is helpful to evaluate the following:

1. How available is the physician? A careful antidepressant drug trial requires frequent contact with the patient, often twice a week or more in the beginning of a new drug.
2. How serious is the risk of suicide? In evaluating this a past history of serious suicidal behavior could provide a strong argument for hospitalization, although the absence of such a history does not mean the absence of current risk. It is also dangerous to assume that because the patient has openly communicated his suicidal intent he won't really do it. The *relationship* between patient and doctor is very important in evaluating the danger of suicide; as long as a strong sense of mutual trust and contact is maintained, the suicide risk is usually manageable. In evaluating suicide risk in depression, it is very important to keep in mind that often the most dangerous period is during the beginning of a drug response, when the patient experiences some return of energy and motivation but is still feeling hopeless and depressed.
3. Are there reliable, willing, and available people in the patient's life who can temporarily take some of the responsibility that otherwise might be borne by the hospital staff? Here, of course, the well-being of the family and their future relationships with the patient also deserve consideration.
4. What are the social, economic, and occupational cost to the patient as a result of being hospitalized—or conversely of being kept out of the hospital? For example, if the patient will lose his job by being hospitalized, more effort would be made to treat on an outpatient basis; on the other hand, in some cases it may be more damaging to the patient's professional well-being for him to continue working while depressed. There is a tendency for the depression per se to color the patient's assessment of his ability to continue functioning on his job. The clinician may have to be careful not to reinforce a self-defeating attitude by a hasty decision to hospitalize.
5. How is hospitalization likely to affect a given patient's response to drugs? Psychiatrists and psychopharmacologists repeatedly have the experience of a patient responding nicely to a drug in the hospital when they had earlier failed to respond to the same

drug as an outpatient (Klein and Davis 1969, Kotin et al 1973). On the other hand, psychiatrists are also well aware that the experience of hospitalization can encourage regression in some patients, contributing to a prolongation of the depression. Knowledge about the personality pattern of the individual patient may help here; for example, a patient with strong dependency needs, who is known to give in easily to feelings of helplessness, might have a negative reaction to hospitalization. On the other hand, for some patients removal from the environment seems helpful in breaking into a depression and allowing drug effects to become established; this should not be surprising, since, as noted earlier, for many the depressive syndrome apparently begins in response to serious ongoing psychosocial stress, often in a marital or family relationship.

Although the role of electroconvulsive therapy in the treatment of depression is beyond the scope of this chapter, a few observations should be made. For a variety of reasons the trend today in the treatment of depression is to try drugs first. Electroconvulsive therapy would generally be reserved for those patients who are not responding to drugs or who have a history of previous depressions unresponsive to drug therapy. It might also be the treatment of choice when an immediate effect is very important, such as in the management of a seriously suicidal, psychotic, or extremely agitated patient, or when one is dealing with a patient so depressed that they are refusing to eat or care for themselves. Although there is no evidence that electroconvulsive therapy achieves a full antidepressant response any faster than antidepressant drugs, it can often break into the patient's severest symptoms after the first few treatments.

The Experimental Approach to the Drug Treatment of Depression

It is of fundamental importance to the successful use of drugs in depression to follow an experimental approach which basically employs a "decision tree" model. By this we mean that one starts with the collection of as much information as possible and then follows a *sequence* of drug trials in which the first drug (treatment of choice) is selected on the basis of past history and diagnostic conclusions made before treatment is initiated; the choice drug for any subsequent trial that might be necessary should be based not only on the information available prior to treatment but also on the nature of the response to the preceding drugs.

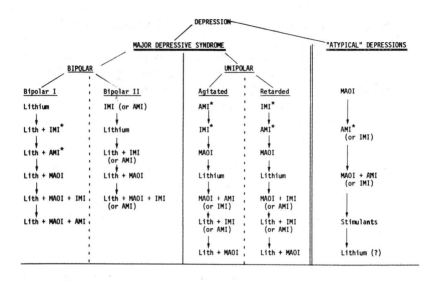

Fig. 2. A drug "decision tree" prototype. IMI—imipramine; AMI
—amitriptyline. Imipramine and amitriptyline were chosen for this illustration because they are the most widely used of the tricyclics. In this prototype, desmethylimipramine, nortriptyline, and protriptyline could substitute for imipramine, while doxepin could substitute for amitriptyline. This
prototype would apply in cases where there is no past history or family
history of specific drug response. In females an incomplete response to
tricyclics may justify an attempt to potentiate with thyroid (and perhaps
estrogen) medication. (The use of stimulants and major tranquilizers in depression is discussed in the next chapter.)

A prototype of a "drug decision tree" is presented in Figure 2; I do
not represent this as the single correct sequence to be followed, but
rather as an illustration of a plan that to a large degree reflects the
experience of the author and much of the literature; the specific data
that bear on choices of individual drugs are discussed elsewhere.
The important point is to have a rational sequential plan in mind at
the outset; in this kind of model the information about lack of response to a drug becomes important in evaluating the likelihood of a
response to the next drug.

The first conclusion to be reached is whether the depression is
sufficiently serious and characteristic in its symptoms to fit the
definition of major depressive syndrome, or whether it is atypical in
one way or another. Only after it has been determined that the patient is suffering from a major depressive syndrome is it meaningful
to classify the episode as unipolar or bipolar. A past history of
mania, severe enough to require hospitalization or definitive an-

timanic treatment, provides an unequivocal basis for designating the patient bipolar; for research purposes this group is referred to as bipolar I. often, however, one encounters a depressed patient with a past history characterized by recurrent depression, interspersed by periods (often brief) of elevated mood, increased activity and energy, overconfidence, moderate irritability, decreased need for sleep, and moderately irresponsible behavior, such as overspending. The patient may or may not report these as "highs"; often the family can provide information which can help distinguish if a "high" should properly be considered abnormal (ie, hypomania) or just a manifestation of normal mood elevation. For research purposes a depressed patient with a past history of hypomania is referred to as bipolar II.

Clearly, the unipolar–bipolar II-bipolar I classification is of great importance to the selection of appropriate drug treatment for a depressed patient. A patient with a clear history of mania generally should be maintained on lithium for preventive purposes. In other words, when approaching the treatment of depression in a bipolar I patient the indication for lithium is already established by the prior history of mania. Therefore, as a general rule, decisions about the antidepressant treatment of bipolar I depression are really decisions about whether to use an additional drug in combination with lithium. Two points favor the approach of starting with lithium alone. First, some depressed patients will respond to lithium alone; for them, beginning with a tricyclic, either alone or in combination with lithium, would subject them to a drug they didn't need. Second, in a bipolar I patient on tricyclics alone there is some risk of precipitating a manic episode; in some instances this occurs very early in the tricyclic treatment. Initiating treatment with the combination of lithium and tricyclics may be indicated, particularly when dealing with a more seriously depressed patient. Specific aspects of the drugs and drug combinations listed in Figure 2 are detailed in the next chapter.

The Therapeutic Alliance in Drug Treatment

Later we will discuss some special issues concerning the interrelationships between psychotherapy and drugs in the treatment of depression—issues that are of most concern to the psychiatrist. At this point, however, it is important to underline a most fundamental concept: for any drug to achieve its full potential in the treatment of the depressed patient, it should be given in the context of a solid and positive doctor-patient relationship—that is, there must be a working therapeutic alliance. In most instances, this is best achieved by approaching the drug trial as an *investigative undertaking*, which depends on *active collaboration* between patient and doctor. It is widely known that controlled double-blind studies of antidepressant drugs consistently report success rates substantially below those reported in open trials (Klein and Davis 1969). In some instances, to be sure, difference reflects bias, at least in part. However, it is also likely that one of the reasons that drugs appear to work better in an open setting is that the positive and reinforcing effects of the therapeutic alliance are able to operate (Sheard 1963).

The physician is in the best position to help the depressed patient when he is able to convey an attitude of serious concern for the individual's suffering (without excessive sympathy), while communicating confidence in his own ability and measured optimism about the *ultimate* outcome of the drug trials. It is very important not to oversell or overpromise results with any particular drug. This is self-defeating, since if the first drug fails to work then the patient's trust is eroded, and the physician feels defeated and discredited —attitudes which, in turn, may be subtly conveyed back to the patient. When a trial with a given drug is viewed by doctor and patient alike as an *experiment*, then even a poor response does not have to be experienced as a defeat but rather as an important piece of new information not available previously that contributes substantially to the rational choice of subsequent drugs. It is helpful to make this explicit to the patient by pointing out that for some groups of antidepressants, nonresponders to drug A are by that fact more likely to be responders to drug B and vice versa.

Another critical aspect of the drug management of depression involves the question of whether the patient is actually taking the drug at all or in the prescribed doses. Large surveys have indicated that up to half of all drugs prescribed by physicians are never taken by the patients (GAP 1975). With depressed patients, there is reason to believe that the illness itself can increase the likelihood of this problem. For the depressed patients' feelings of hopelessness are often powerful; these feelings are often reflected in a pattern of help rejection in which the patient cannot tolerate his own inner awareness of massive needfulness and must reject any help which may remind him of it. Drugs, of course, can become entangled in this hopeless help-rejecting position, and simply not be taken because "they won't work anyway." Often the patient will not make this fully explicit, and only careful and sensitive exploration will uncover that some doses were "forgotten."

For more seriously depressed patients, and for manic patients, it is helpful to include the spouse or other significant family member as an integral part of the therapeutic alliance. It should be kept in mind that in addition to the seriously decreased motivation, depressed patients are preoccupied and often have trouble concentrating and remembering. Therefore, all instructions regarding dosage, time of day, side effects, other drugs, foods, and so forth should be in *writing* and should be reviewed with the patient and the spouse. The patient should be given concrete suggestions on ways to remember his pills; for example, putting all of the pills for the day in a container in the morning and "making up" any that may be found left over that night.

It is very important that the patient know what to expect from the beginning. He should be told first that the drug will probably make him feel *worse* in the beginning, second that he *will have side effects*, some of which almost certainly will decrease as tolerance develops, and third that little or no beneficial effects should be anticipated for at least the first 2 weeks. The patient should be instructed as to which side effects the doctor needs to hear about if they occur, as opposed to those which are more routine and expected.

How Long to Treat?

This question should really be two separate questions: first, how long should a trial of a given antidepressant drug be continued in the absence of a satisfactory response; and second, how long should a successful drug be continued after remission has occurred? The first question is really about what constitutes an adequate trial of an antidepressant drug. It is common to encounter a patient who reports that during a previous depression the physician "tried everything" to no avail; after careful questioning it all too often becomes clear that the physician, in his eagerness to help, has tried a great variety of drugs, but each for only a few days. The lag in the onset of clinical effects is quite variable and depends on a host of factors, including the nature of the specific drug, the dose, the patient's tolerance for side effects, the severity and type of depression, and other individual patient characteristics, such as drug metabolism rates. However, in spite of this variability, there are guidelines which can be followed. As a general rule a drug should be discarded as ineffective if there are *no* indications of improvement after the patient has been on *an adequate dosage of the drug for at least 2 weeks.* If the clinical situation makes it unwise to wait that length of time, then hospitalization and /or electroconvulsive therapy should be considered; in the long run these alternatives are more in keeping with the *patient's* interest than a series of frantic drug "trials," which are uninterpretable.

The fact that at least 2 weeks at adequate therapeutic doses is required for a trial of an antidepressant does not mean that *all* patients require that length of time to show a response. Many patients, particularly those with less serious and less prolonged depressions, show clear signs of improvement within the first week. Controlled studies (Cole 1964, Haskell et al 1975), suggest that improvement in sleep, particularly middle insomnia, is very often the first symptom to improve, and change in this parameter during the first week on a tricyclic has been shown to significantly predict subsequent full response at 3 weeks (Hordern et al 1963). Other reported early signs of antidepressant response include return of appetite, interest in work, and a decrease in suicidal feelings (Klein and Davis 1969).

How long should a drug be continued after remission has been achieved? This question must be separated from the question of what criteria are used for the selection of some patients for *maintenance of prophylactic drug treatment*. Following the successful treatment of a major depressive episode, the medication should be continued for a period of 6 to 12 months, for it is during the initial recovery period that the risk of relapse is high. Systematic follow-up studies support the common clinical experience that recovered patients maintained on drugs for 6 to 12 months after a depression do significantly better than patients withdrawn from drugs shortly after remission is achieved (Klein and Davis 1969).

Sometimes a patient will experience a partial relapse following initial success with an antidepressant even on the dose that had been therapeutic. In this fairly common clinical situation, temporarily increasing the dose (or at times decreasing it) may be sufficient to achieve remission again.

References

Angst J: A clinical analysis of the effects of tofranil in depression. Psychopharmacologia 2:381–407, 1961

Cole JO: The therapeutic efficacy of antidepressant drugs: a review. JAMA 190:448–455, 1964

Group for the Advancement of Psychiatry (GAP): Pharmacotherapy and Psychotherapy: Paradoxes, Problems and Progress. Report No. 93. New York, 1975

Haskell DS, DiMascio A, Prusoff B: Rapidity of symptom reduction in depressions treated with amitriptyline. J Nerv Ment Dis 160:24–33, 1975

Hordern A, Holt NF, Brut CG, Gordon WF: Amitriptyline in depressive states: phenomenology and prognostic consideration. Br J Psychiatry 109:815–825, 1963

Klein DF, Davis JM: Diagnosis and Drug Treatment of Psychiatric Disorders. Baltimore, Williams & Wilkins, 1969

Klerman GL, Cole JO: Clinical pharmacology of imipramine and related antidepressant compounds. Pharmacol Rev 17:101–141, 1965

Kotin J, Post RM, Goodwin FK: Drug treatment of depressed patients referred for hospitalization. Am J Psychiatry 130:1139–1141, 1973

Raskin A, Schulterbrandt MS, Reatig BA, McKeon JJ: Differential response to chlorpromazine, imipramine and placebo: a study of subgroups of hospitalized depressed patients. Arch Gen Psychiatry 23:164–173, 1970

Sheard MH: Influence of doctor's attitude on patient's response to antidepressant medication. J Nerv Ment Dis 136:555–560, 1963

specific antimanic and antidepressant drugs

commentary

Drugs may quite successfully be used in the treatment of mood disorders, but correct diagnosis is essential. Lithium salts are the treatment of choice for manic conditions but blood levels must be carefully monitored to prevent toxic reactions. Antipsychotic drugs may be combined with lithium to obtain speedier calming of a manic patient. Tricyclics are the treatment of choice for depressed patients and there is evidence that some of these drugs are more sedating than others. All these drugs may take days to weeks to produce a discernible improvement. Monoamine oxidase inhibitors are the second choice, although some depressed patients may respond to them better than to tricyclics. Although there is fear of the hepatotoxicity of the monoamine oxidase inhibitors, presently used drugs seem to be relatively safe. Hypertensive crisis due to inhibition of deamination of amines such as tyramine is a bizarre and luckily rare complication of MAOI treatment. Lithium may relieve depressions, particularly the bipolar variety. Antipsychotic drugs may be useful, particularly in patients with psychotic signs. Amphetamine-like drugs may have limited usefulness as a diagnostic predictive agent for imipramine effectiveness. Various combinations of drugs may be helpful as indicated in a decision tree.

specific antimanic and antidepressant drugs

Frederick K. Goodwin, M.D.
Michael H. Ebert, M.D.

Drug Treatment of Hypomania and Mania

The first step in the pharmacologic approach to the treatment of hypomanic and manic disorders is care in proper diagnosis. It is important to emphasize that we are dealing with a spectrum of disorders from mild, transient hypomania to the florid psychosis of full-blown mania. Often serious manic episodes start in a hypomanic phase, and thus, as we shall see, early diagnosis is very important to successful treatment and rapid pharmacologic response. In making the decision to initiate pharmacologic treatment for symptoms in the hypomania-mania spectrum, it is important to make a distinction between a pathologic state of hyperactivity (with mood elevation, grandiosity, irritability, and so forth) and normal swings of mood or other characteristics of an individual that properly belong to the description of certain kinds of personalities. The distinction between mild hypomania and normal mood elevation was detailed in the chapter on diagnosis of affective disorders and this emphasis is repeated here because of the authors' concern that if this distinction is not carefully explored in each individual case, some patients may be placed on lithium for long-term maintenance with absence of demonstrated need.

Lithium and Manic Conditions

True hypomania, or the hypomanic phase of full-blown mania, should be treated promptly with lithium carbonate. When lithium is instituted early in the course of a hypomanic episode, therapeutic response can be expected within a very few days; on the other hand, if treatment is not initiated until full-blown mania has occurred, a response may take considerably longer, and as we will note later, lithium alone may prove to be insufficient in these cases. Depending on the severity of the condition, the initial daily dose of lithium carbonate will vary; for the treatment of hypomania, one would typically start with a dose of 600 mg for the first two days, 900 mg for the next two days, followed by a blood level scheduled on the morning of the fifth day, timed to be drawn between 10 and 12 hours following the last preceding dose. Depending on the findings from this blood level, treatment may be continued at 900 mg a day, and then decreased or increased. Since the dose of lithium required to produce blood levels in the therapeutic range (1.0 to 1.3 mEq per liter for the treatment of mania) vary considerably from one individual to another, it is not possible to give a standard dose or dose range in the absence of information on blood level. The therapeutic-toxic margin of lithium is much more narrow than for other psychotropic drugs, causing serious toxicity at blood levels less than twice the therapeutic level. Therefore, in addition to blood levels, it is important to monitor carefully the signs and symptoms of toxicity through all phases of the initial treatment.

In evaluating dose-blood level relationships, it is important to be aware that a variety of factors influence the blood level on a given dose. The important factors are age and weight of the patient, status of renal function, salt intake, and phase of the illness. Thus younger patients excrete lithium more efficiently than older ones, and heavier patients require more of the drug than lighter ones, particularly when the weight is due to greater muscle mass. Increased salt intake will decrease the effective plasma level on a given dose of lithium by competing with lithium reabsorption in the distal tubule. During mania, the dose-blood level ratio is higher than after the cessation of the manic episode. Thus it may require a very large dose of lithium to achieve a therapeutic blood level in a manic patient, but as soon as the mania begins to respond, the dosage must be adjusted down if elevated blood levels with accompanying toxicity are to be avoided.

In evaluating dose-blood level considerations it is important to distinguish routine side effects from frank or incipient toxicity. A mild tremor, particularly of the upper extremities, is an almost constant concomitant of lithium therapy, particularly in the initial phases and should not constitute a reason for cessation of the drug or dosage reduction. Propanolol, 10 to 40 mg per day, can be used to reduce the tremor if its severity interferes with treatment. Similarly, some initial nausea, mild lethargy, and fatigue might be experienced, and should not be contraindications to continuing the drug. The serious side effects of lithium are predominantly neurologic and can include slurred speech, dizziness, vertigo, incontinence, somnolence, restlessness, confusion, stupor, seizures, and hyperactive reflexes. Leukocytosis is a common concomitant of lithium therapy and is of no apparent consequence (Murphy et al 1971). The more long-term complications of lithium, particularly nontoxic goiter, functional hypothyroidism, and weight gain are more relevant to our later consideration of the long-term maintenance use of this drug.

Antipsychotic Drugs in the Treatment of Acute Mania

If a patient is allowed to go into frank mania, antipsychotic drugs, particularly the phenothiazines and haloperidol are often necessary as an adjunct to lithium. These drugs are particularly useful in rapidly reducing hyperactivity, hyperagression, and severe psychosis. Compared to lithium, they do not have the same degree of selective effects on the core symptoms of mania (Johnson et al 1971). Lithium, although slower to show an initial effect against hyperactivity, eventually has a more specific therapeutic effect on the manic symptoms. Phenothiazines (or haloperidol) should be gradually withdrawn as the acute phase of the illness subsides.

When used in combination with lithium the usual dosage of phenothiazines would be reduced accordingly because of some synergism in regard to sedative and hypotensive effects; here too, individual patient dose titration is required. A recent report of neurologic complications following the combined use of lithium and haloperidol has raised questions about this particular combination (Cohen and Cohen 1974); however, careful independent reanalysis of these cases indicates that other factors were probably responsible for the complications—a conclusion consistent with the bulk of the evidence indicating the safety of this combination (Ayd 1975).

The Drug Treatment of Depression

Tricyclic Antidepressants

By far the most important class of antidepressants used today are the tricyclic antidepressants. The basic constituent of tricyclic antidepressants consists of two benzene rings connected to each other by an ethylene bridge and a nitrogen atom (iminodibenzyl nucleus). This varies only slightly from the basic constituent of phenothiazines, in which two benzene rings are attached by a sulfur and a nitrogen atom. The tricyclic nucleus was synthesized in 1899 by Thiele and Holzinger (Ban 1969), but its clinical usefulness was not explored until the 1950s. The success of chlorpromazine in treating schizophrenic patients led to the testing of various iminodibenzyl compounds in psychiatric patients. Kuhn reported in 1957 that imipramine had a therapeutic effect on patients suffering from depression, rather than schizophrenia. Subsequently a large number of controlled trials have demonstrated the efficacy of imipramine and its derivatives in the treatment of depression (Klein and Davis, 1969).

Table 1 shows the tricyclic antidepressants approved for clinical use in the United States. Desipramine is the demethylated derivative of imipramine, and nortriptyline the demethylated derivative of amitriptyline. Oxidative monodemethylation of the side chain is one of the main pathways of metabolism of imipramine and amitriptyline. Thus, when a patient is taking either of these drugs, desipramine and nortriptyline, respectively, are also present in significant amounts or active metabolites (Fig. 1). The tricyclic antidepressants are thought to exert their therapeutic effects by the inhibition of

TABLE 1
TRICYCLIC ANTIDEPRESSANTS IN CURRENT USE

Compound	Trade Name	Dose Range*
Imipramine	Imipramine Tofranil Imavate Presamine SK-Pramine Janimine	150–300 mg
Desipramine	Pertofrane Norpramine	150–250 mg
Amitriptyline	Elavil Endep	75–300 mg
Nortriptyline	Aventyl	50–150 mg
Protriptyline	Vivactyl	10–60 mg
Doxepin	Sinequan Adapin	150–300 mg

*Doses given are for the acute treatment of depression. Because of individual variability in metabolism, there are some patients who may require (and tolerate) doses outside the usual range.

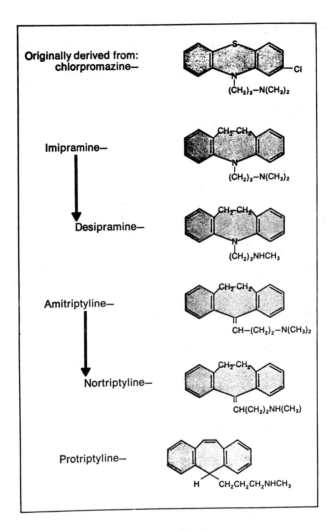

Fig. 1. Tricyclic drugs.

reuptake of neurotransmitter amines at central nervous system presynaptic neurons, as discussed in a previous chapter.* Since reuptake into the presynaptic neuron is a major mechanism for the inactivation of amine neurotransmitters, inhibition of this process has
the effect of potentiating the action of monoamines in the synaptic
cleft.

The tricyclic antidepressants generally take two to three weeks to

*See "Biologic Basis of Drug Action in the Affective Disorders," p. 231.

exert their therapeutic effects on depression, even though some of the side effects of the drug occur immediately. The reason for this delayed action is presently unknown. Studies that have correlated blood levels of tricyclic antidepressants with clinical response indicate that this "lag" cannot be explained entirely on the basis of delayed drug accumulation.* As pointed out in the preceding chapter, the response "lag" can be responsible for therapeutic failures if patients are not treated long enough. The second major source of unnecessary failures is improper dose, generally too low, but sometimes too high. With direct measurement of blood levels not generally available, the dosage must be pushed slowly upwards with an eye on side effects as well as clinical response. The incidence and severity of side effects can give an indirect indication of blood level.

The tricyclic antidepressants would be the treatment of choice for a depression with the "endogenous" characteristics outlined in a previous chapter.† These include sleep disturbance, loss of appetite, weight loss, psychomotor retardation, loss of energy, decreased capacity to feel pleasure, suicidal thoughts, and thought patterns dominated by helplessness, hopelessness, and excessive guilt. In the classification system of the Research Diagnostic Criteria (Spitzer et al 1975), this would represent a major depressive disorder, either unipolar or bipolar. It is important to recognize that a depression with this symptom cluster is likely to respond to an antidepressant, regardless of whether psychodynamic conflicts are or are not thought to be important to its genesis.

Taken as a whole the available body of controlled studies suggests that overall differences between different tricyclic antidepressants are not of major proportion. Nevertheless, more recent evidence supports the common clinical experience of some selectivity. Amitriptyline or Doxepin would appear to be the best choices for patients in whom anxiety and agitation are prominent; this also applies to patients with depressive delusions, particularly older people with involutional syndromes. The greater sedative qualities of amitriptyline and Doxepin recommend their use where sleep disturbance is severe, particularly when sleep is interrupted throughout the night. Imipramine, desmethylimipramine, and protriptyline are felt to have more "activating" and less "tranquilizing" properties than amitriptyline or Doxepin, and may thus have some advantage in patients with prominent psychomotor retardation.

Before starting a tricyclic antidepressant, it is wise to obtain a

*See "Recent Advances in the Drug Treatment of Affective Disorders," p. 275.
†See "Diagnosis of Affective Disorders," p. 219.

complete blood count in all patients. In a patient over 50 years old or when indicated by history, the cardiovascular and renal system should be evaluated by obtaining a BUN, urinalysis, electrocardiogram, and chest film. As noted in a previous chapter, the patient should have a complete physical examination, if he has not had one in the past six months. It is important to obtain a complete history of prior treatment with antidepressants or other psychotropic drugs, focusing on clinical response, side effects, and possibility of hypersensitivity reactions.

Using imipramine as a prototype, for most patients treatment can begin with 50 to 75 mg on the first day administered in divided doses primarily because of side effects. The initial dose can be taken in the evening to observe the severity of side effects before the remainder is given at bedtime. The dose can then be increased at a rate of 10 to 25 mg per day until limited by side effects such as urinary retention, difficulty with visual accommodation, confusion, severe tremors, dizziness, or increased sweating. Mild tremor, dry mouth, constipation, and sedation should not be indications for limiting the dose. The rate and extent of dose increase also depends on the severity of the depression, particularly the extent of functional impairment and suicide potential. Usually after 150 mg per day is reached, it is advisable to wait for five to seven days to evaluate clinical response. If there is no evidence of response at the end of this second week of treatment, the dose should be raised by 25 mg every two to three days, with an upper limit usually reached at 300 mg but with some cases requiring more. (As indicated in the chapter "Recent Advances in the Drug Treatment of Affective Disorders," the optimal and maximal doses may be different for amitriptyline.) The patient should be seen at least twice a week during this time and observed carefully for the severity of side effects. If side effects limit the amount of medication that can be given, the physician can back off on dosage for a week, and then begin to climb upward again. Tolerance usually develops to the side effects of the tricyclic antidepressants, but not to the antidepressant effect. Signs to watch for in terms of a therapeutic response in addition to a clear change in the patient's depressed mood are a normalization of sleep disorder and appetite, a return to normal activity patterns, and a positive change in the patient's dress and appearance.

Although most of the side effects of the tricyclics are anticholinergic, and therefore not related to clinical efficacy, some are secondary to stimulation of the adrenergic system, and may serve as an indication of clinical response to follow. These include tremor, "jitteriness," changes in cold and heat tolerance, and tachycardia.

Some important but more rare complications of tricyclic therapy include hypersensitivity reactions, agranulocytosis, and a mild and transient obstructive jaundice, all of which resolve with cessation of treatment. The case reports of the hematologic and hepatic complication are so few considering the widespread use of the drugs, that it is difficult to tell if the tricyclics are responsible for them.

Even at standard doses the tricyclics have significant physiologic effects on the cardiovascular system, with about 5 percent of treated patients developing postural hypotension and tachycardia. This can become a serious problem in patients with significant cardiovascular or cerebrovascular disease. Disturbances of cardiac rhythm can also occur during tricyclic therapy, although these occur almost exclusively in patients with cardiac pathology or in overdoses. These arrhythmias include extrasystoles of atrial or ventricular origin, atrial fibrillation, and in severe overdoses, ventricular tachycardia. Because of these potentially hazardous cardiovascular effects, tricyclic antidepressants should be administered only with caution to patients with compromised cardiovascular or cerebrovascular status. Myocardial infarction, congestive heart failure, and cerebrovascular accidents have occurred with increased incidence in these patient groups during treatment with tricyclic antidepressants. Tricyclic antidepressants can also cause benign electrocardiographic abnormalities such as widened QRS complexes, depressed S-T segment, and abnormal T waves. On the other hand, it should be kept in mind that the tricyclic antidepressants are prescribed for millions of patients a year with very little toxicity and morbidity.

Monoamine Oxidase Inhibitors

Monoamine oxidase (MAO) inhibitors, the second major class of antidepressants, are underutilized in this country. This appears to be due to fear of serious toxic reactions such as hepatotoxicity, and particularly the hypertensive crisis associated with the ingestion of tyramine containing foods. Although in large studies of mixed groups of patients with major depressions, tricyclics are generally found to be superior to MAO inhibitors, there are certain kinds of depressed patients for whom these drugs may be the treatment of choice.

The mood-elevating properties of this class of drugs were discovered in 1951 during the treatment of pulmonary tuberculosis with isoniazid. After several early trials with isoniazid in depression, its use in psychiatric patients was discontinued because of hepatotoxicity. Antidepressant trials continued in the 1950s with the isopropyl derivative of isoniazid (iproniazid) which proved to be less hepatotoxic and was an effective antidepressant.

Subsequent development of MAO inhibitors for psychiatric use have followed the line of developing compounds with maximal effectiveness and minimal toxicity. Table 2 shows the MAO inhibitors which are in current use in the United States. They can be divided into two classes: hydrazines and nonhydrazines. Free hydrazines are strong reducing agents and extremely toxic, particularly to the hepatic and hematopoetic systems. Various hydrazine derivatives, in which the free hydrazine was blocked, proved to be potent monoamine oxidase inhibitors, and two are currently approved for clinical use, isocarboxazid and phenelzine. There are also some nonhydrazine monoamine oxidase inhibitors; these are phenylethylamine derivatives that bear a structural resemblance to amphetamine. Tranylcypromine is the only member of this group currently on the market. For structures, see Figure 2.

Compared to the tricyclics, there is less solid information available concerning the indications and contraindications for the use of MAO inhibitors as antidepressants. Depressed patients who respond well to MAO inhibitors are described as "atypical" in that they may not have the classical "endogenous" cluster of symptoms. The relationship between the designations of "atypical" and "neurotic" is not clear, but some overlap certainly exists. The potential MAO inhibitor responsive patient is likely to have high levels of anxiety as part of the depression, and may have hypochondriacal, phobic, and obsessive-compulsive features. Rather than the "endogenous" symptoms of middle and late insomnia (with early-morning awakening), the patient complains of excessive sleeping and extreme lassitude. Rather than losing their appetite, these patients eat excessively when depressed, often with a compulsive quality.

TABLE 2
MAO INHIBITORS IN CURRENT USE

Compound	Trade Name	Dose Range*
Hydrazines		
Isocarboxazid	Marplan	10–30 mg
Phenelzine	Nardil	15–75 mg
Nonhydrazine		
Tranylcypromine	Parnate	10–50 mg

*Doses given are for the acute treatment of depression. Some patients may require (and tolerate) doses outside this range.

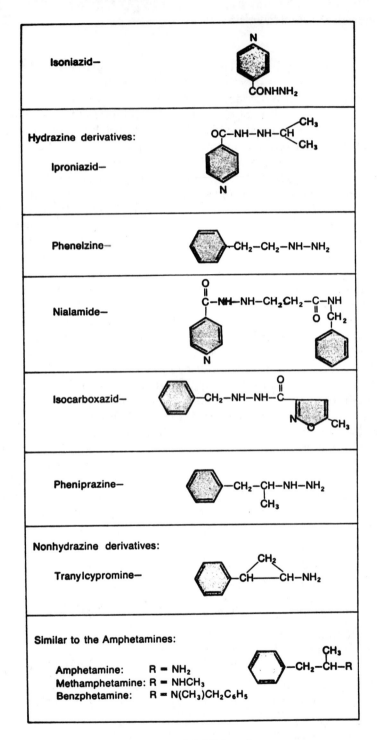

Fig. 2.   MAO inhibitor drugs.

Although there is little systematic data on the question, clinical experience suggests that the patient who will respond to an MAO inhibitor is less likely to respond to a tricyclic and vice versa. Thus, an important group of patients who should be candidates for MAO inhibitors are those who have previously failed to respond to tricyclics. Related to this is the observation that response to either class of antidepressant tends to run in families (Pare et al 1962).

It is important to obtain a medical work-up before starting an MAO inhibitor. This should include a recent physical examination, a chest film and electrocardiogram, a complete blood count, alkaline phosphatase and SGOT, and a urinalysis and BUN. The potency of the MAO inhibitors in current use varies somewhat. It is wise to start with a small test dose and observe the patient for side effects. Then, using phenelzine as an example, dosage could be increased as rapidly as tolerated to 60 to 75 mg per day for the acute treatment of depression, and subsequently lowered in the maintenance period after clinical response has been achieved. These drugs are irreversible blockers of monoamine oxidase. Thus, their clinical effect can last for days to weeks after the administration of the drug in adequate amounts. It is, therefore, rational to give the drug in a single daily dose.

MAO inhibitors interact with mechanisms of blood pressure regulation. All of them can cause hypotension, particularly postural hypotension, in fact, some drugs in this class are used primarily as antihypertensive agents. The most serious cardiovascular complication of MAO inhibition is hypertensive crisis, which occurred with a frequency of 8 percent when the drugs were first introduced. Subsequently, it was postulated that these hypertensive crises were precipitated by the absorption of amines from the diet, particularly tyramine, that are normally deaminated in the gut and liver. Thus, patients under treatment with MAO inhibitors must be cautioned against eating certain foods rich in pressor amines such as cheese, yeast extract, beer, certain wines, sour cream, chocolate, broad beans, chicken livers, pickled herring, avocado, figs, dates, and raisins. The great majority of patients will not have a hypertensive crisis even when these foods are ingested. Thus, in the case of a very favored food (the restriction of which might discourage drug compliance) a trial of small amounts can be undertaken.

The hepatotoxicity of some MAO inhibitors has led to their being removed from the market. Hepatitis was generally associated with hydrazine drugs, rarely with nonhydrazines as well. The reaction is hepatocellular, and is pathologically indistinguishable from viral hepatitis.

The more common side effects of MAO inhibitors are autonomic.

Dizziness, orthostatic hypotension, delayed micturition, dry mouth, and constipation can occur. Occcassionally dermatitis, particularly a maculopapular rash, can occur.

Lithium as an Antidepressant

At first the possibility that lithium might have a role in the treatment of depression was not given very serious consideration primarily because of theoretical considerations. Since mania and depression were generally considered to reflect "opposite" poles of a continuum, it would not be expected that an established antimanic agent would also have antidepressant effects. In fact, the earlier studies of lithium in depression generally reported negative results (Gershon et al 1973). On the other hand, some current theories about manic-depressive illness tend to stress the genetic, biologic, and clinical similarities between the two conditions (Goodwin and Sack 1973), including the frequent coexistence of depressive features during mania (Kotin and Goodwin 1972). Recent evidence on lithium in depression is consistent with this thinking in that it strongly suggests that some patients with major depressive disorders do have an antidepressant response to this drug (Goodwin et al 1969, Mendels et al 1972). However, the total number of patients in these studies is small in comparison with studies of the antidepressant efficacy of the tricyclics or the MAO inhibitors. Overall, in heterogeneous populations of patients with major depressive illness, lithium has a response rate lower than the tricyclic drugs, although there are few studies in which a tricyclic and lithium have been compared in the same population of patients.

The question of subgroup specificity is interesting. In two independent control studies of hospitalized depressed patients, antidepressant responses to lithium were significantly more likely in the bipolar compared to the unipolar groups. (See pp 223 to 224 for a discussion of the unipolar/bipolar dichotomy.) In a related study, those antidepressant responses to lithium which did occur in unipolar patients tended to be associated with a positive family history of mania (Mendels, personal communication).

In initiating the lithium treatment of depression one uses doses somewhat lower than would be appropriate for the treatment of acute mania as described on p 257. It is common clinical experience that the onset of the antidepressant effects of lithium can be quite variable. In general it is advisable to wait somewhat longer than in the case of the tricyclics, since lithium responses in some depressed patients will not become evident until the third or fourth week.

In practice the unipolar/bipolar classification is of great impor-

tance in the selection of the appropriate drug treatment for a depressed patient. A patient with a history of mania should generally be
on prophylactic lithium maintenance. The first issue in the treatment of a depressive episode in such a patient is whether the lithium
level is adequate; sometimes an increase in the lithium dose will be
sufficient to produce an antidepressant response. If the blood level
indicates that a dose increase is not indicated, or if such a move fails
to produce improvement, then it is common to add a tricyclic (or
perhaps a MAO inhibitor). This is discussed further in the section on
drug combinations. When dealing with a "fresh" bipolar-depressed
patient not previously on lithium, some clinicians prefer to start the
treatment with a tricyclic antidepressant or the combination of a
tricyclic with lithium, rather than lithium alone.

Antipsychotic Drugs

Phenothiazines and related antipsychotic agents may be useful in
treating certain types of depression. The depressed patients who are
described as "phenothiazine responsive" are usually those with
high levels of agitation and /or psychotic features. In understanding
the reports of antidepressant effects of phenothiazines (Overall et al
1964), it is important to distinguish between a drug effect on a
specific symptom and a true antidepressant response. Thus, a
phenothiazine may produce clear improvement in symptoms of agitation, sleep, disturbance, and psychosis, and since these features
make up a substantial part of the rating scales for depression, they
would tend to show up as antidepressant effects.

   The phenothiazines seem to have their most rational and secure
place in the management of "involutional depression," that is, agitated depressions in older individuals (predominantly postmenopausal females) with prominent psychotic features, particularly paranoia. When a phenothiazine has been used in a depressed
patient, it is important to discontinue it as soon as possible because
of the potential for exacerbating or contributing to the continuation
of the underlying depressive process.

Use of Stimulants in Depression

The stimulants such as amphetamine and methylphenidate are not
generally useful in the clinical management of a major depressive
episode. Animal studies of the mechanism of action of amphetamine
show that it potentiates adrenergic neurotransmission by release of
norepinephrine and dopamine, blockade of reuptake of amines, and
inhibition of MAO. Thus, according to the catecholamine

hypothesis of depression, it should have antidepressant properties. Clinical research studies have shown that amphetamine has an acute antidepressant and euphoric effect that is short-lived, and that can be blocked by lithium pretreatment (van Kammen and Murphy 1975). This observation has important implications for the neuropharmacology of depression but, unfortunately, does not provide a rapidly acting treatment for depression. Amphetamine has too great a potential for addiction and for increasing psychotic disorganization. Although some clinicians feel that amphetamine has usefulness in the treatment of mild depression, this use is currently not approved because of the potential for addiction.

One interesting new development involves the use of a single dose of amphetamine (30 mg) to depressed patients as a means of predicting subsequent response to imipramine. In one study of hospitalized depressed patients a transient activation-euphoria response to D-amphetamine was highly predictive of a favorable response to imipramine (Fawcett et al 1972).

Combinations of Antidepressant Drugs

Lithium and Tricyclics.   Lithium and tricyclic antidepressants are used frequently in the treatment of patients with bipolar affective disorders. They can be used in the acute management of a depression in a bipolar patient, or in the long-term management of a patient who experiences considerable depressive symptomatology when he is not manic or hypomanic. When using the drugs in combination it may be necessary to give smaller doses of the tricyclics, but there are no serious contraindications to using the two drugs together, and no side effects or complications that do not occur with either drug alone. There is very little systematic information on the differential efficacy of combined lithium-tricyclic versus either drug alone in the treatment of acute depression in a bipolar patient, although anecdotal reports support our clinical experience that this combination can be useful in patients who have failed to show a satisfactory response to a single drug approach. The indication for combined lithium-tricyclics in long-term maintenance treatment of affective illness is not established.

Lithium and MAO Inhibitors.   Lithium and MAO inhibitors can also be used in combination in the management of the bipolar patient. However, this combination is not used frequently, primarily because of the reluctance on the part of most clinicians to use MAO inhibitors. There is some preliminary evidence that this combination is efficacious in a particular subgroup of depressed patients. An open trial of tranylcypromine in combination with lithium led to a clinical response in 16 out of 21 bipolar patients whose depression was previously unresponsive to lithium alone; 11 of these patients had been previously unresponsive to a tricyclic antidepressant. Clinically, the depressions in these patients were characterized by anergia, retardation, hypersomnia, excessive eating, and weight gain (Himmelhoch et al 1972).

Tricyclic Antidepressants and MAO Inhibitors. When these two classes of antidepressants are administered concurrently, a toxic state of central nervous system sympathetic overactivity can occur which may include headache, hypertensive crises (often signaled by headache), hyperpyrexia, convulsions, intracranial hemorrhage, and death. These reactions have occurred principally when the patient is on a large dose of one or both drugs. Because of the possibility of this toxic interaction, product information for tricyclic antidepressants and MAO inhibitors state that the two classes should not be used concurrently. If a patient is to be switched from an MAO inhibitor to a tricyclic antidepressant, 14 days should be allowed to elapse off medication to allow MAO activity to return to normal levels.

In the research setting, and in the hands of experienced psychopharmacologists these combinations can be used safely. When used very cautiously, there are indications that tricyclic-MAO inhibitor combinations can produce antidepressant effects in patients previously unresponsive to either drug individually.

Tricyclic Antidepressants in Combination with Phenothiazines. Combinations of these drugs have been marketed primarily for the treatment of the depressed patient with prominent features of anxiety, agitation, or psychosis, that is, the same indication for which phenothiazines alone have been suggested. The tricyclic-phenothiazine combination used most extensively has been amitripytline and perphenazine. Although controlled studies have not documented that this combination is superior to either drug used alone (Chacon and Downham 1967), in a large clinical trial, there are undoubtedly a mixture of subtypes of unipolar depression, some of which may be differentially responsive to phenothiazines and to tricyclics. It is probably more satisfactory both diagnostically and therapeutically to conduct a trial of one drug at a time, switching to another class if necessary.

The neuropharmacology of the two classes of drugs suggests that they are acting by quite different mechanisms that tend to oppose each other. The antidepressants potentiate catecholamine and indoleamine neurotransmission by several different presynaptic mechanisms, thus increasing the amount of neurotransmitter available to the postsynaptic receptor site. The phenothiazines are thought to exert their central nervous system action by the blockade of adrenergic receptors. Whether this "pharmacologic opposition" is relevant to their combined use in patients is not clear at this time.

References

Ayd FJ: Lithium-haloperidol for mania: is it safe or hazardous? Int Drug Ther Newsletter 10:29–36, 1975

Ban T: Psychopharmacology. Baltimore, Williams & Wilkins, 1969

Chacon C, Downham ET: Amitriptyline and amitriptyline-with-perphenazine in depression: a retrospective study. Brit J Psychiat 113:201–207, 1967

Cohen WJ, Cohen NH: Lithium carbonate, haloperidol, and irreversible brain damage. JAMA 230: 1282–1287, 1974

Fawcett J, Maas JW, Dekirmenjian H: Depression and MHPG excretion: response to dextroamphetamine and tricyclic antidepressants. Arch Gen Psychiat 26:246–251, 1972

Gershon S, Shopsin B: Lithium, Its Role in Psychiatric Research and Treatment. New York, Plenum, 1973

Goodwin FK, Murphy DL, Bunney WE, Jr: Lithium carbonate treatment in depression and mania: a longitudinal double-blind study. Arch Gen Psychiat 21:486–496, 1969

————, Sack RL: Affective disorders: the catecholamine hypothesis revisited. In Usdin G, Snyder S (eds): Frontiers in Catecholamine Research. New York, Pergamon, 1973

Himmelhoch JM, Detre T, Kupfer D, Swantzburg M, Byck R: Treatment of previously intractable depression with tranylcypromine and lithium. J Nerv Ment Dis 155:216–220, 1972

Klein DF, Davis JM: Diagnosis and Drug Treatment of Psychiatric Disorders. Baltimore, Williams & Wilkins, 1969

Johnson G, Gershon S, Burdock E, Floyd A, Hekiman L: Comparative effects of lithium and chlorpromazine in the treatment of manic states. Brit J Psychiat 119:267–276, 1971

Kotin J, Goodwin FK: Depression during mania: clinical observations and theoretical implications. Am J Psychiat 129:679–686, 1972

Kuhn R: Uber die behandlung depressives zustande mit einem iminodibenzylderivat (G-22355). Schweiz Med Wschr 87:1135, 1957

Mendels J: Personal communication

————, Secunda SK, Dyson WC: A controlled study of the antidepressant effects of lithium. Arch Gen Psychiat 26:154–157, 1972

Murphy DL, Goodwin FK, Bunney WE, Jr: Leukocytosis during lithium treatment. Am J Psychiat 127:135–137, 1971

Overall JE, Hollister LE, Meyer F, Kimbell I, Jr, Shelton J: Imipramine and thioridazine in depressed and schizophrenic patients. Are there specific antidepressant drugs? JAMA 189:605–608, 1964

Pare CMB, Rees L, Sainsburg MJ: Differentiation of two genetically specific types of depression by the response to antidepressants. Lancet 2:1340–1343, 1962

Spitzer RL, Endicott J, Robbins E: Research diagnostic criteria. Psychopharm Bull 11:22–25, 1975

van Kammen DP, Murphy D: Attenuation of euphoriant and activating effects of D- and L-amphetamine by lithium carbonate treatment. Psychopharmacologia 44:215–224, 1975

recent
advances
in drug treatment
of affective
disorders

commentary

Mood disorders tend to be cyclical or recurrent; thus prophylaxis is highly desirable. Tricyclics can prevent relapses in unipolar depression and lithium in bipolar, though there is some overlap. A drug decision tree is given (p 248) which programs a logical progression of drug trials until an effective response is achieved. New methods of monitoring blood levels allow one to account for an important factor responsible for effectiveness and toxicity. Individual variability in dose sensitivity is enormous. Furthermore, determination of an individual's optimal plasma level may be necessary for all drugs. Since animal studies show that amitriptyline selectively inhibits 5-hydroxytryptamine uptake, while imipramine affects both 5-hydroxytryptamine and norepinephrine, determination of the particular amine disorder in a patient may help to decide the proper therapy. Some depressed patients who do not respond to tricyclic drugs alone experience relief when triiodothyronine is added to their regime. Potentiation by other hormones and drugs is very likely and deserves further research.

recent advances in drug treatment of affective disorders

Frederick K. Goodwin, M.D.
Michael H. Ebert, M.D.

The Maintenance or "Prophylactic" Treatment of Affective Illness

Lithium

The most important advance in psychopharmacology since the discovery of the tricyclic antidepressants has been the development of "prophylactic" approaches to the long-term management of recurrent affective illness. The potential implications of these developments are enormous considering that major affective illness is essentially a recurrent condition, with evidence that over 95 percent of patients who have been hospitalized for depression or mania will experience a recurrence (see p 223).

Most of the systematic studies of maintenance therapy have involved lithium; these investigations have focused primarily on bipolar patients, a subgroup comprising less than one-third of the affective illness encountered in clinical practice. There is no doubt that the evidence concerning the prophylactic efficacy of lithium is most clear in the case of bipolar illness, because of (a) the relatively large number of patients studied, and (b) the clarity of diagnosis of an illness in which history of mania is the identifying characteristic. In the bipolar group, proper lithium management is associated with the prevention of mania in 85 percent or more of the cases. The depressive episode in bipolar patients on lithium are reduced substantially in frequency, duration, and intensity; in these patients the prophylactic effect against depression is not as dramatic as that against mania, but if reduction in number of hospitalizations is the criterion, then lithium's effect against mania and depression is equivalent.

What about the use of long-term lithium in recurrent unipolar depression? Here the indications are less well established for two reasons: first, the number of patients in whom this question has been studied is smaller; second, the borderlines of the unipolar diagnosis are less well-defined. Most of the studies of lithium maintenance in unipolar depression were done prior to the development of the Research Diagnostic Criteria (p 221), so that it is not always clear just what different investigators have meant by unipolar depression. In order to have a chance to show an effect within a reasonable time, patients were selected for these studies on the basis of having histories of relatively frequent recurrences of depression (in the range of one episode per year or at least two episodes in five years). Thus, the bulk of individuals with depression, who experience episodes less frequently than these criteria, were not included in these studies and therefore conclusions about the prophylactic efficacy of lithium in these patients would not be warranted at this time.

With these limitations in mind it can still be concluded that lithium does have some prophylactic effect in recurrent unipolar depressives as defined above. Thus, if a patient has major affective illness with a unipolar pattern and has relatively rapid recurrences, a prophylactic trial with lithium may be justified. However, other approaches to this problem should also be considered, including the use of maintenance tricyclics.

Tricyclic Antidepressants

Recently the use of maintenance tricyclics in the long-term management of recurrent depression has received attention. In the large National Institute of Mental Health-Veterans Administration collaborative study, conducted over a two-year period, Prien and his associates (1973) concluded that maintenance imipramine was superior to placebo and equivalent to lithium in reducing the relapse rate among unipolar depressives. For the bipolar patients, lithium was superior to imipramine, primarily because of the increased frequency of manic relapses in the patients on imipramine.

General Issues in Maintenance Treatment

The question of who should be on maintenance treatment and for how long is often a very difficult one. Of course in considering the prophylactic treatment of affective illness one must distinguish between a relapse and a new episode. A reasonable rule of thumb is to consider any sustained exacerbation of symptoms as a new episode if it occurs after a symptom-free period of at least six months.

When there is a history of mania the patient should generally be maintained on lithium indefinitely. However, there can be exceptions to this general rule. Based on his extensive long-term follow-up data, Angst feels that patients who experience their first manic episode in the early 20s usually go through a six- to ten-year period during which the chances for recurrence are relatively low (1973). Thus, in such patients it might be justified to discontinue the lithium several months after the episode, particularly if circumstances and patient reliability permit a careful monitoring of symptoms and early intervention when necessary. The fact that this time frame also includes important childbearing years in females provides an additional reason for at least brief periods off lithium, since the drug may have harmful effects on the fetus during the first trimester. In relation to the problem of the patient who wishes to become pregnant, there are other circumstances which might allow the estimation of a relatively "safe" period to be off lithium. Thus, when there has been a history of several episodes that have occurred with a relatively regular pattern, this pattern can be used to predict when the next episode would be likely in the absence of the drug; an "off-drug" period could then be planned. These principles would also apply to situations in which there were other reasons for an "off-drug" period, such as surgery, medical work-ups, and the evaluation and management of possible drug side effects.

A major problem in the long-term use of lithium and the tricyclics is weight gain. Many patients on lithium will experience a weight gain of up to ten pounds, with a smaller proportion (15 to 20 percent) experiencing more serious weight problems which may threaten patient compliance, and at times, even result in discontinuation of the drug. About 5 percent of the patients on long-term lithium therapy will develop a nontoxic goiter which can be treated without discontinuing the lithium. Hypothyroidism, not associated with goiter, can also develop, and can be treated with thyroid hormones. Other long-term effects of lithium have not been documented, although questions have been raised concerning changes in calcium metabolism and possible subtle effects on memory in some individuals.

The lithium blood level for a patient on maintenance treatment should be 0.7 to 1.2 mEq per liter. A practical problem with lithium prophylaxis is to keep the patient on his medication and to maintain interest in regulating the blood level. After a patient's lithium intake is adjusted properly during the initiation of therapy, monthly lithium levels are sufficient. It should be kept in mind that the amount of lithium required to maintain a particular blood level may drop after a manic or hypomanic episode has concluded.

Frequently the manic-depressive patient drifts out of contact with his therapist and takes his lithium irregularly, if at all. A psychodynamic issue in lithium management of bipolar patients is that he may miss his hypomanic phase, feeling that he "needs it" in order to do well. This leads to a desire to stop the lithium in the usually futile hope that he can experience the energizing aspects of hypomania without the full-blown syndrome. Our group has reported the approach of using husband-wife group therapy to follow patients on prophylactic lithium treatment (Davenport et al 1975). We find that this provides an arena to work out some of the psychologic resistance to drug therapy and provides more reliable follow-up of the patient, since the spouse is directly involved in the treatment.

The prophylactic treatment of affective illness is a more complex and demanding task than the acute management of a depressive episode, and is often handled less satisfactorily in clinical practice. It can test the mettle of a flexibly trained psychiatrist in diagnosis, psychopharmacology, and psychotherapy. Often several therapeutic modalities have to be used concurrently to achieve the optimum result.

The Drug Decision Tree

The reader is referred again to the concept of a drug treatment decision tree discussed on page 248. The particular decision tree illustrated there would refer to the treatment of an acute depression, in cases where there is no past history or family history of specific drug response. The physician would decide whether or not the patient met the criteria for a major depressive syndrome as defined in the previous chapter, and from historical information whether the patient was unipolar or bipolar. He would also consider whether the patient has the symptom cluster characteristic of "atypical" depression as defined earlier in the discussion of MAO inhibitors. It should be kept in mind that many patients with depression would not fall into either category, and would not be candidates for drug therapy. The sequence of drug treatments suggested begins with the agent most likely to be efficacious for the particular subcategory of depression. Each vertical sequence then follows a logical progression of drug trials if the patient does not respond to the first treatment.

Blood Levels of Drugs Used in the Affective Disorders

As discussed in the previous chapter, monitoring of drug level in plasma is well established as an integral part of the careful management of lithium therapy. It is no exaggeration to say that blood level monitoring is no less important in the case of tricyclics, and perhaps also the MAO inhibitors. The problem is that reliable and inexpensive assays for these drugs are not yet widely available.

Tricyclic Blood Level Studies.   A detailed review of all of the studies in this area is not appropriate here. However it would be useful to outline several general issues highlighted from this literature. The "steady state" blood level of drug achieved on a standard dose is relatively constant within an individual, but is *highly* variable from one individual to the next (Glassman and Perel 1974). For the two best studied drugs (desmethylimipramine and nortriptyline) this variability is reflected in a *tenfold* or greater range from the highest to the lowest. Thus the individual doses that will be necessary to produce clinical effects in different patients can vary over an enormous range.

In the case of nortriptyline (and presumably also for amitriptyline) recent evidence supports the concept of a "therapeutic window," ie, a relatively narrow range of blood levels of the drug associated with optimal therapeutic response; levels either below or *above* this range are associated with reduced rates of response (Kragh-Sorensen et al 1976). There is less known about the relationship between therapeutic response and blood levels of imipramine and /or desmethylimipramine although the small amount of available data favors a more linear relationship, ie, increasing response rate with increasing blood levels (Walther 1971).

For amitriptyline and nortriptyline, the reduction in response rate with higher doses is consistent with evidence from animal studies that at higher doses these compounds acquire catecholamine-receptor-blocking properties similar to the major tranquilizers (Moeller-Nielsen 1970)—a feature which may contribute to their usefulness against symptoms of anxiety, agitation, and insomnia.

MAO Inhibitors.   In the case of this class of drugs, the compounds themselves have not been the focus, but rather their effects, ie, the degree of inhibition of MAO. Platelet MAO activity has been used as a sensitive bioassay of the effective dose of an MAO inhibitor in a given patient. Some individual variability in dose response relationships has also been noted for these drugs, but the range is not as great as with the tricyclics (Klein and Davis 1969). It has been reported that the rate of response to an MAO inhibitor (Nardil) does not become substantial until greater than 75 percent inhibition of the platelet enzyme has been achieved, and at that this requires different doses in different individuals (Robinson et al 1973).

How might the clinician use this information on blood level-therapeutic response relationships when these assays are not available to him? Given the high degree of variability in dose-blood level ratios, it simply makes no sense to rely on a "standard dose," either in terms of efficacy or safety; each patient must be titrated individually, with careful monitoring of both side effects and clinical response. With imipramine (or desmethylimipramine) and the MAO inhibitors we would suggest a steady increase in dose until clinical response occurs or until limited by major side effects. On the other hand, when using amitriptyline or nortriptyline it would seem justified to work with smaller, more gradual increments (after the first 75 mg) to allow time to evaluate possible response at a lower blood level.

Biologic Predictors of Differential Drug Response

Some interesting correlations between pretreatment biologic variables and subsequent response to antidepressant drugs have occurred as a "spin-off" of research efforts aimed at elucidating biochemical mechanisms in affective illness. It is therefore no surprise that most of these studies have focused on the metabolites of the biogenic amines, since it is around these amine systems that the major hypotheses of affective disorder have been built (p 231). It is not our purpose here to critically review the literature on amine metabolite studies in affective illness. However, the general observation can be made that these studies (both in cerebrospinal fluid and urine) have provided some support for the hypotheses that the function of one or more of these amines may be disordered in some depressed patients. What is striking about these metabolite data is the large degree of *variability* found within a population of depressed patients. Some of this variability may reflect amine differences in different subtypes of depression, particularly differences between unipolar and bipolar depressed patients (p 224). Recently several research groups have examined the possibility that the variability in amine metabolite findings may also prove useful in *predicting* subsequent response to different antidepressant drugs in otherwise homogeneous populations of depressed patients. These studies (Asberg et al 1971, Goodwin and Post, 1975, Maas et al 1972, Beckmann and Goodwin 1975, Schildkraut 1973, Maas 1975) (outlined in Table 1) are of course

TABLE 1
AMINE METABOLITE "SUBGROUPS" IN
DEPRESSION: SOME RELATIONSHIPS TO
PHARMACOLOGIC RESPONSE

Amine Metabolite Subgroups	Drug Response Subgroups
Low 5-HIAA* in the CSF	Poor response to nortriptyline (Asberg et al 1971) or to imipramine (Goodwin and Post 1975)
Low urinary MHPG†	Imipramine response (Mass et al 1972)
	Imipramine response in unipolars (Beckmann and Goodwin 1975)
	Amitriptyline nonresponse (Schildkraut 1973, Beckmann and Goodwin 1975)
Higher urinary MHPG	Amitriptyline response (Schildkraut 1973, Beckmann and Goodwin 1975)
	Imipramine nonresponse (Maas et al 1972, Beckmann and Goodwin 1975)

*5HIAA is 5-hydroxyindoleacetic acid, the major metabolite of serotonin.
†MHPG is 3-methoxy-4-hydroxyphenylglycol, the major metabolite of norepinephrine.

preliminary and so far involve only a relatively small number of patients. Nevertheless the results "make sense" in terms of what is known from animal studies about the differential effects of various tricyclic drugs on different amine neurotransmitter systems in the brain (Table 2). A proper understanding of the clinical findings in Table 1 in terms of the amine specificity data in Table 2 depends on an awareness of the fact that both tertiary amines (imipramine and amitriptyline) are *partially converted* by the liver to the corresponding secondary amines (desmethylimipramine and nortriptyline) so that a patient given imipramine, for example, is really on a combination of imipramine and desmethylimipramine. Although the relative proportion of imipramine or amitriptyline which is demethylated to the secondary amine varies from one patient to the next, there are

TABLE 2
SUMMARY OF EFFECTS OF VARIOUS ANTIDEPRESSANT
DRUGS ON BLOCKADE OF UPTAKE OF BIOGENIC
AMINES*

Drug	Biogenic Amine		
	5-HT	NE	DA
Amitriptyline	+++++†	0‡	0
Nortriptyline	++	++	0
Imipramine	+++	++	0
Desipramine	0	++++	0

*Adapted from Maas JW: Arch Gen Psychiatry 32:1357, 1975
†Indicates most active.
‡Indicates probable lack of activity in vivo at tissue levels clinically achievable.

important overall differences in the two drugs with respect to this. Thus after "steady state" is achieved in a patient on imipramine we find twice as much desmethylimipramine in the CSF as there is imipramine (Goodwin and Muscettola 1975). Although there is less information available for amitriptyline treated patients, an earlier study in plasma indicates the reverse: there was roughly twice as much amitriptyline as nortriptyline (Brathwaite and Widdop, 1971). In other words, the evidence available so far suggests that in the patient imipramine tends to be converted to desmethylimipramine, while amitriptyline tends to stay amitriptyline. With this in mind, let us reexamine Tables 1 and 2. If the pathophysiology of depression in thos patients with low levels of 5-HIAA in the CSF involves serotonin dysfunction, then according to the data outlined in Table 2, they might be expected to respond poorly to nortriptyline, since it is a secondary amine; and for the same reason they might be expected to respond poorly to imipramine, since it is largely converted to the secondary amine, desmethylimipramine. On the other hand, if those patients with low urinary levels of MHPG (the principle metabolite of brain norepinephrine) had depressions related predominantly to norepinephrine dysfunction, they might be expected to respond well to imipramine, but not to amitriptyline since in the former case drug metabolism favors the formation of desmethylimipramine while in the latter case amitriptyline predominates. As yet no

reliable clinical correlates have been uncovered that might differentiate low from high MHPG patients or low from high 5-HIAA patients.

Endocrine Potentiation of Response to Tricyclic Antidepressants

As noted in the chapter on specific antimanic and antidepressant
drugs various types of endocrine dysfunction can sometimes be
found in association with depression. For example, major depression is a relatively frequent concomitant of hypothyroidism,
Addison's disease, or the decreased gonadal functions of the
menopause.

The relationship between thyroid function and depression has
received the most attention. Prange and his associates have shown
that in females, small amounts of triiodothyronine (T_3) can accelerate the antidepressant response to imipramine (Prange et al 1969).
We have extended this work by demonstrating that the addition of
25 μg of T_3 can *potentiate* the action of both imipramine and amitriptyline so that a significant proportion of patients previously considered nonresponders were converted into responders. The majority of these patients were female and had pretreatment thyroid indices in the low range of "normal."

There is no systematic information concerning the potential inter-
relationship between antidepressant treatment and adrenal cortical
hormones; it has been known for some time that individuals with
decreased adrenal cortical function (Addison's disease) may not
have satisfactory antidepressant responses to tricyclics (or to electroconvulsive therapy) until their adrenal cortical dysfunction is
corrected (Fawcett and Bunney, 1967).

In the case of the sex hormones, synthetic estrogens are widely
used to treat the "depressive" symptoms associated with menopause
and there are anecdotal reports that in postmenopausal females,
tricyclic antidepressants can be potentiated by the combined administration of small doses of estrogenic substances (Prange 1971).
However, there is as yet no systematic study of this problem and in
view of the other risk associated with the use of these substances,
they should not be employed in this manner except to correct a
demonstrated deficit syndrome.

A few patients have been given testosterone in association with
tricyclic therapy and a potentiation was reported but in a direction
that suggests that this combination might be dangerous, ie, the patients did have a more rapid and dramatic antidepressant response,
but at the same time the syndrome evolved into a transient paranoid
psychosis (Wilson et al 1974). Further work in this area is indicated.

References

Angst J: Classification and Prediction of Outcome of Depression. Stuttgart, FK Schattauer Verlag, 1973

Asberg M, Cronholm B, Sjoqvist F, Tuck D: Relationship between plasma level and therapeutic effect of nortriptyline. Br Med J 3:331–334, 1971

Beckmann H, Goodwin FK: Central norepinephrine metabolism and the prediction of antidepressant response to imipramine and amitriptyline: studies with urinary MHPG in unipolar depressed patients. Arch Gen Psychiatry 32:17–21, 1975

Brathwaite RA, Widdop B: A specific gas chromatographic method for the measurement of "steady state" plasma levels of amitriptyline and nortriptyline in patients. Clin Chim Acta 35:461–472, 1971

Davenport YB, Ebert MH, Adland ML, Goodwin FK: Lithium prophylaxis: the married couples group. Sci Proc Am Psychiat Assoc 128:66–67, 1975

Fawcett J, Bunney WE, Jr: Pituitary adrenal function and depression. Arch Gen Psychiatry 16:517–535, 1967

Glassman AH, Perel JM: Plasma levels and tricyclic antidepressants. Clin Pharmacol Ther 16:198–200, 1974

Goodwin FK, Muscettola G: Plasma and CSF levels of imipramine and desipramine levels in depressed patients. San Juan, Puerto Rico, Presented at the 14th Annual American College of Neuropsychopharmacology Meeting, 1975

————, Post RM: Amine metabolites in cerebrospinal fluid, brain and urine in the major mental illnesses. In Freedman D (ed): The Biology of the Major Psychoses: A Comparative Analysis. New York, Raven, 1975

Klein DF, Davis JM: Diagnosis and Drug Treatment of Psychiatric Disorders. Baltimore, Williams & Wilkins, 1969

Kragh-Sorensen P, Hansen CF, Baastrup PC, Hvidberg EF: Self-inhibiting acting action of nortriptyline's antidepressive effect at high plasma levels. Psychopharmacologia 45:305–312, 1976

Maas JW. Biogenic amines and depression. Arch Gen Psychiatry 32:1357–1361, 1975

————, Fawcett JA, Dekirmenjian H: Catecholamine metabolism, depressive illness, and drug response. Arch Gen Psychiatry 26:252–262, 1972

Moeller-Nielsen J: Does a true qualitative difference exist in the mode of action of neuroleptics on catecholamine neuron system. In Bobon DP, Janssen PAJ, Bobon J (eds): The Neuroleptics Modern Problems of Pharmacopsychiatry, Vol. 5, Basel, Karger, 1970, pp 68–70

Prange AJ: Proceedings of the Fifth World Congress of Psychiatry. Mexico, 1971, pp 1023–1031

———, Wilson IC, Rabon AM, Lipton MA: Enhancement of imipramine antidepressant activity by thyroid hormone. Am J Psychiatry 126:457–1969

Prien RF, Klett CJ, Caffey EM, Jr: Lithium carbonate and imipramine in prevention of affective episodes. Arch Gen Psychiatry 29:420–425, 1973

Robinson DS, Nies A, Rovaris CL, Lamborn K: Controlled clinical trial of the MAO inhibitor phenelzine in the treatment of depressive-anxiety states. Arch Gen Psychiatry 29:407–13, 1973

Schildkraut JJ: Norepinephrine metabolites as biochemical criteria for classifying depressive disorders and predicting responses to treatment: preliminary findings. Am J Psychiatry 130:695–798, 1973

Walther CJS. Clinical significance of plasma imipramine levels. Proc Roy Soc Med 64:282–285, 1971

Wilson IC, Prange AJ Jr, Lara PP: Methyltestosterone with imipramine in men: conversion of depression to paranoid reaction. Am J Psychiatry 131:21–24, 1974

drug treatment of the hyperactive syndrome in children

commentary

Drug treatment of the hyperactive (sometimes called minimal brain dysfunction) child is important because of the high incidence and deleterious and disruptive nature of this disorder. The syndrome can be diagnosed accurately if parents, teachers, and physicians use the measuring instruments described in this chapter. Possible acute and chronic toxic effects of amphetaminelike drugs (p 467) must be weighed against the long-term debilitating effects of the behavior disorder itself. Treating these children with stimulant medication is favored by numbers of double-blind controlled studies which show improvement in school performance and psychosocial adjustment. In short-term studies, there is little evidence of danger from such drugs. There are no studies as yet showing long-term efficacy and safety, but the ultimate prognosis for the untreated hyperactive child seems rather bleak. Dr. Cantwell compares the relative efficacy of different classes of drugs in treating the hyperactive child and concludes that stiuulants, such as dextroamphetamine and methylphenidate, are the most effective, although tricyclic antidepressants show some promise.

drug treatment of the hyperactive syndrome in children

Dennis P. Cantwell, M.D.

Hyperactive Child Syndrome

This chapter will review general principles of drug treatment of the hyperactive child syndrome and what is known about the safety and efficacy of specific drugs used to treat hyperactive children.

The term *hyperactive child syndrome* describes a heterogeneous group of children with different etiologies for their condition. In some cases the disorder may be due to a structural abnormality of the brain (Werry 1972). In others physiologic arousal of the nervous system may be abnormal (Satterfield et al 1974). In others there may be a genetic basis for this disorder (Cantwell 1975a), while in others there may still be undiscovered important etiologic factors.

Minimal brain damage and *minimal brain dysfunction* are terms often used synonymously with *hyperactive child syndrome*. This has had a number of unfortunate consequences since the above designations have been used in widely divergent ways by different investigators. The same children have been described by different terms and different children by the same terms. Thus research findings cannot be readily compared.

Moreover, these designations imply that brain damage or dysfunction is present, and is presumably etiologic in the hyperactive child syndrome. However, if brain damage is used in its literal sense to mean structural abnormality of the brain, then brain damage syndrome is an inaccurate and misleading term. While some hyperactive children may suffer from frank damage, it is clear that the majority do not (Werry 1972). Likewise most brain-damaged children do not present with the hyperactive child syndrome (Rutter et al 1970a).

Brain dysfunction may be a more accurate term than brain damage to describe children who present with less well-defined disorders manifested by more subtle neurologic signs. These more subtle defects in coordination, perception, or language may only occasionally be associated with actual damage to the brain. However, many hyperactive children do not demonstrate even these subtle neurologic signs. Thus brain dysfunction syndrome is inappropriate in describing the large percentage of hyperactive children who present primarily with behavior abnormalities.

Finally, techniques for the reliable and accurate quantification of brain dysfunction in children are not available. Yet prefixing the word minimal to brain dysfunction implies just such a quantification. It is the author's opinion that the term hyperactive child syndrome should be used to denote a behavioral syndrome only with no implications as to etiology.

Epidemiologic studies indicate that the syndrome may occur in as many as 5 to 10 percent of prepubertal children, with the boy to girl ratio ranging from 4 to 1 to 9 to 1 (Cantwell 1975b).

The cardinal symptoms are hyperactivity, distractibility, impulsivity, and excitability, with the attentional deficit probably being the "core" problem. Associated symptoms that are often, but not necessarily, present include: antisocial behavior, learning disabilities, depression, and low self-esteem.

Follow-up studies of hyperactive children indicate they are prone to develop significant psychiatric and social problems in adolescence and later life. Antisocial behavior, serious academic retardation, poor self-image, and depression seem to be the most common outcomes in adolescence. Alcoholism, sociopathy, hysteria, and possible psychosis seem to be likely psychiatric outcomes in adulthood (Cantwell 1975c).

In beginning a discussion of treatment of the hyperactive child it is well to emphasize that for management purposes, the hyperactive child is best considered a multihandicapped child, requiring a multiple modality treatment approach (Feighner and Feighner 1973). Treatment must be individualized and based on a comprehensive assessment of each child and his family. While evidence for the efficacy of individual psychotherapy with hyperactive children is lacking from studies comparing children receiving psychotherapy with those receiving drug treatment (Eisenberg et al 1965), psychotherapy is indicated for tee secondary emotional symptoms of depression, low self-esteem, and peer relationships. Psychotherapy with these children often requires innovative techniques, such as those described by Gardner (1973). Too often drug treatment is viewed as an "either /or proposition"; that is, either drugs are used or some other modality. Drugs should be used in combination with other modalities needed, based on individual assessment of the child (Satterfield et al 1974).

General Principles of Drug Treatment

1. No medication should be instituted without a comprehensive diagnostic evaluation of the child, including a detailed interview with parents, psychiatric evaluation of the child, information from the school, physical and neurologic examination, and appropriate laboratory studies (Cantwell 1975d).
2. An old and tried drug should be used in place of a new one, unless there is a great deal of experimental evidence showing the superiority of the newer medication (Eisenberg 1968).
3. Baseline assessments of the child's behavior that are expected to be affected by the medication must be obtained systematically. The same instruments should be used to record the same behaviors at regular intervals during the course of treatment. Response to treatment is probably best singly evaluated by the physician from reports of behavior at school. However the more standardized ratings made by different observers in different settings, the greater the likelihood that the physician will obtain a true picture of the effect of medication. The author recommends that the physician use the Conners Parent Symptom Questionnaire (PSQ), the Conners Teacher Questionnaire (TQ), the Conners Abbreviated Symptom Questionnaire (ASQ), and the Rutter-Graham Psychiatric Rating Scale for children as baseline and followup measures to judge the effectiveness of the medication (Department of Health, Education, and Welfare 1973). The Conners Teacher Questionnaire seems to be the most widely used teacher evaluation procedure for hyperactive children. Normative data are available; it has been shown to clearly distinguish normal children from hyperactive children and to be quantitatively very sensitive to the behavioral effects of psychotropic drugs (Sprague et al 1974, Sprague and Werry 1974).

Ten items on the PSQ and TQ are identical and have been combined to form an Abbreviated Symptom Questionnaire (ASQ), which can be used by the physician to obtain frequent follow-up assessments of the child from both parents and teachers. This abbreviated scale has been found to have almost the same sensitivity in obtaining statistically significant differences in psychotropic drug studies with hyperactive children (Sprague and Werry 1974).

The Rutter-Graham Rating Scale contains specific items of behavior to be rated, based on observation of the child during the interview or on what the child has to say during the interview. In epidemiologic studies, this scale has been shown to be a valid and reliable indicator of psychiatric illness in children (Rutter et al 1970b).

4. Side effects should be assessed and monitored in the same systematic fashion as expected behavioral effects of the medication. There are systematic rating sheets for side effects to be completed by parents and to be asked of the children, which are quite effective for this purpose (Gofman 1973).

5. The initial dose should be the smallest available dose of the medication being used. A knowledge of the duration of action of the medication is necessary in order to know whether to prescribe the drug on a once-a-day basis or two- or three-times-a-day, depending on how long the physician wishes the medication to be effective. Starting with the low dose, the physician should then titrate the medication and raise the dose until either clinical improvement is noted or side effects occur, which necessitate discontinuation of the drug. At present there are no laboratory or other measures against which one can titrate the medication. The physician must use his clinical judgment based on the information he obtains from the parents, the school, and from his own observation of the child.

While there are rough guidelines that can be used for optimal dose of individual drugs on a milligram per kilogram body weight basis, this is a controversial area. For example, Wender (1971) has advocated a high dose of 1.5 mg /kg of D-amphetamine and a high dose of 4.6 mg /kg of methylphenidate. Sprague and his colleagues have conducted laboratory studies showing that teacher ratings show an increased improvement in behavior ratings up to doses of 0.70 and 1.00 mg /kg of methylphenidate. However, this dose is double that at which the peak enhancement of cognitive performance occurs (Sprague and Sleator 1973).

It is well to remember that children considered nonresponders to medication often simply have not been given an effective dose (Conners 1972, Wender 1971). Tolerance does develop (Arnold 1973), and just as the amount of medication that an individual child might require is highly idiosyncratic, so is the development of tolerance.

6. All children should be given a drug-free trial at some time during the course of a year if they are on medication chronically. There

are several ways to do this. One is by substituting placebo without letting the child or the schoolteacher know and obtaining a rating scale to see if behavior has deteriorated. Another is to let the child go back to school in September without being on medication, and after several weeks obtain a rating scale to see how it compares with that obtained at the end of the school year when he was on medication. If it looks like the child no longer requires medication, he should be followed more closely to see if his behavior deteriorates over time. Abstinence syndromes do not seem to develop during a drug-free trial.

At present there is no good method for determining when a child should be taken off medication completely, other than by clinical judgment. Certainly the popular idea that the hyperactive child syndrome disappears and medication has a "reverse effect" at puberty has never been established scientifically. The medication should not be stopped because a child reaches a certain age, but only when the clinical picture indicates the child no longer requires it.

7. A good deal of *psychotherapy*, using the term in the broad sense, must be done with both the child and the parents in conjunction with the use of medication. At the very least, the treating physician should help the hyperactive child understand the nature of his difficulties and how the medication (and other therapeutic intervention) is intended to help the child help himself. The role and action of the medication in his life then can make more sense to the hyperactive child and he will hopefully see the medication as one of his tools, not something forced on him by his parents, his teachers, or his doctor (Wender 1971).

The parents should also be prepared in a rational way for a trial of any medication and possible failure of that trial. Expected side effects should also be gone over in great detail and the parents encouraged to observe their child carefully for any likely side effects. The time invested in this type of preparation of the child and his family will reap its benefits should medication have to be changed or should dosage have to be changed over a long period of time in order to find the optimal dose of the optimal drug for each child.

8. An important and often neglected part of the physician's work in treating hyperactive children with medication is establishing contact with the school. The physician should make direct contact with the child's teacher, either in person or over the phone. Without cooperation from the school in reporting both positive and negative effects of the medication, it is the author's opinion that it is impossible to effectively manage a hyperactive child on

any medication. The teacher is likely to be the only person to see the child regularly in a group setting, where he is required to do the same tasks as a large number of his peers of the same age. Thus in a sense the teacher is in a position to compare the performance of the hyperactive child with a nonhyperactive control group on a daily basis. This is not meant to imply that the teacher has control of either the prescribing or the regulation of medication dosage, but that the physician needs to be in contact with the teacher so that he can make proper adjustments in the dose of medication.

Specific Drugs Used to Treat Hyperactive Children

Most of the literature on treatment of the hyperactive child syndrome consists of reports of drug treatment. Since several critical reviews of this voluminous literature are available (Conners 1972, Werry and Sprague 1972), only selected aspects of clinical importance will be discussed here.

Central Nervous System Stimulants

The central nervous system stimulants, methylphenidate and D-amphetamine, are currently the drugs of choice in the treatment of hyperactive children. Improvement in behavior can be expected in 5 to 10 percent (Cantwell 1975e).

The therapeutic properties and side effects of the two medications are very similar. They both seem to act by potentiating norepinephrine and dopamine at central synapses (Ferris et al 1972). The latency of onset of action for both stimulants is approximately 30 minutes, with a 3- to 6-hour duration of action. Methylphenidate must be given at least twice a day to ensure an effective dose throughout the school day. If D-amphetamine is given in the long-acting spansule, it need be given only once a day. Both drugs decrease hyperactivity and impulsivity and increase attention span. The total amount of bodily activity may actually be increased by the stimulants. The crucial change is an increase in *directed* or *controlled* motor activity. The stimulants have also been shown to produce small improvements in tests of general intelligence and visual motor perception and to enhance performance in learning tasks (Werry et al 1970). Memory for material learned while under the drug persists when medication is stopped; thus state dependency does not occur (Sprague 1972). Most hyperactive children who respond to one stimulant will respond to the other, but certain hyperactive children respond only to one (Winsberg et al 1974).

Anorexia, insomnia, headache, stomachache, nausea, tearfulness, and pallor are common side effects with both stimulants, but anorexia and insomnia seem more frequent and more severe with D-amphetamine. While it is generally stated that stimulants are not thought to produce euphoria in children, there has been very little systematic work on the effects of stimulant medication on mood. Long-term use of stimulants is known to produce depression in adults. This side effect is rarely mentioned in the literature on stimulant drug treatment of hyperactive children. However, the author has had several children who developed mild to moderate depressive episodes during the course of treatment with both methylphenidate and amphetamine. These episodes required cessation of or a reduction in the dose of stimulant plus the use of imipramine, following which the depression lifted. Since depression in children may be difficult to detect, particularly in a child who was previously hyperactive, it should be looked for systematically in children receiving stimulant medication. Children who suddenly develop a dysphoric mood, whether constant, intermittent, or fluctuating, and who also present with a marked change in behavior, such as loss of self-confidence, withdrawal from social intercourse, school refusal, and somatic symptoms should be suspected of having a depressive disorder.

There does not seem to be a predilection for hyperactive children, who have been medicated, to become drug abusers (Freedman 1971). There is some suggestion that suppression of weight and height may occur with prolonged use of D-amphetamine, and suppression of weight, but not height, with methylphenidate (Safer and Allen 1973). However, the results are inconsistent. The effects on growth seem to be related to the anorexia caused by the medication. The children simply eat less while on the medication, and return to previous growth patterns has been demonstrated when the children are taken off the drug (Safer and Allen 1973, Schain and Reynard 1975). Repeated measurements of height and weight of all children on medication should be charted on standard growth curves.

In children in whom weight loss becomes a significant problem some simple measures might be tried. Having the child eat a large breakfast before giving him his medication in the morning and/or having him eat a large supper when the effect of the medication has generally worn off has been found to be effective by the author. Also, if the child can be maintained off medication on weekends and during the summer, his appetite will usually improve, helping to alleviate some of the effects of decreased appetite that occur when the child is on medication. It is possible that appetite stimulants might also be tried. However the author is unaware of any systematic studies in which this has been done.

Clinical experience suggests that most side effects of medication usually subside with time (Eisenberg 1972). However, more systematic investigations of long-term effects of the use of stimulant medications are sorely needed.

Little is known about the predictors of treatment response or about the mechanism of action of stimulant drugs. The presence of "organic factors" has been claimed by a number of authors (Satterfield 1973) to predict a good response to stimulant treatment, but the findings have not always been consistent (Werry 1968).

In one of the few attempts to discover clinical predictors of response, Barcai (1971) found both the clinical interview and a "finger twitch test" to be useful in differentiating responders to amphetamine from nonresponders. With the child sitting opposite the examiner, hands hung between his knees in a normal position with the fingers moderately flexed, the interval between the start of the test and the time of the first twitch of a hand or finger was recorded. The finger twitch appeared in all nonresponders after 25 seconds and in 18 of 21 positive or equivocal responders before 25 seconds had elapsed. Items from the clinical interview with the child found most helpful in differentiating responders from nonresponders were the presence, in the drug responders, of: excess body movements, poor language ability, lack of ability to abstract and use imagination constructively, lack of adjustment to the values of society, and lack of planning ability.

Satterfield (1973) found that drug response was unrelated to family background while Conrad and Insel (1967) found that children whose parents were rated as "grossly deviant" or "socially incompetent" were less likely to respond positively to medication, even in the presence of other factors that tended to predict a good response. Other authors have noted that the attitude of the family to the child's taking medication is likely to affect treatment response. However, few studies have attempted to look at family variables in a systematic way.

In a series of studies, Satterfield and his associates (Satterfield et al 1974) found nine predictors of response to methylphenidate: low skin conductance level, high amplitude electroencephalogram, high energy in the low frequency band of the electroencephalogram, large amplitude evoked cortical response, slow recovery of the evoked response, an abnormal electroencephalogram, four or more "soft signs" on neurologic exam, more behavioral abnormalities reported by the teacher, and age (older children had a better response). Six of these predictors were electrophysiologic measures consistent with the hypothesis that the pathophysiology of most children with the hyperactive child syndrome is a low central nervous system arousal level.

Wender (1971) has proposed that the metabolism of the central neurotransmitters, serotonin, norepinephrine, and dopamine is abnormal in hyperactive children. He feels that the biochemical abnormality affects the behavior of these children by impairing the reward mechanism and the activating system of the brain. Thus he hypothesizes that these children have a diminished capacity for positive and negative affect, which he terms *anhedonia*. The differential effect of the two isomers of amphetamine, L-amphetamine and D-amphetamine, on the behavior of hyperactive children (Arnold et al 1973) offers indirect evidence that in some hyperactive children the disorder is mediated by dopaminergic systems and in others by norepinephrinergic systems. More direct studies of a possible metabolic abnormality have been limited. Wender et al (1971) failed to detect any difference in the metabolites of serotonin, norepinephrine, or dopamine in the urine of hyperactive children as compared to a group of normal children. However, the study population was very heterogeneous. Wender (1969) did find very low concentrations of serotonin in the blood platelets of three hyperactive children, all of whom were from the same family. In the rest of the study population the platelet serotonin levels were normal or in the borderline range. Coleman (1971) demonstrated low platelet serotonin concentrations in 88 percent of 25 hyperactive children. The two most hyperactive children in the group were studied in a research ward. Interestingly the serotonin concentration rose toward the normal range and the hyperactivity of the children lessened during the hospital stay. When both children returned home, the serotonin values dropped to prehospitalization levels and hyperactivity increased. Urinary monoamine metabolites in both of these children remained within normal limits during their hospital stay. Rapoport et al (1970) did find an inverse relationship between the degree of hyperactive behavior and urinary norepinephrine excretion within a group of hyperactive boys, but the mean 24-hour urinary catecholamine excretion did not differentiate the hyperactive group from a normal comparison group. In addition, there was an inverse relationship between response of the hyperactivity to D-amphetamine and urinary norepenephrine levels.

More systematic research in this area is sorely needed, with careful, comprehensive consideration of stimulus factors, response parameters, and social, familial, and organismic factors that might be related to treatment response (Conners 1972).

Other stimulants have also been tried. Magnesium pemoline (Cylert) is a weak central nervous system stimulant which has the advantage of a long duration of action so that one daily dose is sufficient. Preliminary results indicate that it decreases hyperactivity and produces improvement on the Performance Scale of the

WISC (Conners et al 1972; Millichap 1973). Deanol also acts as a central nervous system stimulant, possibly by being converted to acetylcholine within neurons. A recent review of the literature indicates that the better controlled studies with Deanol tended to show little or no drug effect and it is no longer considered to have any value in the treatment of hyperactive children (Conners 1973). Coffee (with caffeine the presumed active ingredient) twice a day has been reported to be as effective as methyphenidate in one study (Schnackenberg 1973). Preliminary results of well-controlled studies using caffeine tablets fail to substantiate this finding (Garfinkel et al 1975). The side effects of these central nervous system stimulants are similar to those of methylphenidate and D-amphetamine.

Antidepressants

The tricyclic antidepressant imipramine (Tofranil) has been found to be effective with 45 to 85 percent of hyperactive children by different investigators (Waizer et al 1974, Rapoport et al 1974). Mean doses in these studies ranged from 50 to 175 mg per day and this could explain the differences in results. However, the mean dose in the Huessy and Wright (1970) study was only 50 mg per day and they were able to employ a single bedtime dose with the therapeutic effect being evident the next day. This is distinctly different from the antidepressant effect of these medications, which take 2 to 3 weeks to occur. This nighttime dosage schedule offers a distinct advantage if future studies support the efficacy of imipramine. However, there is some indication that the likelihood of toxicity from imipramine is increased by a single dose at nighttime (Winsberg et al 1976). Main side effects include anorexia, nausea, weight loss, insomnia, and dry mouth. The results of the above studies are promising and in the future imipramine may be one of the major drugs used to treat hyperactive children. However, as of yet imipramine is not approved by the FDA for use with children under the age of 12, except for enuresis. Moreover, due to recent reports of EKG abnormalities in children treated with imipramine (Winsberg et al 1975) the FDA has decided to approve investigational protocols for the use of imipramine only within certain dose ranges for children of specified body weights, with regular EKG monitoring recommended.

Sedatives

There is general agreement that sedatives such as phenobarbital are usually contraindicated for hyperactive children (Conners 1972).

Antipsychotic and Antianxiety Agents

The rather large literature on the use of antipsychotic and antianxiety agents consists of mostly uncontrolled studies and contradictory findings (Sprague and Werry 1971). There is general agreement that the major tranquilizers produce deleterious effects on learning and cognitive functioning (Conners 1971).

Thioridazine (Mellaril) appears to be the most effective of the phenothiazines used with hyperactive children, although it has been used primarily in hyperactive children who are also mentally retarded and/or have demonstrable brain damage. By and large the phenothiazines are not as effective as the stimulant medications when used alone and are potentially more toxic (Conners 1972).

Antihistamines

Although the antihistamine diphenhydramine (benadryl) has been advocated by some (probably due to its sedative effect), the efficacy of this medication with hyperactive children has not yet been proven in a comparative trial using objective measures of evaluation (Fish 1975).

Anticonvulsants

The anticonvulsants are useful for the treatment of children with hyperactivity only if they also have epileptic seizures. There is no evidence that in the absence of seizure activity anticonvulsants are indicated for hyperactive children who have abnormal electroencephalograms. All drugs should be used to treat illnesses, not abnormal laboratory tests (Cantwell 1975e).

Lithium Carbonate

Lithium carbonate has been tried with varying success by several investigators (Greenhill et al 1973), but it is not as effective as the stimulants in treatment of the usual hyperactive child. In the extremely rare case of mania presenting with hyperactivity in a prepubertal child, lithium carbonate may be the treatment of choice.

Unanswered Questions About the Hyperactive Child Syndrome

While there is a large literature on the hyperactive child syndrome, there are a number of important unanswered questions about the syndrome that future investigations should focus on. Among these are the following:

How can children with the syndrome be divided into meaningful subgroups whose conditions differ in etiology, prognosis, and response to treatment?

What percentage of children with the hyperactive syndrome recover completely and at what age do they do so?

What are the factors within the child, within his family, or within his social milieu that predict which hyperactive child will develop into a healthy adult and which child will manifest in later life social and psychiatric pathology?

What treatment modalities influence the later life development of the hyperactive child and how do they do so?

These questions can only be answered by careful, long-term, prospective studies of large groups of hyperactive children, viewed from several different theoretical frameworks at several different points in time. The rewards from such investigative efforts should be great. In the meantime we must use all the therapeutic modalities at our disposal to intervene in children with this syndrome to prevent the poor outcome that now seems to be prevalent in a significant number (Cantwell 1975c). Although there is good evidence from double-blind controlled studies that stimulant medication is quite effective in reducing the maladaptive behavior and in improving learning in hyperactive children, none of these studies has demonstrated long-term efficacy or long-term safety. This is a critical research area for the future (Cantwell 1975c).

Summary

A critical review of the literature dealing with treatment of the hyperactive child reveals the following:

1. Central nervous system stimulants are effective for some symptoms with some children over the short term. Methylphenidate (Ritalin) seems to be the drug of choice with the amphetamines next in line.
2. Other drugs, in general, have not been found to be as effective as the stimulants, though the tricyclic antidepressant imipramine shows promise.
3. Little is known about how to predict whether an individual child will respond to a particular drug. However, several studies of groups of children indicate that there are neurologic, neurophysiologic, and family factors that are important predictors of response.

4. More information is needed about the long-term efficacy and safety of the medications currently used to treat hyperactive children.
5. Studies of other treatment modalities used with hyperactive children are fewer in number than the reports of drug studies and little is known about their long-term effects.
6. Involvement of the family is critical to the success of any management program with hyperactive children, but familial factors are rarely mentioned in studies of treatment.
7. Successful management of an individual hyperactive child will involve the use of multiple treatment approaches.

References

Arnold L: The art of medicating hyperkinetic children: A number of practical suggestions. Clin Pediatr 12:35–41, 1973

Barcai A: Predicting the response of children with learning disabilities and behavior problems to dextroamphetamine sulfate: The clinical interview and the finger twitch test. Pediatrics 47:73–80, 1971

Cantwell D: Familial genetic research with hyperactive children. In Cantwell D (ed): The Hyperactive Child: Diagnosis, Management and Current Research. New York, Spectrum, 1975a, pp 93–105

———: Epidemiology, clinical picture and classification of the hyperactive child syndrome. In Cantwell D (ed): The Hyperactive Child: Diagnosis, Management and Current Research. New York, Spectrum, 1975b, pp 3–15

———: Natural history and prognosis in the hyperactive child syndrome. In Cantwell D (ed): The Hyperactive Child: Diagnosis, Management and Current Research. New York, Spectrum, 1975c, pp 51–64

———: Diagnostic evaluation of the hyperactive child. In Cantwell D (ed): The Hyperactive Child: Diagnosis, Management, and Current Research. New York, Spectrum, 1975d, pp 17–50

———: A critical review of therapeutic modalities with hyperactive children. In Cantwell D (ed): The Hyperactive Child: Diagnosis, Management and Current Research. New York, Spectrum, 1975e, pp 173–189

Coleman M: Serotonin concentrations in whole blood of hyperactive children. J Pediatr 78:985–990, 1971

Conners CK: Deanol and behavior disorders in children: A critical review of the literature and recommended future studies for determining efficacy. Psychoparmacology Bulletin, Department of Health, Education, and Welfare, 1973, pp 188–95

———: Pharmacotherapy of psychopathology in children. In Quay H,

Werry J (eds): Psychopathological Disorders of Childhood. New York, Wiley, 1972, pp 316–348

——: Recent drug studies with hyperkinetic children. J Learn Disabil 4:476–483, 1971

——, Taylor E, Meo G, Kurtz M, Fournier M: Magnesium pemoline and dextroamphetamine: A controlled study in children with minimal brain dysfunction. Psychopharmacologica 26:321–336, 1972

Conrad W, Insel J: Anticipating the response to amphetamine therapy in the treatment of hyperkinetic children. Pediatrics 40:96–99, 1967

Department of Health, Education, and Welfare: Psychopharmacol Bull (Special Issue: Pharmacotherapy of children), 1973

Eisenberg L: The hyperkinetic child and stimulant drugs. N Engl J Med 287:249–250, 1972

——: Psychopharmacology in childhood: A critique. In Miller E (ed): Foundations of Child Psychiatry. New York, Pergamon, 1968, pp 625–641

——, Conners C, Sharpe L: A controlled study of the differential application of outpatient psychiatric treatment for children. Jpn J Child Psychiatry 6:125–132, 1965

Feighner A, Feighner J: Multi-modality treatment of the hyperkinetic child. Am J Psychiatry 131:459–463, 1974

Ferris RM, Tang, FLM, Maxwell RA: A comparison of the capacities of isomers of amphetamine deoxypipradol and methylphenidate to inhibit the uptake of tritiated catecholamines into rat cerebral cortex slices, synaptosomal preparations of rat cerebral cortex, hypothalamus and striatum and into adrenergic nerves of rabbit aorta. J Pharmacol Exp Ther 181:407–416, 1972

Fish B: Drug treatment of the hyperactive child. In Cantwell D: The Hyperactive Child: Diagnosis, Management and Current Research. New York, Spectrum, 1975, pp 109–127

Freedman D: Report on the conference on the use of stimulant drugs in the treatment of behaviorally disturbed young school children. Washington DC, Department of Health, Education and Welfare, 1971

Gardner RA: Psychotherapy of the psychogenic problems secondary to minimal brain dysfunction. Int J Child Psychother 2:224–256, 1973

Garfinkel B, Webster C, Sloman L: Methylphenidate and caffeine in the treatment of children with minimal brain dysfunction. Am J Psychiatry 132:723–728, 1975

Gofman H: Interval and final rating sheets on side effects. Psychopharmacology Bulletin (Special Issue: Pharmacotherapy of Children). Washington DC, U.S. Government Printing Office, 1973, pp 182–187

Greenhill L, Rieder R, Wender P, Buchsbaum M, Zahn T: Lithium carbonate in the treatment of hyperactive children. Arch Gen Psychiatry 28:636–640, 1973

Huessy H, Wright A: The use of imipramine in children's behavior disorders. Acta Paedopsychiatr 37:194–199, 1970

Millichap J: Drugs in management of minimal brain dysfunction. Ann NY Acad Sci 205:321–334, 1973

Rapoport J, Quinn P, Bradbard G, Riddle K, Brooks E: Imipramine and methylphenidate treatments of hyperactive boys. Arch Gen Psychiatry 30:789–793, 1974

———, Lott I, Alexander D, Abramson A: Urinary noradrenaline and playroom behaviour in hyperactive boys. Lancet 2:1141, 1970

Rutter M, Graham P, Yule W: A Neuropsychiatric Study in Childhood. Philadelphia, Lippincott, 1970a

———, Tizard J, Whitmore K: Education Health and Behaviour: Psychological and Medical Study of Childhood Development. New York, Wiley, 1970b

Safer D, Allen R: Long-term side effects of stimulants in children. Presented at 126th annual meeting of the American Psychiatric Association, 1973

Satterfield J: EEG issues in children with minimal brain dysfunction. Semin Psychiatry 5:35–46, 1973

———, Cantwell D, Satterfield B: Pathophysiology of the hyperactive child syndrome. Arch Gen Psychiatry 31:839–844, 1974

Schain R, Reynard C: Observations on effects of a central stimulant drug (methylphenidate) in children with hyperactive behavior. Pediatrics 55:709–716, 1975

Schnackenberg RC: Caffeine as a substitute for Schedule II stimulants in hyperkinetic children. Am J Psychiatry 130:796–798, 1973

Sprague R: Psychopharmacology and learning disabilities. J Operational Psychiatry 3:56–67, 1972

———, Sleator E: Effects of psychopharmacologic agents on learning disorders. Pediatr Clin North Am 20:719, 1973

———, Werry J: Psychotropic drugs and handicapped children. In Mann L, Sabatino D (eds): Second Review of Special Education. Philadelphia, JSE Press, 1974, pp 1–50

———, Werry J: Methodology of psychopharmacological studies with the retarded. In Ellis N (ed): International Review of Research in Mental Retardation, Vol 5. New York, Academic, 1971, pp 147–219

———, Christensen D, Werry J: Experimental psychology and stimulant drugs. In Conners CK (ed): Clinical Use of Stimulant Drugs in Children. The Hague, Excerpta Medica, 1974, pp 141–164

Waizer J, Hoffman SP, Polizos P, Engelhardt DM: Outpatient treatment of hyperactive school children with imipramine. Am J Psychiatry 131:587–591, 1974

Wender PH: Minimal Brain Dysfunction in Children. New York, Wiley, 1971

————: Platelet serotonin level in children with "minimal brain dysfunction." Lancet 2:1012, 1969

————, Epstein R, Kopin I, Gordon E: Urinary monoamine metabolites in children with minimal brain dysfunction. Am J Psychiatry 127:1411–1415, 1971

Werry J: Studies on the hyperactive child. IV. An empirical analysis of the minimal brain dysfunction syndrome. Arch Gen Psychiatry 19:9–16, 1968

————, Sprague R: Psychopharmacology. In Wortis J (ed): Mental Retardation IV. New York, Grune, 1972, pp 63–79

————, Sprague R, Weiss G, Minde K: Some clinical and laboratory studies of psychotropic drugs in children: An overview. In Smith WL (ed): Drugs and Cerebral Function. Springfield, Ill., Thomas, 1970, pp 134–144

Winsberg B, Yepes L, Bialer I: Psychopharmacological management of children with hyperactive /aggressive /inattentive behavior disorders: A guide for the pediatrician. Clin Pediatr, 15:471–477, 1976

————, Goldstein S, Yepes LE, Perel JM: Imipramine and electrocardiographic abnormalities in hyperactive children. Am J Psychiatry 132:542–545, 1975

————, Press M, Bialer I, Kupietz S: Dextroamphetamine and methylphenidate in the treatment of hyperactive /aggressive children. Pediatrics 53:236–241, 1974

drug treatment
of anxiety

commentary

The incidence of anxiety in our population, although common, is hard to determine because it is a subjective feeling. Anxiety can be measured by a number
of psychologic tests of varying reliability and validity and can coexist with mental
or physical illness. It is the most common symptomatic drive for psychotherapy,
but for most patients who have neither the time, money, nor inclination for
psychotherapy, a combination of support and pharmacotherapy is the treatment
of choice.

Today, the benzodiazepines, particularly diazepam (Valium), appear to be
preferred, since they are more effective and safer than other sedative hypnotic
drugs. They do not eliminate anxiety but do reduce its unpleasantness.
Whenever possible the cause of anxiety should be identified and dealt with, but
antianxiety drugs often provide welcome relief.

Dr. Rickels has drawn upon his extensive experience in dealing with this
symptom in describing the uses and limitations of the antianxiety drugs. Sleep
disturbances are another manifestation of anxiety and are treated with the
same drugs (p 327). Small wonder that the benzodiazepines are the most
widely prescribed drugs in the world today.

drug treatment
of anxiety*

Karl Rickels, M.D.

Each year millions of patients visit physicians for relief of tensions, fears, worries, anxieties, and depression. Most physicians have found psychopharmacologic agents, prescribed within the context of supportive, manipulative, ventilating or nonexploratory, as well as dynamic and insight-oriented psychotherapy, most useful for alleviating these disturbing emotions. Psychopharmacologic agents do not, of course, represent a panacea for all neurotic ills. They do not, for example, directly affect the psychodynamic and environmental factors responsible for emotional problems; they do not, at least in a direct sense, affect the characterologic or personality side of the patient (Joyce 1971). By relieving symptoms of anxiety, tension, and depression, however, they often render a patient less miserable and able to cope with intra- and extrapsychic stress more appropriately.

To achieve good therapeutic results it is of utmost importance that psychopharmacologic agents be prescribed appropriately. The physician who uses these agents to achieve unobtainable goals rather than for symptomatic relief or as a vehicle of rejection rather than within the context of a supportive relationship, will see only few beneficial effects. In other words, drugs must be prescribed for the right reasons. To achieve good results it is equally important that the physician be knowledgeable about psychopharmacologic agents. Even if prescribed for the right reasons, the wrong agent or the right

*This work was supported by USPHS research grants 17H-08957 and 17H-08958.

agent, given in the wrong treatment regimen, will not prove helpful to the patient.

This paper deals with the use of antianxiety agents in nonpsychotic anxiety, including the "garden variety of anxiety" commonly seen in psychiatric but even more often in nonpsychiatric practice.

What Is Anxiety?

Anxiety is perceived as a subjective feeling of heightened tension and diffused uneasiness, defined as the conscious and reportable experience of intense dread and foreboding, conceptualized as internally derived and unrelated to external threat. It is not merely fear because it lacks a specific object. It is a painful dread of situations which covertly symbolize unconscious conflict and impulses.

The many symptoms of anxiety are attributable to the fact that anxiety, more than any other type of emotional disorder, can induce widespread physiologic changes. Anxiety is perceived as a threat arising primarily from within, triggering somatic and visceral responses through the autonomic nervous system and the hypothalamic-pituitary-endocrine system (Lader 1974). Frequently some remembrance of a past threat, triggered by some unrecognized present situation, signals a feeling tone and somatic responses of the past fearful state.

Anxiety can be partly bound by such mechanisms as phobias, obsessions, and conversions or it can be diverted into the soma, leading to somatization. In fact, pure anxiety states are relatively rare because such syndromes as depression, hysteria, hypochondriasis, somatization, phobias, and obsessional thinking are often concomitantly present. Also, in my experience the acutely ill, anxious, or depressed neurotic patient is actually in the minority and the more chronically ill neurotic patient is more and more frequently seen.

Anxiety can be operationally defined in terms of scores on such patient-completed checklists as the Hopkins Symptom Checklist (HSCL) (Derogatis et al 1974) and on such physician scales as the Hamilton Anxiety (Hamilton 1959) or Physician Anxiety Questionnaire (Rickels and Howard 1970).

How Drugs May Be Used to Alleviate Anxiety

The combination of support and pharmacotherapy seems to be the treatment of choice for millions of patients who cannot deal with their emotions in a verbal or symbolic way, ie, who cannot think in abstract terms, or who cannot tolerate the emotional intimacy of the transference-countertransference relationship in psychotherapy. It also represents an appropriate first treatment approach for all anxious patients who have not responded to some supportive intervention or with patients who do not respond to pharmacologic treatment in family practice and are referred for psychiatric consultation. Talking with a friend, a priest, or a physician is often of great help to many who suffer from anxiety and, in fact, may be all that is needed by some, particularly those who suffer from a rather acute situational anxiety episode. More often, however, anxious patients need something more, that is, they need additional pharmacologic treatment, at least for a limited period of time.

Drugs not only bring about change through their pharmacologic effects but also induce psychologically based improvement by serving as an indication to the patient of the doctor's knowledge and interest in him. In other words the doctor helps, and this realization leads to psychologic improvement (Rickels 1968).

Regrettably, pure obsessive-compulsive, dissociated, and phobic states, as well as conversion hysteria, either fail to respond or respond only mildly to antianxiety agents. Such treatment modalities as behavior modification and psychotherapy, with or without the concomitant use of medication, have also proven relatively unsuccessful in these conditions.

Antianxiety Drugs

Pharmacologic Actions

The newer antianxiety agents, such as meprobamate and chlordiazepoxide, have pharmacologic effects resembling the older sedatives. They depress the central nervous system to various degrees, depending on dosage. Mild depression often results in the desired therapeutic effect, that is, relief of anxiety occurs, which may or may not, depending on dosage, be accompanied by some degree of impairment in various psychologic functions. Larger doses may cause sleep, and toxic doses produce coma. Many of these drugs are anticonvulsive by virtue of depressing the motor cortex. Blockage of spinal cord internuncial neurons, as well as sedative effects, contribute to varying degrees of muscle relaxant action. Overdoses are usually manifested by weakness, lack of coordination, and placidity.

The newer antianxiety agents differ somewhat in their pharmacologic action from the antihistamines or phenothiazines and the differences are of clinical importance. The phenothiazines have unique pharmacologic properties and produce a somewhat different type of sedation from the other antianxiety agents. Antihistamines are also anticholinergics and, like the phenothiazines, produce a different type of sedation. These differences may limit their clinical acceptance by patients but at the same time militate against the possibility of serious abuse.

Clinical Efficacy and Safety

Table 1 gives the antianxiety agents most widely used today. Most clinicians would agree that the order of efficacy for these agents ranges from the barbiturates, through meprobamate, to the benzodiazepine derivatives, probably the most effective antianxiety agents today (Rickels 1968, Klerman 1974).

Hydroxyzine, an antihistamine with sedative properties, has generally been found rather disappointing unless given in daily doses of 400 mg, a regimen associated with marked sedation (Rickels 1968). Chlormezanone appears closer in clinical efficacy to the barbiturates

TABLE 1
MINOR TRANQUILIZERS (ANTIANXIETY DRUGS)

Antianxiety Agent		Total Daily Dose (mg) (divided in 2 to 4 doses)
Substituted Propanediols (glycol or glycerol derivatives)		
Meprobamate	(Miltown, Equanil)	800–3200
Tybamate	(Solacen)	750–3000
Benzodiazepines		
Chlordiazepoxide	(Librium)	15–100
Diazepam	(Valium)	5–60
Oxazepam	(Serax)	30–120
Clorazepate	(Tranxene)	15–60
Diphenylmethane Antihistamines		
Hydroxyzine	(Atarax, Vistaril)	100–400
Miscellaneous Compounds		
Chlormezanone	(Trancopal)	200–800
Barbiturates		
Phenobarbital		60–150
Butabarbital	(Butisol)	60–150

than to the benzodiazepines (Rickels et al 1974), and tybamate seems effective only in rather severe neurotic disorders and is not very widely used. Chlorazepate, the most recently introduced antianxiety agent, is claimed to be equal in effect to diazepam but produces fewer side effects (Cooper et al 1973). Whether these findings can be confirmed, or will prove simply dosage related, has yet to be demonstrated.

In regard to the clinical safety of antianxiety agents, it should be mentioned that the concomitant use of alcohol is often considered an important public health problem. The minor tranquilizers, given in conventional doses, apparently do not potentiate the already present detrimental effects of alcohol, as assessed in a number of behavioral and cognitive measures (Kielholz et al 1967). In contrast, a recent study did show that diazepam enhanced the effects of alcohol in a 40-minute driving test (Linnoila and Hakkinen 1974). Like most other studies in which the combined effects of alcohol and antianxiety drugs was tested, however, this study was carried out only in nonanxious patients. It should be noted that untreated anxiety may also result in seriously impaired driving ability. In general, and at least according to presently available evidence, it seems possible that too much clinical importance has been attached to the dangers of combining alcohol, lightly consumed, with antianxiety agents, taken according to regular drug-usage patterns.

Turning now to such aspects of clinical safety as suicide potential, withdrawal reactions, and addiction, it should be noted that the newer antianxiety agents are clearly superior to the barbiturates. In fact, an individual would find it practically impossible to kill himself with the benzodiazepines alone. There have been some reports of withdrawal reactions for the newer antianxiety agents (Rickels 1968) but only for patients treated for long periods of time, with excessive doses, and only when medication is stopped abruptly (Covi 1973). A certain, even if mild, potential for addiction does exist for the newer antianxiety agents (Rickels 1968) but is probably to be expected only in those patients previously addicted to the barbiturates, opiates, or alcohol. Habituation may even be limited within these individuals, as the newer antianxiety agents do not provide comparable gratification, since euphoria is usually absent.

Warnings concerning the abuse of various antianxiety agents continue to be issued despite clinical evidence of their relative safety. In the opinion of this investigator, it is time to dispel the myth that the unsuspecting patient must be protected from the careless prescribing of dangerous drugs likely to produce lifelong addiction. The newer antianxiety agents, so widely prescribed by physicians, are simply not dangerous, and indeed have a low addiction potential.

Also, extensive experience in the drug treatment of neurotic patients indicates that these individuals take *less* not *more* medication than prescribed. To discourage the use of an effective agent because a very limited group of patients, such as heroin addicts or alcoholics, may misuse such a drug seems indefensible.

Furthermore, it seems to this investigator that far too much importance is attached to warnings about the "psychologic dependence" patients may develop with antianxiety agents. Granting that some patients may come to use these agents as an occasional crutch, is this necessarily so harmful? Such dependency is clearly less expensive and may even be less hazardous than reliance on a physician's continued support. Freud's "psychoanalysis interminable" comes to mind. Dependent persons will simply depend on something or someone for support, and taking an occasional pill for emotional problems hardly seems cause for great concern.

Barbiturates

A frequent question confronting the physician treating anxiety is whether or not the newer, more expensive tranquilizers do indeed differ from such older sedatives as phenobarbital. Figure 1 gives representative data on this question from a large-scale study comparing diazepam, the most effective agent in the study (Hesbacher et al 1970b). Similar results have been observed when global improvement obtained with chlordiazepoxide, the barbiturates, and placebo, is compared. In fact this order of efficacy is probably found in most published studies to date.

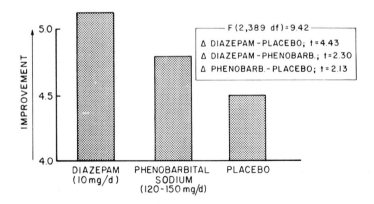

Fig. 1.   Global clinical improvement after two weeks of treatment.

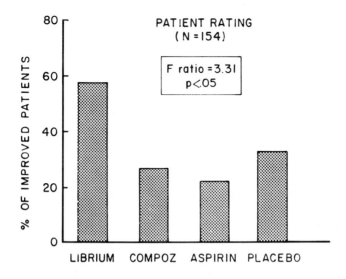

Fig. 2.   Patients rated as moderately or markedly improved.

Besides their lesser efficacy, the barbiturates possess several other disadvantages that render them less appropriate for the treatment of anxiety than the newer antianxiety agents. Compared to the minor tranquilizers, particularly to the benzodiazepines, barbiturates produce more frequent and more severe sedative side effects (Hesbacher et al 1970a), are considerably more toxic, stimulate microsomal liver enzymes, are much more successful suicide agents (Berger 1967, Hollister 1966), and have a higher dependency and addiction potential.

Over-the-Counter Sedatives

A discussion of antianxiety agents would be remiss without some comparison of their short-term effectiveness to that of the over-the-counter (proprietary) sedatives. In a 2-week double-blind trial conducted by this research group (Rickels and Hesbacher 1973), chlordiazepoxide (30 mg /day) was demonstrated to be far more effective than a widely used proprietary daytime sedative, as well as aspirin and placebo (Fig. 2). The latter three agents, in fact, produced a rather similar and very minimal degree of improvement. In contrast, 60 percent of patients on chlordiazepoxide reported moderate or marked improvement after only 2 weeks of treatment. The lesson is clear: proprietary sedatives are no replacement for antianxiety agents (see p 345).

Phenothiazines and Other Antipsychotic Drugs

Phenothiazines are used primarily in the treatment of prepsychotic and psychotic patients and only infrequently for neurotic patients. In fact, in most neurotic anxiety conditions these neuroleptics are generally prescribed only if established antianxiety agents, such as meprobamate, chlordiazepoxide, or diazepam, have proven ineffective. Even in the lower doses used for neurotic patients, phenothiazines may produce disturbing side effects, including mild symptoms of akathisia or inner restlessness, thereby increasing rather than decraasing the patient's anxiety. In addition, long-term use of these agents involves the danger of irreversible tardive dyskinesia.

Other Drugs Used in Anxiety

Beta-adrenergic blocking agents are proposed for the symptomatic treatment of anxiety, particularly in England (Ramsay et al 1973, Lader 1974) but have yet to be approved for anxiety in the United States. While these agents do effect a demonstrable decrease in heart palpitations, which may or may not be related to anxiety, there is little direct evidence of their anxiolytic properties, and this investigator questions their utility.

There is clinical evidence that the tricyclics, and imipramine in particular, are effective in certain "panic anxiety" states (Klein 1964).

Antianxiety Agents in Anxious Depression

About 70 percent of all neurotic depressed patients can be classified as anxious depressed. It is of considerable clinical interest, then, that such minor tranquilizers as meprobamate and the benzodiazepines (diazepam, in particular), given in relatively high daily dosages, as well as a number of phenothiazines, have been found effective in alleviating anxious depression (Hollister et al 1971, Rickels et al 1967, 1973). In fact, a trial of about 4 weeks with a minor tranquilizer such as diazepam may represent the most appropriate treatment approach for depressed patients who suffer from concomitant symptoms of anxiety and agitation but not retardation. Should such treatment prove unsatisfactory, the more powerful and relatively more toxic antidepressants could then be prescribed.

Response of Specific Symptoms to Antianxiety Drugs

Based largely on research conducted with the Hopkins Symptom Checklist (HSCL) (Derogatis et al 1974) in a variety of anxious samples, it has been found that antianxiety agents are considerably more effective in alleviating symptoms of anxiety and somatization than in relieving obsessive-compulsive (performance difficulty) and interpersonal sensitivity complaints. Similarly, Klerman and associates (1974), in a study comparing drug therapy and psychotherapy in depression, reported that drugs are not very effective in improving interpersonal disturbances, and that psychotherapy appears a more effective modality for patients who suffer from maladaptive behavior patterns. Present evidence thus suggests that the response to antianxiety agents is likely to be particularly good in patients who are initially higher in anxious and somatic complaints and lower in obsessive-compulsive and interpersonal sensitivity symptoms.

The effect of the benzodiazepines, particularly chlordiazepoxide, on another symptom dimension, namely, hostility, should also be mentioned here. Several studies conducted with normal volunteers have reported that chlordiazepoxide caused increases in hostility, as measured with the Buss-Durkee Hostility Inventory (DiMascio et al 1969). Within anxious patients, however, this group has found that hostility and irritability, as rated by both patient and physician, are reduced significantly more by chlordiazepoxide than by placebo (Rickels and Downing 1974). This differential reduction was found to occur in relatively high as well as low anxious patients.

Comments on the Appropriate Prescribing of Antianxiety Agents

A flexible approach, based on the individual patient's needs, is urged for antianxiety drug treatment. For example, antianxiety agents should be titrated for the individual patient, as drug plasma levels, assessed for the same doses, may vary widely from patient to patient (Greenblatt and Shader 1974). Within this context, it should be noted that sedative side effects often decrease, without dosage adjustment, within a few weeks, allowing for increases in dose at this time in patients who do not begin to show improvement.

The choice of a specific antianxiety agent is largely empirical, and most physicians, quite correctly initiate treatment with agents most familiar to them. As noted earlier, however, the barbiturates should not be considered the drugs of first choice. At present, the benzodiazepines, primarily chlordiazepoxide and diazepam, as well as meprobamate, represent the antianxiety agents of choice.

Drug treatment should be employed only when warranted by the patient's degree of disability or discomfort and should be primarily symptom oriented. Duration of treatment should be influenced by duration of symptoms. Thus, many more acutely ill anxious patients

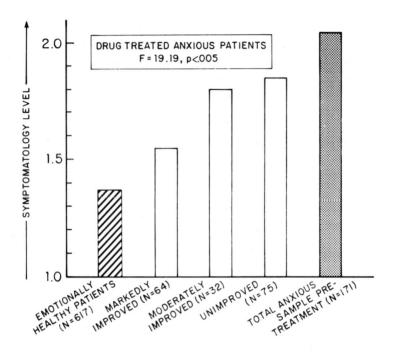

Fig. 3. Symptom levels reached by drug-treated anxious patients: HSCL total score.

may require treatment for only a few weeks, as anxiety complaints are often short-lived and of a situational nature. Within these acutely anxious patients, the main function of drug treatment is generally to render the patient less miserable until his anxiety attack runs its course.

More chronically anxious patients, however, often require longer periods of treatment. Indeed, there is considerable clinical evidence to suggest that many anxious patients show a low tendency to improve over conventional short treatment periods, even when effective medications are used. Figure 3 gives representative data on chlordiazepoxide-treated patients from a 4-week trial in which study medication was consistently and significantly demonstrated superior to placebo. It will be noted that many patients have shown little improvement, and that those reporting marked improvement, as a group, failed to reach symptom levels of "emotionally healthy" patients from the same treatment setting. In fact, according to most clinical trials of 4 to 6 weeks duration, rarely do more than 40 to 50 percent of anxious patients come close to reaching normal symptom levels.

There is also evidence to suggest that many anxious patients continue to remain relatively symptomatic for some time after participating in short-term trials. Thus, 6-month follow-up data for a large sample of patients showed that no further improvement had occurred for the group as a whole since the end of their clinical trials. Indeed, slight improvement at 6 months was noted only for those patients who had reported no improvement with study treatment, and many of these patients had received subsequent psychiatric intervention. Moderately improved patients reported no further improvement, and most disturbing, markedly improved patients had become somewhat more symptomatic. Data such as these suggest that many anxious patients have relatively enduring symptoms for which short-term drug treatment appears inadequate.

What can the physician do to bring about improvement in those patients who remain far from symptom-free following short-term drug treatment? Should he continue the same agent in a different regimen, try a new agent, or turn to some form of nondrug treatment? How soon should alternative drug or nondrug treatment be instituted in patients reporting no improvement or only minimal improvement with a given agent? How long should treatment be continued, and at what dosages, in order to maintain improvement in those patients who do experience moderate-to-marked relief of their symptoms? It is indeed regrettable that no data are currently available to answer these most important questions. These data can only be obtained from studies evaluating the efficacy of long-term antianxiety drug treatment in securing maximal improvement for the chronically anxious patient. The need for such maintenance studies cannot be overstated.

Some suggestions related to the drug treatment of chronically anxious patients are offered here. First, this investigator is convinced that many anxious patients do, in fact, require a more protracted course of pharmacologic treatment than is generally provided. Some may even need a form of maintenance treatment similar to that of diabetics receiving insulin. Within such patients, the physician may periodically discontinue medication in order to determine whether anxiety does return and further medication is needed. It should be emphasized that the longer the patient is treated with minor tranquilizers, the more carefully he should be monitored for possible mild withdrawal symptoms or dependency effects when medication is temporarily discontinued. Also, physicians can practically eliminate withdrawal symptoms by decreasing medication in two or three steps.

It is also true that some anxious patients who fail to respond to drug treatment within conventionally short periods of time may need such nondrug approaches, either alone or in combination with drug treatment, as family therapy, marriage counselling, or group or individual psychotherapy. Present findings suggest that this may be particularly appropriate for patients who are only mildly anxious, who are high in obsessive-compulsive and performance difficulty complaints, and who have marked problems in their interpersonal relations. The clinician should also consider whether some patients who are not responding well to antianxiety agents are actually latent depressives who might be better treated with antidepressants. In fact, it is a good practice to review the diagnosis of any patient who does not respond to antianxiety agents within a reasonable period of time in order to determine whether an underlying depression, a pseudoneurotic schizophrenic or pan-neurotic illness, or some major characterologic problem has been overlooked.

Nondrug Factors in Drug Therapy

Research has clearly established that many nonpharmacologic factors have a profound impact on the outcome of pharmacologic

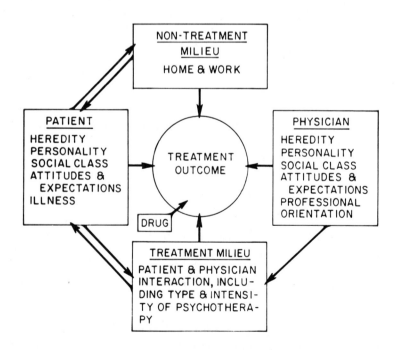

Fig. 4.   Nonspecific variables in drug therapy.

TABLE 2
CONSISTENT REPLICATED PREDICTORS OF IMPROVEMENT IN PATIENTS TREATED WITH DIAZEPAM (10-20 MG/DAY) (N = 184) OR CHLORDIAZEPOXIDE (40-60 MG/DAY) (N = 254) BASED ON ZERO ORDER CORRELATIONS

Patient	Illness and Treatment Related
Employed	Acute duration
More educated	None or few previous drugs
Expects drug treatment	Good response to previous drugs
Knows problems are emotional	No concurrent medical illness
Married	Precipitating stress present
Female without menopause or hysterectomy	

Physician	Presenting psychopathology HSCL
Good prognosis	Low in obsessive-compulsive
Feels comfortable with patient	Low in interpersonal sensitivity
Feels comfortable prescribing drugs	Low in depression
	High in anxiety
	High in somatization

treatment. Figure 4 summarizes some of the patient, physician, treatment milieu, and nontreatment milieu factors which almost invariably occur in endless combinations and affect treatment response. Since anxiety is often characterized by fluctuating symptoms and a high placebo response, these nondrug factors are particularly important for response to antianxiety agents. Indeed, any attempt to predict how anxious, neurotic patients will respond to drug treatment must take these factors into account.

Considerable research effort has been directed toward determining which nondrug factors predict a positive response to antianxiety agents. Table 2 summarizes some of the more consistent and replicated predictors that have emerged from correlational analyses conducted with patients treated in short-term trials with the two most widely used benzodiazepines, namely, chlordiazepoxide and diazepam. It will be noted that the predictors obtained often tend to be interrelated, eg, "employed" and "more educated," "acute duration," and "none or few previous drugs." The interrelated nature of nondrug factors makes accurate assessment of their independent contributions to treatment outcome most difficult. More research is clearly needed in this area, and research directed toward determining which factors predict better response to some agents than to others should prove of particular interest to the clinician. Even so, the data presented in Table 2 are not without value to the practicing physician.

For example, they indicate to the physician that he can expect good results with antianxiety agents, and with the benzodiazepines in particular, in patients who are relatively well educated and employed, who know that their problems are emotional and expect drug treatment, and who have received few previous drugs and reported a good prior drug response. He may expect even better results if he feels comfortable with the patient and has a positive attitude toward prescribing drugs. These data also support previously reported findings by showing that best results are to be obtained in patients high in anxious and somatic complaints and low in obsessive-compulsive, interpersonal sensitivity, and depressive symptoms.

In addition, these data indicate to the physician which patients may not benefit greatly from the routine prescribing of antianxiety agents. Thus, the physician may decide that minor tranquilizers alone, without additional supportive therapy or perhaps the assistance of social agencies, will be of little help to patients who are poorly educated, unemployed, and possibly living in dire social and economic circumstances. Also, the physician may make an effort to instill more appropriate attitudes and expectations before prescribing antianxiety agents to patients who believe that their problems are physical rather than psychologic, who expect nondrug treatment, or who have negative drug treatment expectations because of past drug experiences. In these ways, the physician may use a knowledge of nondrug factors to obtain a favorable response in patients who might otherwise have responded poorly to antianxiety drugs.

In conclusion, the minor tranquilizers, particularly the benzodiazepines, chlordiazepoxide, and diazepam, as well as meprobamate, represent safe and effective agents for the symptomatic treatment of neurotic anxiety. Yet, even in clinical trials demonstrating their significant superiority to placebo, it has been observed that only a minority of drug-treated anxious patients generally report marked improvement. The majority of anxious patients appear to remain relatively symptomatic following short periods of drug treatment and many fail to show any improvement at all. In addition, those patients who do report marked improvement in 4- to 6-week drug trials often fail to reach the symptom levels of normal persons, and have a tendency to become more symptomatic again over time.

To this investigator, these data suggest that many patients treated with antianxiety agents for conventionally short periods of time represent chronically anxious patients who cannot be expected to improve with such inadequate treatment. Indeed, it seems that an often unwarranted concern for protecting the anxious patient from over-medication may have created an atmosphere in which physicians often tend to undertreat the anxious patient. The result is that many anxious patients do not obtain maximal drug benefits. What is needed is not more cautious but more appropriate drug usage.

References

Berger FM: The role of drugs in suicide. In Yochelson L (ed): Symposium on Suicide. Washington D.C., George Washington University, 1967

Cooper AJ, Magnus RV, Rose M, et al: Controlled trial of dipotassium chlorazepate ('Tranxene') in anxiety. Br J Psychiatry 123:475–476, 1973

Covi L, Lipman RS, Pattison JH, Derogatis LR, Uhlenhuth EH: Length of treatment with anxiolytic sedatives and response to their sudden withdrawal. Acta Psychiat Scand 49:51–64, 1973

Derogatis LR, Lipman RS, Rickels K, Uhlenhuth EH, Covi L: The Hopkins Symptom Checklist (HSCL): a measure of primary symptoms dimensions. In Pichot P (ed): Psychological Measurements in Psychopharmacology. Modern Problems in Pharmacopsychiatry, Basel, Karger, 7:79–110, 1974

DiMascio A, Shader RI, Harmatz J: Psychotropic drugs and induced hostility. Psychosomatics 10:46–47, 1969

Greenblatt DJ, Shader RI: Benzodiazepines in Clinical Practice. New York, Raven, 1974

Hamilton M: The assessment of anxiety states by rating. Br J Med Psychol 32:50–55, 1959

Hesbacher PT, Rickels K, Gordon PE, et al: Setting, patient and doctor effects on drug response in neurotic patients: I. Differential attrition, dosage deviation and side reaction responses to treatment. Psychopharmacologia 18:180–208, 1970a

———, Rickels K, Hutchison J, et al: Setting, patient, and doctor effects on drug response in neurotic patients: II. Differential improvement. Psychopharmacologia 18:209–226, 1970b

Hollister LE: Overdoses of psychotherapeutic drugs. Clin Pharmacol Ther 7:142–146, 1966

———, Overall JE, Pokorny AD, Shelton J: Acetophenazine and diazepam in anxious depressions. Arch Gen Psychiatry 24:273–378, 1971

Joyce CRB: Can drugs affect personality? In Ramsey IT, Porter R (eds): Ciba Foundation Symposium on Personality and Science. London, Churchill Livingstone, 1971, pp 65–72

Kielholz P, Goldberg L, Obersteg J, et al: Circulation routière, tranquillisants et alcohol. Hyg Ment 2:39–60, 1967

Klein DF: Delineation of two drug-responsive anxiety syndromes. Psychopharmacologia 5:397–408, 1964

Klerman GL: Psychotropic drugs as therapeutic agents. Hastings Center Studies 2:81–93, 1974

———, DiMascio A, Weissman M, Prusoff B, Paykel ES: Treatment of depression by drugs and psychotherapy. Am J Psychiatry 131:186–191, 1974

Lader M: The peripheral and central role of the catecholamines in the mechanisms of anxiety. Int Pharmacopsychiat 9:125–137, 1974

Linnoila M, Häkkinen S: Effects of diazepam and codeine, alone and in combination with alcohol, on simulated driving. Clin Pharmacol Ther 15:368–373, 1974

Ramsay I, Greer S, Bagley C: Propranolol in neurotic and thyrotoxic anxiety. Br J Psychiatry 122:555–560, 1973

Rickels, K: Anti-neurotic agents: Specific and non-specific effects, In Efron DH, Cole JO, Levine J, Wittenborn JR (eds): Psychopharmacology: A Review of Progress, 1957–1967. Public Health Service publication 1836, 1968, pp 231–247

———, Chung HR, Feldman HS, et al: Amitriptyline, diazepam, and phenobarbital sodium in depressed outpatients. J Nerv Ment Dis 157:442–451, 1973

———, Downing RW: Chlordiazepoxide and hostility in anxious outpatients. Am J Psychiatry 131:442–444, 1974

———, Hesbacher PT: Over-the-counter daytime sedatives: A controlled study. JAMA 223:29–33, 1973

———, Howard K: The physician questionnaire: A useful tool in psychiatric drug research. Psychopharmacologia 17:338–344, 1970

———, Pereira-Ogan JA, Case WG, et al: Chlormezanone in anxiety: A drug rediscovered? Am J Psychiatry 131:592–595, 1974

———, Raab E, De Silverio R, Etemad B: Drug treatment in depression: antidepressant or tranquilizer? JAMA 201:675–681, 1967

hypnotic and sedative agents

commentary

Anxiety and insomnia are two symptoms very commonly encountered in medical practice. The sedative hypnotic agents are used to treat these symptoms, in lower sedative doses for anxiety and in higher hypnotic doses for insomnia. These drugs include ethyl alcohol, the barbiturates, meprobamate, and a variety of nonbarbiturates, including chloral hydrate and the benzodiazepines. All have the properties of inducing a pleasant state of drunkenness characterized by incoordination, disequilibrium, nystagmus and dysarthria, and electroencephalographic changes when sufficiently high doses are reached; all are pleasantly reinforcing so that patient cooperation in taking them is generally not a problem—stopping may be. Tolerance and dependence are the main problems associated with the popular sedative hypnotic drugs.

A variety of other drugs used to induce sleep includes bromides, phenothiazines, antihistamines, anticholinergics, and others. These can induce sleep, but their side effects are either unpleasant or dangerous, and patients do not prefer them even though they are commonly found in over-the-counter preparations (p 345).

Dr. Jaffe gives us a comprehensive account of the uses and dangers of drugs in treating anxiety and insomnia.

hypnotic and sedative agents

Jerome H. Jaffe, M.D.

This chapter discusses the uses of a chemically heterogeneous group of drugs generally referred to as the sedative-hypnotics. This group included such drugs as the barbiturates, chloral hydrate and its derivatives, paraldehyde, ethylchlorvynol, ethinamate, meprobamate, glutethimide, methyprylon, methaqualone, and certain benzodiazepines, especially flurazepam and nitrazepam. At low doses, these compounds have in common the capacity to produce the type of reversible general depression of the central nervous system that is associated with feelings of relaxation and drowsiness; at slightly higher doses they induce sleep, and at still higher doses they produce severe central nervous system depression and coma. While the precise mechanisms by which this diverse group of drugs exerts their actions is uncertain, it is probable that they depress tissue excitability through an action on the cell membrane. Transmission at synaptic junctions seems particularly sensitive to this action, and synapses in both the central and autonomic nervous systems are affected (Harvey 1975, Byck 1975, Greenblatt and Shader 1974).

Until quite recently the preponderant view was that within this broad and diverse grouping there was no clear distinction between antianxiety, sedative, and hypnotic drugs; with proper adjustment of dose any drug could be used to produce a reduction of anxiety, a state of sedation or, with somewhat higher doses, induction of sleep (Hollister 1972, Greenblatt and Shader 1972). Furthermore, all of these compounds seem to share other common effects on the central nervous system and on behavior, such as muscle relaxation and the disinhibition of behavior that has been suppressed by punishment

(Harvey 1975, Greenblatt and Shader 1974, McMillan 1975). They also share a generally similar pattern of side effects and psychomotor impairment. Such a view would imply that despite chemical heterogeneity, these drugs may all act in a similar fashion, and that whatever differences exist are due to variations in absorption, metabolism, and central nervous system distribution.

Some studies, however, suggest that differences between certain classes of drugs, eg, the barbiturates and the benzodiazepines, may be qualitative as well as quantitative and that the benzodiazepines may be exerting some of their effects on different neurotransmitters or neuronal systems (Greenblatt and Shader 1974). For example, the antianxiety effects of the benzodiazepines seem to be accompanied by less drowsiness than older agents. The benzodiazepines also seem to produce less respiratory depression for a given degree of sedation than the barbiturates (Greenblatt and Shader 1974, Gasser et al 1975), an effect that is of some practical importance in view of the frequency with which hypnotic drugs are used in suicide attempts.

Some researchers and clinicians now feel that the use of the older sedative-hypnotics (barbiturates, glutethimide, and others) should be restricted primarily to the management of insomnia. And there are some researchers who feel that even for the treatment of insomnia, certain benzodiazepine derivatives, such as flurazepam, are significantly superior to the barbiturates (Greenblatt and Shader 1974, Kales and Kales 1974, Kales et al 1975). Koch-Weser and Greenblatt (1974) have expressed the view that the barbiturates and, by inference, closely related sedative-hypnotics are "obsolete." Given the weight of opinion, the possible uses of these older drugs in treating anxiety will not be discussed here (p 309). Some of these drugs are used in treating motor disorders (p 127).

The benzodiazepines are already the most commonly prescribed drugs in the United States, and, at present, it seems likely that the benzodiazepines will be used increasingly for the treatment of anxiety to the exclusion of other sedative-hypnotics (p 309). Whether further research will strengthen the argument that certain of the benzodiazepines ought to replace the barbiturates and older hypnotics even in treating insomnia remains to be seen. For the present, however, the older drugs are likely to be widely used as hypnotics, and the clinician should be aware of some of the factors that enter into the selection of a specific therapeutic agent, the various complications that may arise with each, and the basic principles involved in the management and prevention of sedative-hypnotic dependence.

Insomnia

The discovery that there are several distinct phases of natural sleep, each with its own distinctive pattern of electroencephalographic activity, muscle tone, and extraocular eye movements opened the way for methodic research on sleep and its disorders (p 105). Subsumed under sleep disorders are problems as diverse as insomnia, somnambulism, and enuresis (p 105). At some point about one-third of the general population is affected by insomnia. The problem is generally divided into three major types or patterns: (a) trouble falling asleep; (b) waking up during the night; and (c) early final awakening. Some people have more than one type at a time. While insomnia tends to affect both sexes about equally, it is more common in older patients than in younger ones (Kales et al 1974).

In terms of causality, Kales and his co-workers (1974) have described four major classes of insomnia: (a) situational; (b) medical; (c) psychologic; and (d) drug withdrawal. Insomnia may occur in response to stressful situations or in response to changes that are disruptive of established patterns—the latter may include the altered diurnal activity patterns that occur with travel across time zones. Insomnia is also common in conditions associated with pain and discomfort. In addition, even when pain is not present, sleep disturbance often accompanies emotional reactions to the presence of serious medical disorders and their limitations. Paroxysmal nocturnal dyspnea and hypoxic conditions associated with transient apnea during sleep can also disrupt normal sleeping patterns.

A number of psychiatric disorders have sleep disturbances as a major symptom. For example, decreased sleep is a hallmark of manic episodes; early-morning awakening is a classic sign of endogenous depression, and severe sleep disturbances are also common in acute schizophrenic reactions. Sleep problems are a major complaint in patients with acute or chronic anxiety. Often there is no distinction between the insomnia seen as a response to stressful situations and that which is an aspect of an anxiety state.

Finally, insomnia may accompany a reduction in dosage or abrupt withdrawal of chronically administered sedative-hypnotic and antianxiety drugs. Drug withdrawal insomnia may also be seen for varying periods (days to weeks) after withdrawal of opiate drugs and not uncommonly after detoxification from a period of chronic alcohol use.

Alcohol, and all of the sedative-hypnotics in appropriate doses, have the capacity to reduce that phase of sleep characterized by rapid extraocular movements (REM). When these drugs are abruptly

withdrawn, there tends to be a rebound increase in the REM phase of
sleep associated with vivid dreams and increased frequency of
dreaming. Just how this phenomenon is related to withdrawal insomnia is not entirely clear. However, it does seem clear that regardless of the original cause of the sleep disturbance, people who are
prescribed sedative-hypnotics over a period of several weeks may
find it difficult to stop the prescribed hypnotic agent abruptly for at
least two reasons: (a) their original sleep disturbance problem may
still be present and (b) they may experience a special time-limited
insomnia that corresponds to the period of hypnotic withdrawal.

Management

Even for so simple a problem as insomnia a good history is important, and it is sometimes possible to help the patient get a better
night's sleep without prescribing a hypnotic. Some patients, for example, may be having difficulty falling asleep because they have
recently increased their intake of caffeine. Some clinicians have
noted that patients who in their youth were able to tolerate caffeine
and still sleep, lose their ability to do so as the years go by (Hollister
1972). Other medications that may interfere with sleep include sym-
pathomimetics used in treating asthma and appetite suppressants
(Hollister 1972). Sometimes changing these medications entirely or
avoiding them during the latter part of the day will alleviate the
insomnia.
   It is usually important to encourage the development of a regular
ritual associated with going to sleep. This may include a variety of
methods aimed at minimizing stimulation and increasing relaxation. Bedtime is not the time for exercise, heated discussions, or
work requiring concentration and difficult decisions. A warm bath
or shower and a boring book (as opposed to an interesting late show
on TV) are good inducers of sleep. More recently there has been
increased interest in special relaxation techniques, such as yoga and
transcendental meditation; and some workers feel that insomniacs
can be trained to relax through use of a variety of biofeedback techniques. Through a process of conditioning any regularly followed
bedtime ritual will enhance the effects of any hypnotics used and
may help bridge over the periods when it is necessary to interrupt
the use of hypnotics.
   Some patients who complain of insomnia may be suffering from
depression, but they may not spontaneously discuss other manifestations of depression or even be consciously aware of just how depressed they have become (p 219). It is useful to note that certain
of the tricyclic antidepressants have hypnotic properties. Some pa-

tients prescribed antidepressants (eg, 25 to 50 mg amitriptyline) may experience some improvement in sleep almost immediately even though the antidepressant action may not occur for 1 to 2 weeks after therapy is initiated. However, the sleep disturbance may not respond to tricyclics alone and some patients may require a hypnotic as well.

When the sleep disturbance is due to an emerging schizophrenic reaction or manic disorder, the appropriate medication (eg, phenothiazines or lithium) may not alter the syndrome for several days. If the physician judges that the disorders are mild enough in form not to require hospitalization, the use of a hypnotic may be required until the primary medication takes effect.

Available Hypnotic Agents

While it is probable, as pointed out earlier, that all hypnotics share similar mechanisms of action, there are significant differences among the drugs in the way they are absorbed, distributed, metabolized, and excreted, which give rise to differences in dose, onset and duration of action, the probability of unwanted side effects, the risk of nonprescribed self-medication, the likelihood of clinically significant interactions with other drugs, and consequences of deliberate overdosage.

Unlike the central nervous system, which seems to respond to this diverse group in a very similar fashion, the liver, the site for metabolic alteration of these compounds, responds very distinctly to the different chemical classes. It is convenient to categorize the commonly used hypnotics into several major groups: (a) the barbiturates; (b) the chloral derivatives (chloral hydrate, chloral betaine, and triclofos sodium); (c) piperidinediones (methyprylon, glutethimide); (d) carbamates (meprobamate, ethinamate); (e) benzodiazepines (especially flurazepam, nitrazepam, and triazolam); (f) miscellaneous (paraldehyde, methaqualone, ethchlorvynol). The more common tradenames for these drugs and their average hypnotic dose are shown in Table 1.

Other drugs sold over-the-counter or sometimes prescribed to induce sleep in special situations include ethyl alcohol (in the form of wine, beer, or whiskey), certain antihistamines with sedative actions, certain tricyclic antidepressants (eg, amitriptyline), and some phenothiazines (eg, chlorpromazine, thioridazine).

At therapeutic dose levels all of the drugs shown in Table 1 are metabolized according to first-order kinetics. That is, the amount of drug metabolized over a given period of time depends on its plasma

TABLE 1
DOSAGE AND BIOLOGIC HALF-LIFE OF SOME COMMONLY USED HYPNOTICS

Generic Name	Common Trade Name	Average Hypnotic Dose*	Biologic Half-life (hr)*	Comment
Amobarbital sodium	Amytal sodium	100–200 mg	16–42	—
Pentobarbital sodium	Nembutal sodium	100–200 mg	21–42	—
Phenobarbital	Luminal	100–200 mg	24–96	—
Secobarbital	Seconal	100–200 mg	20–28	—
Chloral hydrate	Noctec, Somnos	0.75– 1.5 g†	8	‡,
Chloral betaine	Beta-Chlor	0.874– 1.74 g†	—	‡,§,//
Triclofos sodium	Triclos	1.5– 1.75 g	—	‡,§,//
Meprobamate	Miltown, Equanil	800 mg	10	—
Ethinomate	Valmid	0.5–1.0 g	—	#
Ethchlorvynol	Placidyl	0.5– 1.0 g†	5.6	—
Glutethimide	Doriden	500–1000 mg	10– 13	**
Methyprylon	Noludar	200–400 mg	4	—
Methaqualone	Sopor, Quaalude	150–300 mg†	2.6	††
Flurazepam	Dalmane	15–30 mg†	50–100	—
Nitrazepam	Mogadon	—	21– 25	‡‡
Triazolam	—	0.4– 0.8 mg	—	‡‡

*Dosages and ranges for biologic half-lives in table have been obtained by combining data from various references. In most cases the half-life is before enzyme induction. Repeated use may shorten half-life through enzyme induction. (See bibliography, including Morris [1972], Medical Letter [1972] and Sunshine [1975].)

†Lower dosage thought to be of marginal efficacy; higher dosage is often required.

‡Causes gastric irritation.

§With repeated administration, trichloracetic acid may build up, altering metabolism of anticoagulants and other drugs.

//Half-life assumed to be similar to chloral hydrate: side effects also similar since drug acts via same active metabolite.

#Reported to have relatively short duration of action.

**Erratic absorption from the gastrointestinal tract.

††Plasma levels decay in a biphasic manner; the half-life of the fast component is approximately 0.9 hr and the slow one 16 hr.

‡‡Not generally available in the United States.

concentrations, and increases as the plasma level increases. The rate at which the body metabolizes the drug is usually expressed in terms of biologic half-life, the time required to metabolize half of the drug in the body. After four half-lives, the process is 94 percent complete. Since a number of the drugs discussed here have half-lives significantly longer than 8 hours when these drugs are given once a day, there will be an accumulation of the drug in the body. The accumulation will continue until the amount of drug eliminated by the body during the 24-hour interval between doses just equals the dose administered. At this point an equilibrium or a steady state has been reached.

The longer the half-life, the greater the accumulation that will occur before a steady state is reached. The time required to reach the steady state depends solely on the half-life. In general, with repeated administration the steady state level is reached after five to six elimination half-lives, eg, if a drug has a half-life of 30 hours, the steady state will be reached after 150 to 180 hours. However, the plasma concentration reached at the steady state depends on the maintenance dosage as well. For a drug with a long half-life, administered once a day, the plasma level reached at the steady state can be approximated by multiplying the level produced by a single dose, by the biologic half-life in days, and the number 1.44. A drug with a half-life of 2 days, for example, would reach a mean plasma level of 2 × 1.44 or 2.88 times higher than the mean level produced by the first dose. And it follows from the previous rule that for a drug with a half-life of 2 days it would take about 10 to 12 days to reach this steady state level (Fingl and Woodbury 1975). However, for most of the drugs in Table 1, repeated administration will result in enzyme induction which will shorten the half-life, so that the steady state reached will be less than would be predicted from the plasma levels reached after the first dose.

It can be seen from Table 1 that a number of the drugs used as sedative-hypnotics will accumulate to some degree. This is not necessarily a serious disadvantages since many patients with insomnia are chronically anxious and may obtain some relief of anxiety during the day as a result of residual levels of the drugs used for inducing sleep. Certainly such accumulation would seem to occur with the benzodiazepines. Residual hypnotic, after a single dose, or the accumulation of the hypnotic after multiple doses, is probably an important factor in producing complaints of the side effects of hangover and drowsiness during the next day. It would seem, however, that considerable central nervous system tolerance to the effects of hypnotic drugs develops in most patients, since not all patients complain of progressively increasing sedation. To the contrary, many patients find that after a few weeks of use, low doses of pentobarbital have largely lost their hypnotic effects; this decreasing effect of low doses of pentobarbital with time has been confirmed in laboratory studies (Kales et al 1975).

The Process of Selection

The barbiturates can be subdivided on the basis of their duration of action into three subgroups: (a) the long acting; (b) intermediate and short acting; and (c) ultrashort acting. A few of the more commonly used barbiturates and other sedative-hypnotics are shown in Table 1.

The intermediate to short-acting barbiturates—pentobarbital and secobarbital—can be thought of as the standard hypnotics against which the advantages and disadvantages of other hypnotics are usually measured. These barbiturates are well and quickly absorbed after oral administration and the effects are apparent within 30 minutes. In patients having insomnia without complicating medical or psychiatric disorders, the usual dose of 100 mg of pentobarbital or secobarbital produces a demonstrable decrease in latency to sleep and the number of awakenings and an increase in total sleep time. The barbiturates suppress the REM phase of sleep as well as sleep Stages 3 and 4. Similar effects on sleep latency, number of awakenings, and stages of sleep are seen with chloral hydrate (1000 mg), glutethimide (500 mg), and methaqualone (150 or 300 mg).

With repeated administration over as short a period as 1 to 2 weeks, tolerance seems to develop to the hypnotic effectiveness of these dose levels (Kales and Kales 1974, Kales et al 1975). It is not clear whether this tolerance is due to more rapid metobolism or to adaptation in the central nervous system, but both phenomena are probably involved. Some patients, either as a result of previous experience with hypnotic drugs or as a result of natural tolerance, may require a somewhat higher than average initial dose of barbiturates (eg, 150 to 200 mg pentobarbital). The problem of patients who seek increases in dosage for other reasons is described below.

Flurazepam (15 to 30 mg) is about equieffective with the aforementioned drugs in decreasing latency to sleep and decreasing the number of awakenings, but the drug does not lose its effectiveness to the same extent over a period of 4 weeks. This does not necessarily mean that no tolerance develops. Flurazepam has an active metabolite with a half-life of 50 to 100 hours, and with daily administration the metabolite builds up, reaching the steady state anywhere from 8 to 16 days after the drug is started. It is more likely that rising plasma levels overcome the effect of tolerance development. Low doses of flurazepam have slight suppressant effects on the REM phase of sleep over the first few days, but with continued administration a definite effect on REM sleep occurs. It has also been noted that flurazepam is not as effective as a hypnotic on the first night or two as it is on later nights—an effect that is predictable from its pharmacokinetics (Greenblatt and Shader 1974, Kales et al 1975).

Since there is known to be cross-tolerance between drugs in the sedative hypnotic group, it is not useful to switch from one to another, and it is probably not overly useful to switch to a benzodiazepine. In order to restore a measure of central nervous system sensitivity to the hypnotics, it is necessary to interrupt hypnotic administration for a period of a week or two; this may require a period of gradual reduction. During the period when no hypnotics are given, it may be helpful to try drugs with sedative properties that do not exhibit cross-tolerance with the sedative-hypnotic group (eg, amitriptyline, thioridazine).

For the patient who has difficulty in getting to sleep, but little difficulty staying asleep, a drug with a short half-life (eg, methyprylon, chloral hydrate) would be a better first choice than one likely to have effects that carry over into the day. Contrary to the view that pentobarbital and secobarbital are short-acting barbiturates, sensitive measures can detect impairment of performance for 18 to 20 hours after a 200-mg dose.

While it is likely that many of the complaints of hypnotic hangover are due to the continued presence of the hypnotic in the body, it has been difficult to demonstrate that drugs with the shortest half-lives produce the lowest incidence of such complaints (Greenblatt and Shader 1972, Harvey 1975). However, all other factors being equal, it would seem logical to look for the shortest acting drug if the problem is primarily sleep induction and if the patient complains about "morning-after" effects.

Drugs with very short half-lives are also appropriate for the patient who awakens early and is unable to get back to sleep, but is reluctant to take hypnotics like pentobarbital because of the possibility of hangover. There is a possibility, however, that the shorter acting drugs may have a higher abuse potential than drugs such as flurazepam.

For the more typical patient who has problems getting to sleep and staying asleep, the drugs with somewhat longer half-lives are indicated.

Side Effects

While the most common side effects of hypnotic drugs are drowsiness, fatigue, headache, and dizziness, some hypnotics produce effects less typical. For example, chloral hydrate and its derivatives produce gastric irritation; other drugs have been associated with skin eruptions. While severe overdosage with any of the hypnotics produces severe depression and coma, different effects are sometimes seen. For example, with toxic doses of methaqualone hyperreflexia, myoclonus, and frank convulsions may occur. With the benzodiazepines, cumulative effects may not be seen for 2 weeks; the biologic half-life of certain hypnotics (eg, amobarbital, diazepam) may be prolonged in the elderly.

Drug Interactions

With the exception of the benzodiazepines, all of the hypnotic drugs appear to stimulate hepatic enzymes that metabolize anticoagulants or interfere, in other ways, with the effects of anticoagulant drugs. Enzyme induction may also accelerate the metabolism of other drugs, such as diphenylhydantoin and tricyclic antidepressants, necessitating increased doses of these agents. The impairment of skilled motor performances by alcohol and codeine are accentuated when combined with the sedative-hypnotics (Linnoila et al 1974).

This point needs to be considered when using drugs that have cumulative effects. On the other hand, at doses of 30 to 60 mg, codeine is synergistic with pentobarbital in including sleep (Belleville et al 1971); aspirin in doses of 650 to 950 mg appears to have some sedative actions and when combined with either low doses of chloral hydrate or certain antihistamines, is slightly more effective than placebo in inducing sleep (Wolff 1974, Smith et al 1974).

Drugs with Hypnotic Effects That Do not Exhibit Cross-Dependence

Although controlled studies of over-the-counter drugs (containing scopolamine and the antihistaminic methapyralene) have not shown them to be effective in reducing anxiety, at least two controlled studies have shown that over-the-counter hypnotics with similar ingredients are somewhat better than placebo in inducing sleep in patients with insomnia (Wolff 1974, Smith et al 1974). However, the slight effect was clearly less than that produced by 100 mg of pentobarbital.

The usual doses of amitriptyline (Elavil) are often, if not invariably, accompanied by sedative effects (Hollister 1972). In patients with depressive symptoms this effect is often sufficient, so that it is

unnecessary to prescribe an additional hypnotic for the sleep disturbances that often accompany depression. The phenothiazine drugs,
chlorpromazine or thioridazine, in doses of 50 or 75 mg orally, also
produce considerable drowsiness, and these drugs have been prescribed in situations where the physician felt that more conventional
hypnotics are contraindicated. While the tricyclic antidepressants
and the phenothiazines are generally prescribed for depression and
schizophrenia, respectively, there may be occasions where they can
be helpful in other situations. Since these substances show no
cross-tolerance to the sedative-hypnotics shown in Table 1, it may be
possible to reduce the rate at which tolerance develops by periodically substituting one of the former for the more conventional hypnotics for a week or two. However, both the tricyclics and
phenothiazines have relatively long half-lives and patients may
complain of sedative side effects the following day.

Sedative Dependence

Another problem with many of the drugs shown in Table 1 is the
possibility that some patients may begin to use them in inappropriate amounts or in inappropriate situations. As mentioned previously some patients who begin to increase their dose (eg, 100 mg to
200 mg of phenobarbital) may not be developing patterns of drug
abuse but may be telling the physician that they still have insomnia
and that they have become tolerant to the effects of the original dose.
Other patients may begin to use their prescribed hypnotic drug to
relieve anxiety during the day or as a substitute for alcohol-induced
intoxication. All of the intermediate and short-acting barbiturates, in
appropriate doses (usually about double the dose needed for hypnotic effect), will produce a state of intoxication somewhat similar to
that produced by alcohol and which is considered pleasurable by
some individuals. In general, appropriate doses (generally higher
than needed for inducing sleep) of most of the other drugs listed in
Table 1 will also produce such an effect. However, they do not all do
so to the same degree. For example, phenobarbital is not reported to
produce the kind of intoxication or euphoria produced by the short-
or intermediate-acting barbiturates. Whether this is due to the
slower rate of absorption of phenobarbital, a slower onset of action,
or to some more basic difference in action is not clear. But it does
seem clear that barbiturate and sedative abusers rarely consider
phenobarbital as a drug worthy of self-administration.

  With a few notable exceptions, most of the drugs listed in Table 1
have been self-administered without medical supervision to induce

euphoria or intoxication or to substitute for alcohol, and cases of physical and psychologic dependence have been reported. Some drugs listed in Table 1 have had notable cycles of popularity as self-administered drugs for intoxication. The abuse of methaqualone (Quaalude), for example, was widespread in 1970 to 1972. Whether its popularity faded spontaneously or was related to the more stringent Federal regulations introduced in 1973 is not yet clear. A somewhat similar epidemic of glutethimide abuse occurred soon after that drug was released as a nonbarbiturate. It might be noted that both methaqualone and glutethimide appear to have rather short durations of action.

With respect to abuse potential, some of the benzodiazepines seem to have special advantages. To date flurazepam (Dalmane) has not been reported to be a drug that induces either marked euphoria or a sense of pleasurable intoxication. Neither has chlordiazepoxide (Librium) been notable as a drug of abuse, although a few such cases have been reported. Diazepam (Valium), on the other hand, is widely prescribed and has been self-administered for the induction of intoxication, although it seems to be less of a problem in this respect than the short-acting barbiturates. Since it has not been suggested that these two benzodiazepines act at different sites, it is possible that differences in abuse potential are due, at least in part, to differences in onset of action—that of diazepam being relatively more rapid than that of flurazepam.

There is a distinct possibility that other factors being equal, rapidity of onset of effects and a short duration of action are prime factors in determining whether a given drug in this group will be abused and will lead to dependence. Rapid onset of action produces a rapid reinforcement of the drug-taking behavior, and the short duration will ensure that such behavior will occur frequently (if intoxication is to be maintained) and will be reinforced frequently. However, it is worth emphasizing that "other factors" are probably not equal—the drugs in Table 1 do not appear to produce identical degrees of euphoria or, if they do, the euphoria produced is in some cases accompanied by other effects that reduce the abuse potential of the drug. Furthermore the availability of different drugs is not the same. Just where each of the drugs fits in the continuum between pentobarbital and secobarbital on one extreme and flurazepam and phenobarbital on the other, cannot be stated with precision.

While there is usually no difficulty in recognizing the extreme forms of sedative-hypnotic dependence, there is no sharp line that separates inappropriate and excessive use of these drugs from the more obvious cases of sedative addiction. It is important to recognize that in the context of dependence, alcohol and the drugs in Table 1 are largely addictive and interchangeable. A number of studies have demonstrated that the drugs shown in Table 1 exhibit cross-dependence; ie, one drug can substitute for another in preventing the central nervous system depressant withdrawal syndrome. These drugs are also cross-dependent with alcohol, and from this characteristic, their utility in preventing or treating the alcohol withdrawal syndrome is derived (Jaffe 1975).

Chronic use of any one hypnotic agent in ordinary dosage is not indicative of a problem. But when an individual is combining modest doses of antianxiety drugs with daily use of 5 or 6 ounces of alcohol, plus regular use of hypnotic drugs, a clinically significant degree of physical and, probably, psychologic dependence may be present. At these levels, the individual might experience moderate withdrawal symptoms if this combination of medications is abruptly discontinued or the doses are sharply reduced (Jaffe 1975).

The older views of sedative-hypnotic dependence evolved from studies of severely physically dependent addicts in whom abrupt withdrawal often produces not merely severe insomnia and anxiety but also autonomic disturbances, convulsive seizures, delirium, and, in extreme cases, hyperthermia, collapse, and death. As a general rule withdrawal syndromes develop more rapidly after the discontinuation of drugs with short half-lives, and because of slow metabolism and excretion such syndromes may not be seen for several days after the longer-acting drugs are discontinued. Based on such observations, the standard therapeutic approach was hospitalization, stabilization on sufficient barbiturate (or other hypnotic) to produce mild intoxication, and very gradual withdrawal of the hypnotic drug. The rate of reduction is usually 100 mg per day of phenobarbital or the equivalent of another hypnotic (Jaffe 1975).

It is possible to stabilize patients on phenobarbital. This involves converting the patient's total sedative dosage into hypnotic units (equivalent to 100 mg of pentobarbital) and substituting 30 mg of phenobarbital for each such unit. The total daily dose of phenobarbital is divided into four doses; the total is then reduced by 30 mg per day. For example, a patient taking 600 mg of secobarbital (6 pentobarbital units), 800 mg meprobamate (1 unit), and 1000 mg of glutethimide (2 units) would be given 9 × 30 or 270 mg of phenobarbital in four divided doses (Smith and Wesson 1971).

More recently there has been a recognition that milder degrees of sedative-hypnotic dependence are quite common and range from the hypnotic drug withdrawal insomnia described previously to states of anxiety and tremulousness that have their onset several days after a chronically administered antianxiety agent is discontinued. When the patient is considered reliable, withdrawal as an outpatient is possible. It generally involves stabilizing the patient on one of the sedative-hypnotic (or antianxiety) drugs listed in Table 1 and then slowly reducing the daily dose over a period of several weeks. Drugs with long half-lives, such as phenobarbital or one of the benzodiazepines, are superior for this purpose because their pharmacokinetics provides for a very gradual reduction in plasma levels and minimizes the likelihood that they, too, will become drugs of abuse. The rate of reduction is usually about 30 mg of phenobarbital per day or its equivalent in benzodiazepines.

Drug-withdrawal insomnia is managed in a similar fashion; the patient is switched to a long-acting drug like flurazepam, and the dosage reduced by about one clinical dose per week. The patient should be warned to expect some increased frequency of dreaming (Kales et al 1974).

Overdose

A major limitation in the use of intermediate or short-acting barbiturates and most of the other hypnotics shown in Table 1 is the possibility that some patients may save their prescription until they have enough to make a suicidal gesture or a genuine suicidal attempt. Overdosage with barbiturates or related hypnotics is the most common method of attempting suicide and is one of the most frequent causes of successful suicide. For several reasons (in part due to inherent properties of the drugs and in part due to the use of lower initial dosage because therapeutic effects depend on the gradual accumulation of the drugs), the likelihood of successful suicide with the benzodiazepines is lower than it is with the barbiturates or with any of the other classes of drugs shown in Table 1 (Greenblatt and Shader 1972, 1974). This distinguishing characteristic of certain benzodiazepines has increased their popularity as hypnotics for patients with depressive symptomatology. Another way to reduce the probability of a successful suicide (other than to prescribe no hypnotic drug at all) is to prescribe no more than one week's supply of a hypnotic and to write the prescription so that it cannot be renewed without a physician's approval.

It would seem good practice to carefully monitor the amount of drug used and prescription renewals even when the drugs prescribed are benzodiazepines.

References

Bellville JW, Forrest WH, Shroff P, Brown BW: Hypnotic effects of codeine and secobarbital and their interaction in man. Clin Pharmacol Ther 12:607–612, 1971

Byck R: Drugs and the treatment of psychiatric disorders. In Goodman LS, Gilman A (eds): The Pharmacological Basis of Therapeutics, 5th ed. New York, MacMillan, 1975, pp 152–200

Fingl E, Woodbury DM: General Principles. In Goodman LS, Gilman A (eds): The Pharmacological Basis of Therapeutics. New York, MacMillan, 1975, pp 1–46

Gasser JC, Kaufman RD, Bellville JW: Respiratory effects of lorazepam, pentobarbital and pentazocine. Clin Pharmacol Ther 18:170–174, 1975

Greenblatt D, Shader R: Drug Therapy: Benzodiazepines, Part One. N Engl J Med 291:1011–1015, 1974

———: Drug Therapy: Benzodiazepines, Part Two. N Engl J Med 291:1239–1243, 1974

———: The clinical choice of sedative-hypnotics. Ann Intern Med 77:91–100, 1972

Harvey SC: Hypnotics and sedatives. In Goodman LS, Gilman A (eds): The Pharmacological Basis of Therapeutics, 5th ed. New York, MacMillan, 1975, pp 102–123

Hollister LE: Psychiatric and neurologic disorders. In Melmon KL, Morrelli HF (eds): Clinical Pharmacology. New York, MacMillan, 1972, pp 453–511

Jaffe JH: Drug addiction and drug abuse. In Goodman LS, Gilman A (eds): The Pharmacological Basis of Therapeutics. New York, MacMillan, 1975, pp 238–324

Kales A, Kales JD, Bixler EO: Insomnia: An approach to management and treatment. Psychol Ann 4:28–44, 1974

———, Kales JD: Sleep disorders—recent findings in the diagnosis and treatment of disturbed sleep. N Engl J Med 290:487–499, 1974

———, Kales JD, Bixler EO, Scharf MB: Effectiveness of hypnotic drugs with prolonged use: Flurazepam and pentobarbital. Clin Pharmacol Ther 18:356–363, 1975

Koch-Weser J, Greenblatt DJ: The archaic barbiturate hypnotics. N Engl J Med 291:790–791, 1974

Linnoila M, Hakkinen S: Effects of diazepam and codeine, alone and in combination with alcohol, on simulated driving. Clin Pharmacol Ther 15:4, 368–373, 1974

McMillan DE: Determinants of drug effects on punished responding. Fed Proc 34:1870–1879, 1975

Medical Letter on Drugs and Therapeutics (Reference Handbook). New Rochelle, New York, The Medical Letter, Inc., 1973, p 9

Morris RN, Gunderson GA, Babcock SW, Zaroslinski JF: Plasma levels and absorption of methaqualone after oral administration to man. Clin Pharmacol Ther 13:719–723, 1972

Smith GM, Coletta CG, McBride S, McPeek B: Use of subjective responses to evaluate efficacy of mild analgesic-sedative combinations. Clin Pharmacol Ther 15:118–129, 1974

Smith DE, Wesson DR: Phenobarbital technique for treatment of barbiturate dependence. Arch Gen Psychiatry 24:56–60, 1971

Sunshine A: Comparison of the hypnotic activity of triazolam, flurazepam hydrochloride and placebo. Clin Pharmacol Ther 17:573–577, 1975

Wolff BB: Evaluation of hypnotics in outpatients with insomnia using a questionnaire and a self-rating technique. Clin Pharmacol Ther 15:130–140, 1974

nonprescription psychotropic drugs

commentary

Numerous over-the-counter (proprietary) pharmaceutical preparations, available without prescription in drug stores and supermarkets, are sold as treatments for anxiety, tension, and insomnia. These preparations are forcefully promoted by their manufacturers, and extensively used by the American public. Most over-the-counter psychotropic drugs contain methapyrilene, scopolamine, bromides, or some combination of these. Controlled studies demonstrate that these preparations are no more effective than placebo, and clearly less effective than standard prescription psychotropic drugs. In addition to being ineffective, proprietary psychotropics are potentially hazardous. Individuals suffering from anxiety or insomnia are encouraged to seek medical help rather than resorting to self-medication with over-the-counter drugs.

nonprescription psychotropic drugs

David J. Greenblatt, M.D.
Richard I. Shader, M.D.

Recently much attention and concern has been focused upon the widespread and possibly excessive use of psychotropic drugs in the Western world (Boe 1971, Greenblatt and Shader 1971, Lennard et al 1970, Parish 1971, Rucker 1974). Drugs available only by prescription have received the most attention, but data from several sources suggest that the use of proprietary or over-the-counter psychotropic agents, available without prescription in drug stores and supermarkets, also is extensive (Erikson 1973, Greenblatt et al 1975, Parry et al 1973). This chapter will consider clinical aspects of the use of proprietary psychotropic drugs by ambulatory adults. Ethanol, caffeine, and nicotine clearly qualify as nonprescription psychotropic drugs (pp 407, 451, and 483). Furthermore, a number of old-time medicinal tonics and elixirs, such as many of the Lydia Pinkham products, contained high concentrations of ethanol, which undoubtedly contributed to their therapeutic effects. However, this discussion will be limited to tablet and capsule preparations promoted specifically for the relief of nervousness, tension, and insomnia.

Self-Medication

Reasons for Self-Medication

American adults commonly resort to pharmacologic solutions for problems associated with anxiety, tension, and insomnia. Numerous surveys of the extent of psychotropic drug prescribing and use suggest that 15 percent or more of American adults take antianxiety or hypnotic drugs (Gottschalk et al 1971, Greenblatt et al 1975, Manheimer et al 1968, Mellinger et al 1971, Parry et al 1973). These data could be interpreted as depicting drug overuse and misuse, indicating that drugs are a crutch for emotional problems of which neither physicians nor patients are willing or able to work toward more lasting, satisfactory solutions. On the other hand, widespread use of psychotropic agents could indicate that they provide a highly satisfactory and effective means of coping with common emotional problems (Balta 1975, Gardner 1974). Regardless of how the findings are interpreted, the extensive use of psychotropic drugs is a fact (Blackwell 1973, Greenblatt and Koch-Weser 1975). Furthermore, it is clearly in the interest of the pharmaceutical industry to promote, sustain, and even to broaden the use of psychotropic drugs. Accordingly, billions of dollars are spent annually on drug advertising in medical publications and on detailing of drugs by trained salespersons. This effort is unquestionably effective. Advertising and detailing are more important determinants of physicians' prescribing habits than are rational, objective evaluations of drug efficacy and safety (Greenblatt and Shader 1971, Miller 1974). Factors that influence physicians' drug prescriptions are likely to influence the public's consumption of drugs as well. Only a recluse could avoid the constant barrage of advertising in the popular media, promoting a variety of over-the-counter tablets, capsules, potions, droplets, ointments, creams, jellies, and aerosol sprays as the final solution for the bodily dysfunctions of humanity, including insomnia, anxiety, fatigue, headache, arthritis, muscle strain, nausea, abdominal pain, constipation, diarrhea, hemorrhoids, acne, psoriasis, nasal congestion, asthma, edema, dysmenorrhea, and vaginal odor. The consumption of nonprescription psychotropic drugs undoubtedly reflects the widespread expectation reinforced by pharmaceutical promotion that the use of such preparations is a satisfactory method of dealing with problems of insomnia and anxiety.

Extent of Self-Medication

Reliable assessment of the extent of nonprescription psychotropic drug use is a difficult task. Partly because no government agency is concerned with monitoring or regulating the use of these drugs, no single source can provide adequate data on the kinds of preparations available and on how widely they are used. Although many studies have addressed the problems of drug dispensing and consumption, most of these deal only with prescription drugs for which much more reliable data are available.

Two studies did consider the use of proprietary psychotropic drugs. Parry and associates (1973) interviewed 2552 adult Americans to determine their use of psychotropic drugs in the year prior to the interview. Over-the-counter hypnotics or tranquilizers were reportedly used by 7 percent of men and 10 percent of women. Usage was considerably higher among adults under 30 years of age and among those living on the West Coast of the United States. A majority of users found the preparations provided little or no benefit and took the drugs only sporadically. The authors conclude that over-the-counter preparations are less commonly used and less effective than prescription psychotropic drugs and constitute only an alternative pharmacologic method of dealing with anxiety and insomnia for individuals unwilling or unable to obtain more effective prescription drugs from a physician. Greenblatt and associates (1975) reported a study by the Boston Collaborative Drug Surveillance Program in which approximately 25,000 hospitalized medical and surgical patients were interviewed to determine their use of psychotropic drugs in the 3 months prior to admission. Fifteen percent of this population sample reportedly took psychotropic drugs; proprietary preparations for the treatment of nervousness or insomnia were used by 1 percent of the sample. Again usage was more common among female than among males, but further details are not available.

Despite differences in population samples and methodology, both of the studies suggest that proprietary psychotropic drugs are widely used by American adults, although they are less extensively taken and probably less effective than prescription drugs.

Preparations Available for Clinical Use

The production of proprietary medications is essentially unregulated by the Federal government. Preparations appear and disappear from the commercial market, and the components of a given preparation frequently are changed without announcement. There is no single reliable compendium of available products. Table 1 lists 41 proprietary hypnotics and tranquilizers that are or have been available during the last decade. The list is probably incomplete and not entirely accurate, but it indicates that many preparations with similar or identical composition have been marketed.

Antihistamines and belladonna alkaloids are the most common components of nonprescription psychotropic drugs. Eighty percent of the preparations listed in Table 1 contain an antihistamine (usually methapyrilene) and 58 percent contain a belladonna derivative (usually scopolamine). These two pharmacologic agents can be sold

TABLE 1
COMPOSITION OF PROPRIETARY HYPNOTICS AND TRANQUILIZERS

Preparation	Belladonna alkaloids*	Antihistamines†	Bromides‡	Analgesics§	Vitamins	Other
Alva-Tranquil		+	+	+	+	
Asper-Sleep	+	+				
Compoz	+	+				
CVS sleep capsules	+	+				
Devarex	+	+				
Dormirex	+	+				
Dormatol	+	+				
Dozar		+				
Ethased	+					Passion flower Ethaverine
Ex-Tension			+			
Hypno-Bromic	+		+			Chloral hydrate
Mason's timed sleep capsules	+			+		
Narkine			+			Chloral hydrate

Product						Other ingredients
Neo Nyte				+		
Nervine	+			+		
Neurosine	+		+		+	Cascara sagrada
Nite Rest			+		+	
Nytol		+		+		
Osco sleep tablets		+	+			
Paradorm		+	+		+	
Pasitabs		+		+		
Pheno-Bromide			+	+		Phenobarbital
Professional sleeping pill	+		+	+		
Quietabs		+	+	+	+	Passion flower
Quiet world		+	+	+	+	
Rexall sleep capsules			+	+	+	
Rexall sleep tablets		+	+	+		
Sedacaps			+	+		
Sedaflora				+	+	Passion flower, Phenobarbital, Valerian extract
Sedatabs		+		+		Glyceryl guaiacolate

TABLE 1 *(cont.)*

Preparation	Components					
	Belladonna alkaloids*	Antihistamines†	Bromides‡	Analgesics§	Vitamins	Other
Seedate	+	+				
Sleep-Aid		+				
Sleep-Eze	+	+				
Sleeprin	+	+	+			
Slumba-Tabs	+	+	+			
Somets	+	+				
Sominex	+	+	+			
Somnicaps		+				
Sta-Kalm	+	+			+	Passion flower
Tranquileez		+		+	+	
Transil	+	+	+	+	+	Passion flower

*Usually scopolamine hydrobromide or scopolamine aminoxide hydrobromide.
†Usually methapyrilene hydrochloride.
‡As the sodium, potassium, or ammonium salt.
§Usually salicylamide.

without prescription not because they are particularly mild or safe, but simply because they appeared in clinical medicine prior to the modern era of stringent drug regulation (Hodes 1974). Nine preparations in Table 1 contain bromide salts, and a few others contain small quantities of barbiturates or chloral derivatives. In many cases vitamins, analgesics, and other components are thrown in, but it is safe to assume that whatever sedative or tranquilizing activity these preparations have is attributable to their content of antihistamine, belladonna, or bromide.

Pharmacologic Properties

Methapyrilene.   Methapyrilene is one of a number of antihistaminic compounds available for clinical use without prescription. On the basis of its ethylenediamine structure, methapyrilene is chemically related to tripelennamine and pyrilamine (Tempero and Hunninghake 1970). Drugs of this class have mild sedative and anticholinergic properties as well as antihistaminic effects. Unfortunately, very little is known about the absorption, distribution, and metabolism of methapyrilene by the human body.

Scopolamine.   Scopolamine, or hyoscine, is a naturally occurring plant alkaloid. Both scopolamine and its cogener, atropine, can be extracted from *Atropa belladonna* and a number of other plants of the Solonaceae family (Greenblatt and Shader 1973, Shader and Greenblatt 1972). Owing to their peripheral cholinergic blocking properties, atropine and scopolamine have a variety of legitimate uses in clinical medicine. The legendary intoxicant properties of the belladona alkaloids, however, have been known for centuries and far antedate the understanding of their legitimate medical uses (Greenblatt and Shader 1973, Shader and Greenblatt 1972).

It is classically taught that scopolamine has greater sedative and hallucinogenic effects than atropine. More recent studies suggest that the two compounds differ only in milligram potency and in pharmacokinetic properties. In low doses both atropine and scopolamine produce drowsiness, inattention, incoordination, and impairment of memory (Crow and Grove-White 1973, Drachman and Leavitt 1974, Greenblatt and Shader 1973, Itil 1966, Ketchum et al 1973, Longo 1966, Safer and Allen 1971, Shader and Greenblatt 1972). Electroencephalographic studies reveal an effect consistent with generalized sedation, not unlike that produced by other sedative hypnotic drugs (Itil 1966, Domino and Corssen 1967). At higher doses, atropine and scopolamine cause restlessness, agitation, and delirium rather than sedation.

The human pharmacokinetic properties of atropine are reasonably well established (Kalser 1971), but scopolamine has received little study. One report (Bayne et al 1975) suggested that oral scopolamine is rapidly absorbed in the blood. The plasma half-life was found to be approximately 1 to 2 hours, but this is probably an overestimate since samples were taken only for 6 hours after the dose. Urinary excretion of intact scopolamine accounted for only 4 to 5 percent of the oral dose, suggesting that hepatic metabolism is the major route of scopolamine elimination (Bayne et al 1975).

Bromide.   Sodium, potassium, and ammonium salts of inorganic bromide have been in clinical use for more than a century (Woodbury 1972). Bromide salts have central depressant and anticonvulsant properties. Bromides now are generally found only as components of proprietary hypnotics and tranquilizers, although an occasional patient with epilepsy may respond to bromide therapy.

The pharmacokinetic properties of bromide in humans resemble those of chloride (Woodbury 1972). The ion is completely absorbed when given by mouth, unmetabolized by the body, and excreted unchanged by the kidney. The rate of bromide excretion is very slow. One study suggested that the excretion half-life in humans is approximately 12 days. This indicates that bromide will slowly accumulate in the body if given on a chronic basis (Greenblatt and Koch-Weser 1975). Plateau levels are reached only after 60 to 90 days of repeated use. The mean steady-state blood concentration during chronic therapy will be approximately 18 times greater than the mean concentration after the first dose (Greenblatt and Koch-Weser 1975). This is a considerable degree of accumulation and is further discussed below.

Clinical Efficacy

Nearly two decades ago Lasagna (1956) pointed out the lack of adequate data substantiating the clinical efficacy of proprietary psychotropic drugs. This unfortunate situation still holds true. Only a few controlled studies evaluate the effectiveness of nonprescription hypnotics and tranquilizers. In 1955 Straus and associates compared the hypnotic efficacy of 50 mg of methapyrilene to that of phenobarbital and placebo in a crossover study. They found that methapyrilene was significantly more effective than placebo, as judged by observer ratings and subjective self-ratings. In a more recent study Teutsch and co-workers (1975) reported that 50 mg of methapyrilene was no more effective than placebo, whereas 50 mg of diphenhydramine (Benadryl) was significantly superior to placebo. Kales and associates (1971) investigated the effects of two tablets of Sominex and placebo in volunteers with insomnia, using all-night electroencephalographic recordings. They were unable to demonstrate that Sominex produced any significant beneficial effects on any clinically relevant sleep parameters. Rickels and Hesbacher (1973) compared the daytime antianxiety efficacy of placebo with that of Compoz, a proprietary tranquilizer and chlordiazepoxide (Librium), a benzodiazepine antianxiety agent of established clinical value. Approximately 120 anxious neurotic outpatients were randomly assigned to treatment with one of these three preparations in a double-blind noncrossover study. At the end of the 2-week trial, subjects receiving chlordiazepoxide experienced significantly more symptomatic improvement than those receiving placebo, whereas Compoz was no more effective than placebo. Furthermore, side effects were reported more frequently by patients taking Compoz than by those taking chlordiazepoxide or placebo.

The results of controlled studies are consistent with the epidemiologic findings of Parry and associates (1973), suggesting that proprietary psychotropic drugs are of dubious clinical efficacy. If the modern federal requirements for effectiveness of prescription drugs were applied to these nonprescription preparations, it is very unlikely that any of them would qualify for marketing.

Unwanted Effects

Since nonprescription psychotropic drugs almost always are taken without the supervision of a physician, the side effects of these preparations seldom come to his attention. Accordingly, there is very little reliable data on unwanted effects of nonprescription psychotropic drugs after therapeutic doses. As with other central depressant drugs, unwanted drowsiness, fatigue, or hangover are probably the most common adverse effects, but the frequency of these manifestations is not established. Symptoms of peripheral cholinergic blockade can be produced by small doses of belladonna alkaloids and antihistamines. These include dry mouth, tachycardia, blurring of vision, constipation, and voiding difficulties. In most cases anticholinergic effects are troublesome but not serious. They may be of greater concern in patients with untreated glaucoma, prostatic hypertrophy, or intestinal obstruction which is present or impending. In some susceptible individuals, proprietary psychotropic drugs, particularly when excessive doses are taken, can cause agitation, confusion, and delirium consistent with "atropine psychosis."

Intentional overdosage of nonprescription hypnotics and tranquilizers is of increasing concern, both in the United States and in other parts of the world. For pleasure-seeking drug users, proprietary psychotropics are inexpensive, readily available, and fully legal hallucinogens. They also are commonly taken for self-destructive purposes by depressed individuals. Although deaths have been attributed to overdosage with such drugs (O'Dea and Liss 1953), serious poisoning fortunately appears to be rare. Intoxicated individuals usually are found to be confused, agitated, and delirious, with widely dilated and unresponsive pupils, tachycardia, dry mouth and mucous membranes, flushed skin, and reduced motility of bowel and bladder (Greenblatt and Shader 1973, Greiner 1964, Landauer and Csillag 1971, Leff and Bernstein 1968, Owens et al 1971, Shader and Greenblatt 1972, Thakkar and Lasser 1972, Ullman and Groh 1972). In most cases the syndrome is short-lived and relatively benign. Physostigmine salicylate, a nonquaternary cholinesterase inhibitor, is established as the specific antidote, which can be administered to patients with more serious poisoning (Ullman and Groh 1972).

Acute intoxication with bromides is rare. More common is the insidiously developing syndrome of bromism, which occurs as bromide accumulates in the body during chronic use. Manifestations usually include nonspecific signs of chronic central depressant drug use, such as drowsiness, fatigue, and incoordination. Occasionally toxic psychoses occur. Bromism continues to be a drug-induced disease of current concern (Carney 1971, Fried and Malek-Ahmadi 1975, Stewart 1973).

Conclusion

Numerous hypnotic and tranquilizing preparations are available without prescription in drug stores and supermarkets. They are forcefully promoted and extensively used. Controlled clinical trials and epidemiologic studies suggest that they are less effective than prescription psychotropic drugs and probably no more effective than placebo. Acute and chronic intoxication with such preparations is of considerable medical and social concern. Legislative action is needed to bring the manufacture, promotion, and distribution of nonprescription psychotropic drugs under more stringent control. At the same time public educational efforts intended to discourage the use of these preparations should be undertaken by the medical profession and by allied social and community agencies.

References

Balter MB: Coping with illness: choices, alternatives, and consequences. In Helms RB (ed): Drug Development and Marketing. Washington, American Enterprise Institute Center for Health Research, 1975, pp 27–45

Bayne WF, Tao FT, Crisologo N: Submicrogram assay for scopolamine in plasma and urine. J Pharm Sci 64:288–291, 1975

Blackwell B: Psychotropic drugs in use today. The role of diazepam in medical practice. JAMA 225:1637–1641, 1973

Boe S: The increasing use of prescription and over-the-counter psychoactive drugs by adults in the U.S. J Drug Issues 1:286–294, 1971

Carney MWP: Five cases of bromism. Lancet 2:523–524, 1971

Crow TJ, Grove-White IG: An analysis of the learning deficit following hyoscine administration to man. Br J Pharmacol 49:322–327, 1973

Domino EF, Corssen G: Central and peripheral effects of muscarinic cholinergic blocking agents in man. Anesthesiology 28:568–574, 1967

Drachman DA, Leavitt J: Human memory and the cholinergic system: a relationship to aging? Arch Neurol 30:113–121, 1974

Erikson CK: Sleep aids and other sedatives. In Griffenhagen GB, Hawkins LL (eds): Handbook of Non-Prescription Drugs. Washington, American Pharmaceutical Association, 1973, pp 51–53

Fried FE, Malek-Ahmadi P: Bromism: recent perspectives. South Med J 68:220–222, 1975

Gardner EA: Implications of psychoactive drug therapy. N Engl J Med 290: 800–802, 1974

Gottschalk LA, Bates DE, Fox RA, et al: Psychoactive drug use. Patterns found in samples from a mental health clinical and general medical clinic. Arch Gen Psychiatry 25:395–397, 1971

Greenblatt DJ, Koch-Weser J: Clinical pharmacokinetics. N Engl J Med 293:702–705, 964–970, 1975

———, Shader RI: Meprobamate: a study of irrational drug use. Am J Psychiatry 127:1297–1303, 1971

———, Shader RI: Drug therapy: anticholinergics. N Engl J Med 288:1212–1215, 1973

———, Shader RI, Koch-Weser J: Psychotropic drug use in the Boston area: a report from the Boston Collaborative Drug Surveillance Program. Arch Gen Psychiatry 32:518–521, 1975

Greiner TH: A case of "psychosis" from drugs. Texas State J Med 60:659–660, 1964

Hodes B: Nonprescription drugs: an overview. Int J Health Sci 4:125–130, 1974

Itil TM: Quantitative EEG changes induced by anticholinergic drugs and their behavioral correlates in man. Rec Adv Biol Psychiatry 8:151–173, 1966

Kales J, Tan T-L, Swearingen C, Kales A: Are over-the-counter sleep medications effective? All-night EEG studies. Curr Ther Res 13:143–151, 1971

Kalser SC: The fate of atropine in man. Ann NY Acad Sci 179:667–683, 1971

Ketchum JS, Sidell FR, Crowell EB, Aghajanian GK, Hayes AH: Atropine, scopolamine and ditran: comparative pharmacology and antagonists in man. Psychopharmacologia 28:121–145, 1973

Landauer AA, Csillag ER: Alleged hallucinogenic effect of a toxic overdose of an antihistamine preparation. Med J Aust 1:653–654, 1971

Lasagna L: Across-the-counter hypnotics: boon, hazard of fraud? J Chron Dis 4:552–554, 1956

Leff R, Bernstein S: Proprietary hallucinogens. Dis Nerv Syst 29:621–626, 1968

Lennard HL, Epstein LJ, Bernstein A, et al: Hazards implicit in prescribing psychoactive drugs. Science 169:438–441, 1970

Longo VG: Behavioral and electroencephalographic effects of atropine and related compounds. Pharmacol Rev 18:965–996, 1966

Manheimer DI, Mellinger GD, Balter MB: Psychotherapeutic drugs. Use among adults in California. Calif Med 109:445–451, 1968

Mellinger GD, Balter MB, Manheimer DI: Patterns of psychotherapeutic drug use among adults in San Francisco. Arch Gen Psychiatry 25:385–394, 1971

Miller RR: Prescribing habits of physicians: a review of studies on prescribing drugs. Drug Intell Clin Pharm 7:492–500, 557–564, 1973; 8:81–91, 1974

O'Dea AE, Liss M: Suicidal poisoning by methapyrilene hydrochloride, with documentation by paper chromatography. N Engl J Med 249:566–567, 1953

Owens H, Crist T, Brenner WE: Methapyrilene toxic psychosis mimicking eclampsia. NC Med J 32:18–20, 1971

Parish PA: The prescribing of psychotropic drugs in general practice. J R Coll Gen Pract 21 (Suppl 4):1–77, 1971

Parry HJ, Balter MB, Mellinger GD, Cisin IH, Manheimer DI: National patterns of psychotherapeutic drug use. Arch Gen Psychiatry 28:769–783, 1973

Rickels K, Hesbacher PT: Over-the-counter daytime sedatives: a controlled study. JAMA 223:29–33, 1973

Rucker TD: Drug use: data, sources and limitations. JAMA 230:888–890, 1974

Safer DJ, Allen RP: The central effects of scopolamine in man. Biol Psychiatry 3:347–355, 1971

Shader RI, Greenblatt DJ: Belladonna alkaloids and synthetic anticholinergics: use and toxicity. In Shader RI: Psychiatric Complications of Medical Drugs. New York, Raven, 1972, pp 103–147

Stewart RB: Bromide intoxication from a nonprescription medication. Am J Hosp Pharm 30:85–86, 1973

Straus B. Eisenberg J, Gennis G: Hypnotic effects of an antihistamine —methapyrilene hydrochloride. Ann Intern Med 42:574–582, 1955

Tempero KF, Hunninghake DB: Antihistamines. Postgrad Med 48:149–155, 1970

Teutsch G, Mahler DL, Brown CR, et al: Hypnotic efficacy of diphenhydramine, methapyrilene and pentobarbital. Clin Pharmacol Ther 17:195–201, 1975

Thakkar MK, Lasser RP: Scopolamine intoxication from nonprescription sleeping pill. NY State J Med 72:725–726, 1972

Ullman KC, Groh RH: Identification and treatment of acute psychotic states secondary to the usage of over-the-counter sleeping preparations. Am J Psychiatry 128:1244–1248, 1972

Woodbury DM: Bromides. In Woodbury DM, Penry JK, Schmidt RP (eds): Antiepileptic Drugs. New York, Raven, 1972, pp 519–527

psychotherapeutic drugs in aging

commentary

Even though the Fountain of Youth has not yet been tapped, and the anatomic changes during aging are largely irreversible, there is still reason to hope that drugs may help to relieve some of the age-related changes in mental functioning. Psychiatric depression is one of the most common age-related mental disorders, and considerable progress has been made with the use of antidepressant drugs (see p 241). The usefulness of cognitive-acting drugs is still in the realm of research. Although circulatory disorders are age-related, it is unlikely that vasodilators provide much help, since their action is primarily on the peripheral circulation. Medical control of atherosclerosis has still not been achieved, though it is the major cause of death and the subject of active investigation. The following drugs are discussed, but none of them—neither the sympathomimetic amines, analeptics, vasodilators, anticoagulants, procaine, local anesthetics, hydrogenated ergot alkaloids, hyperbaric oxygenation, vitamins, nor adrenergic blocking agents—has unequivocally been shown to provide therapeutic improvement of cognitive disorders. There is some hope that hormones may be useful. Androgens and estrogens do provide replacement therapy, but there is danger of possible carcinogenic side effects. The efficacy and toxicity of drugs is influenced by age-related changes in metabolism and drug disposition processes.

psychotherapeutic drugs in aging

Carl Eisdorfer, Ph.D., M.D.
Robert O. Friedel, M.D.

Background

The population of older Americans, that is, those 65 years of age and older, is increasing at a more accelerated rate than that of the population at large. Persons past the age of 65 now comprise about 21 million Americans, those above age 60, about 27 million, and their number (and proportion of the population) will continue to grow for at least two decades. The extent of emotional disorders, significant enough to be labeled psychiatric disease, probably ranges from 20 to 45 percent among aged persons in the community. In a recent survey of nursing home patients, the prevalence of conditions that could be identified as requiring psychiatric intervention ranged from 62 percent upward (Office of Secretary, HEW 1975).

It is no surprise, therefore, that there is reported to be extensive use of psychopharmacologic agents by aged patients, especially those in supervised residential settings. A recent statement indicates that 75 percent of all nursing home patients are receiving at least one such medication (Nursing Home Care in US 1974).

This chapter will give a brief review of the information available in geriatric psychopharmacology, identify factors affecting drug efficacy as these involve the elderly, and discuss the special problems encountered in the use of psychotropic drugs for older patients.

Pharmacokinetics

The pharmacokinetics of any drug involves absorption, distribution, metabolism, receptor state activity, and elimination. An identical dose of diazepam will result in lower blood concentration and longer blood half-life in elderly versus younger patients (Garattine et al 1973). These age-related changes are probably secondary to decreased drug absorption, metabolism, and drug elimination in the elderly (Bender 1974). With advancing age, lean body mass is replaced by fat (Gregerman and Bierman 1974), which also affects distribution and acts further to increase retention of lipid-soluble psychotropic drugs. On clinical grounds, several investigators have suggested the presence of absorption difficulties in older patients such that the use of alternative routes of delivery, such as liquid concentrate or parenteral administration, may yield differences in action.

As demonstrated with analgesics (Bellville et al 1971), age dependent changes in drug activity can occur as a result of altered receptor sensitivity without change in the drug level in blood or tissue. Frolkis et al (1972) performed a number of studies indicating that there is greater sensitivity to neurotransmitters and that as much as 20 to 50 percent less neurotransmitter substance is required to initiate endorgan response in the aged organism.

Side Effects

The widespread clinical impression that aged patients are more susceptible than young patients to adverse drug reactions (side effects) from most classes of drugs is probably accurate. In a review of the records of both psychiatric and general medical inpatients, Hurwitz (1969) found side effects in 21.3 percent of patients age 70 to 79, compared to 7.5 percent for patients 40 to 49 years, and 3.0 percent for those 20 to 29 years. Women had a higher risk of side effects than did men. These figures are consistent with those of Learoyd (1972) who noted that, of the patients admitted to his psychogeriatric ward, 16 percent presented disorders directly attributed to undesirable side effects of the psychoactive drugs they had received prior to admission. Among the major categories of adverse effects were drug intoxications with increased lethargy; confusion and disorientation; paradoxic behavioral reactions, such as restlessness, agitation, and aggressions; and medical effects such as hypotension, respiratory depression, and urinary retention. Common offenders included various antipsychotic, antidepressant, and antianxiety agents, often prescribed in a multiple drug regimen.

Antipsychotic Drugs

The Diagnostic and Statistical Manual of Mental Disorder (DSM-II) (APA, 1968) defines *psychosis* broadly. The term applies to the patient with an acute schizophreniform illness and no evidence of dementia, as well as to the patient with a chronic dementia (organic brain syndrome) without hallucinations, or illogical thinking, but who is crippled by general intellectual impairment. Compounding the problem are three groups of elderly psychotic patients: those with long-standing chronic schizophrenia; those with dementia who have developed schizophreniform symptoms; and those with chronic dementia without schizophreniform symptoms, but who show behavior (agitation, irritability, assaultiveness, and so forth) that causes marked distress to themselves or to those in their environment.

Impressionistic reports of efficacy for many antipsychotic drugs have appeared, claiming the relief of almost any imaginable behavioral symptom of elderly patients. Fortunately, some controlled studies are also available. Honigfeld et al (1965) demonstrated that phenothiazines were decidedly superior to placebo in treating such areas as motor disturbances, conceptual disorganization, manifest psychosis, and personal neatness. Haloperidol, for example, is effective in alleviating agitation, overactivity, and hostility in patients with chronic organic brain syndrome. Chlorpromazine and thioridazine are also useful in the treatment of organic brain syndrome.

In balance, it appears that the antipsychotic drugs in adequate dosage are probably effective for symptom relief in both elderly chronic schizophrenics and behaviorally disturbed patients with chronic organic brain syndrome, especially if the patients are acutely disturbed. Such effects, however, are less consistent than in younger patients. The paranoid schizophreniform psychosis of later life, so-called paraphrenia, is allegedly responsive to antipsychotic drugs (Post 1965); but no clinical studies with this difficult group of patients have been reported and there is no evidence that these drugs are effective for reversal of memory impairment, confusion, or intellectual deterioration in the patient with a chronic organic brain syndrome. There is also no evidence at this time that one antipsychotic agent is more effective than another in this age group.

Adverse Effects

Short-term use of antipsychotic drugs may lead to peripheral and central anticholinergic effects and undesirable medical and neurologic effects (see p 211). Paradoxically, increased confusion in patients treated with antipsychotic agents, especially if an antiparkinsonian agent is administered concurrently, is usually secondary to central anticholinergic toxicity (Yousef et al 1973). This phenomenon is common in the elderly patient, particularly if some

Clinical Psychopharmacology

degree of organic dementia is also present. It is crucial to realize that increased confusion in a patient receiving antipsychotic agents may well be an adverse drug effect, and temporarily discontinuing all medications with anticholinergic activity (antipsychotic agents, antiparkinsonian agents other than levodopa, and tricyclic antidepressants) should be considered. Although antipsychotic medication has not been associated with striking cardiotoxicity in elderly patients, electrocardiogram abnormalities have been seen and caution must be observed.

The recent recognition of tardive dyskinesia as an adverse effect of the administration of antipsychotic drugs is especially pertinent to the elderly patient. This syndrome of buccofaciolingual involuntary movements, occasionally accompanied by choreoathetoid movements of the extremities and trunk, is reported more commonly among elderly patients. This is both because of a heightened incidence of extended antipsychotic drug administration in elderly chronic schizophrenics, but may be related to the physiognomic relationship that ill-fitting dentures or the edentulous state bears to this syndrome. Although professionals may tend to dismiss cosmetic factors as unimportant to the elderly patient, advancing age is often accompained by a heightened self-consciousness of unattractive physical appearance, and may lead to social withdrawal and despondency in the case of a severe tardive dyskinesia. Steps to reduce the incidence of this phenomenon in elderly patients include reduction of dosage to the lowest level clinically possible, as well as trials without medication. Anticholinergic medications may actually increase the intensity duration and perhaps appearance of tardive dyskinesia (see pp 127, 213).

Antidepressants

Depression is the most common psychiatric illness of the elderly. Unfortunately, much depressive illness is overlooked or accepted as "just growing old," because of the similarity of depressive symptomatology to the common stereotype of the withdrawn, listless, pessimistic elderly person. To further complicate diagnosis, depression can mimic dementia in the older patient (Post 1965), with transient confusion, disorientation, and impaired intellectual function accompanying the affective episode. This "pseudodementia" will clear as the depression responds to treatment. There is, however, a risk that untreated depression may lead to secondary nutritional deficiency disease, institutional placement, social isolation, and a deepening withdrawal syndrome.

A further barrier to the detection of depression in the elderly is the high incidence of masked depression, presenting as somatic complaints or hypochondriasis. DeAlarcon (1964) found hypochondriac symptoms to be more common among the aged as the first manifestation of depression in 29.1 percent of 152 depressed patients over the age of 60 years admitted to the Bethlem Royal Hospital. Somatic complaints typically preceded the appearance of overtly depressive symptoms in these patients by 2 to 3 months. Only 20 percent of these patients had a history of excessive bodily preoccupation in earlier life.

Antidepressant drugs include the monoamine oxydase inhibitors, the tricyclics, and for our purposes in this context, stimulant medications (pp 277, 467). Of the classes of antidepressant drugs available, the monoamine oxidase inhibitors appear least suitable for use in the elderly. While they are effective drugs, their capacity to produce both hypotensive and hypertensive episodes, the latter usually precipitated by ingestion of foods rich in tryamine, is especially hazardous in elderly patients with already compromised cardiovascular systems.

Stimulants, especially sympathomimetic drugs such as methylphenidate and D-amphetamine, have received some attention as geriatric antidepressants. Some clinicians have successfully used them over brief periods of time for the treatment of mild depressions. However, adverse effects of these agents with time include dysphoric mood, irritability, anorexia and weight loss, and production or exacerbation of paranoid symptoms with extended use. These drugs should be avoided in patients with a history of paranoid ideation or drug abuse.

The tricyclic antidepressants are effective agents and are widely used with the elderly. Few clinical studies have specifically examined their efficacy in the depressed geriatric patient (Chien et al 1973). Numerous studies (Davis 1974) have indicated that the antipsychotic drugs are effective in the treatment of agitated depressions, perhaps more so than the tricyclic antidepressants. For elderly depressed patients, controlled trials of various tricyclic antidepressants and antipsychotic agents with demonstrated potency are clearly needed.

Side Effects

Those adverse reactions with special relevance for the elderly will be mentioned here (see also p 259). Orthostatic hypotension is a greater hazard, and those elderly with circulatory problems must be instructed to change from a supine to a sitting or standing position slowly and with careful attention to the onset of dizziness. Like some phenothiazines, tricyclic antidepressants block the action of guanethidine, a frequently used antihypertensive medication for the aged. The peripheral anticholinergic actions of the tricyclics can delay or halt micturition, produce constipation, or precipitate acute glaucoma. Implications are obvious for the elderly patient. Dryness of the mouth, although usually benign, may lead to water intoxication in patients on diuretics. The risk of producing a central anticholinergic confusion syndrome is especially high in elderly patients with a chronic organic brain syndrome. Because of cardiac toxicity, tricyclic antidepressant agents must be administered cautiously to elderly patients.

Antimanic Drugs

Lithium carbonate is effective in the treatment of acute mania and lowers the incidence of exacerbations of manic depressive disease. This illness may first be detected in later life and certainly continues into old age in patients who had developed the disease earlier. Prien et al (1974) found lithium equally efficacious in elderly and young patients, supporting the clinical impression that lithium is useful in elderly manic patients.

Elderly patients develop lithium central nervous system and neuromuscular toxicity at lower serum levels than do young patients (Van Der Velde 1971). Furthermore, the half-life of lithium increases from 24 hours for the middle-aged adult to 36 or 48 hours for the elderly persons (Davis 1974), and even longer if glomerular filtration rate is seriously impaired. Toxic levels for aged individuals may be reached quickly, thus low dose levels (600 to 900 mg per day for the acutely manic patient) and careful monitoring of serum levels and clinical status are recommended. However, lithium levels of 1.0 to 1.5 mEq per liter must be achieved in order to give manic patients a fair therapeutic trial on this medication.

The most common hazard in administering lithium to the elderly patient is the effect of body sodium depletion on lithium metabolism. Many elderly patients are on sodium restricted diets, and as body sodium is depleted, the kidney avidly retains lithium, rapidly leading to excessive serum lithium concentrations. Aldactone does not cause lithium retention and is probably the best diuretic to use with lithium. Lithium directly suppresses thyroid function and can produce hypothyroidism, the latter often mimicking depression or dementia in the elderly patient (Eisdorfer and Raskind 1975).

Antianxiety Drugs and Hypnotics

Although barbiturates and nonbarbiturate hypnotics are generally prescribed for sleep, and the antianxiety agents (benzodiazepines and alcoholgylycols) for the relief of daytime anxiety and agitation, they are often prescribed for overlapping effects and hence will be discussed together (pp 105, 327).

Although the barbiturates were without serious competition as hypnotic and sedative agents for many years, reports of excessive sedation, motor incoordination, and paradoxic excitement in elderly patients have appeared. In a widely quoted article, Dawson-Butterworth (1970) stated that barbiturates were "absolutely contraindicated in the geriatric population."

Despite similarities between the side effects of benzodiazepines and barbiturates in the elderly, the former class of drugs has several practical and theoretical advantages. The low incidence of drug dependence with benzodiazepines, and the diminished probability that an overdose will prove fatal are significant advantages. Of importance for elderly patients, who often receive multiple drugs, is the absence of documented significant effects upon hepatic microsomal enzyme systems, thus sparing metabolism of other drugs, such as tricyclic antidepressants and oral anticoagulants.

We should mention the most commonly used drug in this class, ethanol (see pp 407). This drug, in the form of moderate doses of beer and wine, appears to reduce disturbing behavior and to increase social interaction in institutional settings (Chien 1971). It is also a socially acceptable reinforcer in behavioral approaches to the treatment of behavioral disorders in the elderly (Mishara and Kastenbaum 1974) and in changing role relationships in an inpatient setting.

Cognitive Acting Drugs

Intellectual impairment has always been regarded as an inevitable concomitant of normal aging. Recent longitudinal studies (Eisdorfer and Wilkie 1973, Baltes and Labouvie 1973) suggest that such decline is not as predictable as was thought and, for certain abilities, may not occur at all until shortly before death (Jarvik and Cohen 1973).

Memory loss and intellectual impairment are, however, among the hallmarks of senile brain syndrome, and perhaps for this reason cognitive acting drugs are often referred to as *geriatric* drugs. The search for an agent that may reverse or retard intellectual impairment and behavioral regression is intense, and a wide range of medications have been investigated for properties as geriatric drugs.

Stimulants and Analeptics

The amphetamines methylphenidate, deanol, pipradrol, pentylenetetrazol, and magnesium pemoline have been reported to increase activity level, alertness and attention to stimuli, to improve recall and recognition, to counteract lethargy, and to stimulate circulation and respiration. However, promising early positive findings have not been supported by later controlled research (Gilbert et al 1973).

Vasodilators

These medications (nicotinyl alcohol, papaverine, cyclandelate, isoxsuprine, hexobenidine) relax the smooth muscle of blood vessel walls in the peripheral circulation and possibly in the cerebral vessels. Hypothetically, this effect would be to decrease ischemic changes in brain tissue by increasing blood flow and by increasing oxygenation of brain tissue. This presumed effect has not yet been convincingly demonstrated.

Terry and Wisniewski (1972), among others, have proposed that senile dementia is not different from Alzheimer's disease of later onset, and that neither disease is primarily of vascular origin. British data report that less than 50 percent of dementias are vascular in origin (Kay 1975). Thus, the efficacy of vasodilator treatment for chronic organic brain syndrome in the aged rests upon questionable, albeit logical, clinical grounds.

Papaverine, an alkaloid derivative of opium with vasodilator properties, has produced general improvement in behavior in association with increased cerebral blood flow and decreased arterial resistance. However, significant intellectual improvement has not been consistently demonstrated (Lu et al 1971).

Cyclandelate is similar in its action to papaverine. In both uncontrolled and controlled studies (Ball and Taylor 1967), positive findings have been reported including one (Smith et al 1968) in which patients improved on long-term memory, verbal expansiveness, reasoning, and orientation. The group consisted in the main of mildly impaired patients.

Hydergine

This drug, consisting of three hydrogenated alkaloids of ergot, has been reported to increase cerebral blood flow and oxygen uptake by direct action on ganglion cell metabolism, without producing hypotension (Emmengger and Meier-Ruge 1968). The majority of controlled studies against placebo have been positive (Roubicek et al 1972). Improvement has been noted in attitude, activities of daily living, and somatic complaints, but not quantitatively in cognitive functions. In Roubicek's study (1972), improvement was most marked for symptoms associated with depression (emotional withdrawal, depressive mood, motor retardation, blunted affect, activity, wakefulness), whereas cognitive functions were not demonstrably improved. Perhaps the efficacy of hydergine is a result of antidepressant activity. Pacha and Salzman (1970) found hydergine to inhibit reuptake of norepinephrine in vitro, a property compatible with antidepressant effects.

Anticoagulants

Walsh and Walsh (1972), using bishydroxycoumarin in uncontrolled studies, claimed remarkable improvements in intellectual function. The action is presumed to be due to decreased sludging of blood. More controlled studies, however, have been less encouraging. Lukas et al (1973) compared an oral anticoagulant to papaverine over a 4-month period in small groups of patients with organic brain syndrome. No significant differences were found between the two groups and both groups showed significant deterioration in the Graham-Kendall test of organic abnormalities. In a year-long, double-blind study, Ratner et al (1972) found no difference in 24 of 25 variables reflecting cognitive functions and mental changes. However, the anticoagulant groups showed a trend toward less deterioration than the control group. The potential hazards of anticoagulation in aged subjects appear to be a legitimate deterrent to the use of this approach.

RNA-like compounds

RNA and DNA have been administered to patients, with conflicting reports of significantly positive intellectual changes (Cameron et al 1963, Kral et al 1967).

Procaine and Gerovital

For years, a buffered form of procaine, developed in Romania, has been promoted enthusiastically as an antiaging medication. It is usually given intramuscularly three times a week for 12 weeks. Many uncontrolled studies have found it effective in the treatment of a broad spectrum of physical and mental disorders associated with aging. Procaine was studied intensively in England, Canada, and in the United States by controlled studies, which were mostly negative (Kral et al 1962), with some exceptions. For a time, Gerovital (European procaine) was discredited. Recently, however, interest has been revived after it was found to be a reversible inhibitor of monoamine oxidase (MacFarlane and Besbris 1974) in the rat liver and thought to be more stable in solution than procaine. Sakalis et al (1974) found Gerovital (H_3) to have a mild euphoriant effect in 10 senile-arteriosclerotic patients with features of depression, which suggests a possible antidepressant effect for the drug. In view of the data reported by Nies et al (1973), indicating increased levels of monoamine oxidase in the aging central nervous system, the potential effectiveness of a mild reversible monoamine oxidase-inhibitor holds some promise.

Hyperbaric Oxygenation

Following remarkably positive findings by Jacobs and her associates (1969) of the effectiveness of pure oxygen administered under high pressure (100 percent at 2.5 atmospheres absolute for 3 hours a day for 15 days) in improving memory and other cognitive functions, other investigators undertook to replicate their findings. Neither Goldfarb and his associates (1972) nor Thompson and collaborators (Thompson, personal communication) have been able to confirm their findings.

Vitamins

Lehmann and Ban (1969) suggest from clinical experience that the B vitamins and vitamin C are helpful in demented patients and are nontoxic. Altman et al (1973) found administration of a vitamin B complex-vitamin C combination strikingly effective in the reduction of excitement and agitation in patients with organic brain syndrome. They hypothesized that institutionalized elderly may be deficient in vitamin C. Cognitive function per se was not tested. This interesting finding deserves further study. The therapeutic use of vitamins, where medically indicated, particularly among the elderly with poor nutritional habits, should not be overlooked.

Gonadal Hormones

These have also been suggested as therapeutic for elderly patients with cognitive deterioration. Michael (1970) administered conjugated equine estrogen to a group of elderly women in a nursing home in a 38-month placebo-controlled trial. The estrogen group showed significant behavioral improvement compared to placebo, but drop-out rate was very high. Lifshitz and Kline (1961) compared estrogen to placebo for 15 months in a large group of chronically demented men. Disappointingly, the only significant difference between groups was a higher mortality in the estrogen-treated group. Further work in the area, however, may prove profitable.

Beta-Adrenergic Blockage

Eisdorfer, Nowlin, and Wilkie (1970) had administered propranolol, a beta-adrenergic blocking agent, to aged nonpatient volunteers and found that performance on serial rote learning improved, while the level of free fatty acids decreased. This suggests a facilitory effect on cognitive function of decreased autonomic nervous system arousal.

Conclusion

Psychopharmacologic treatment should be a part of a comprehensive treatment program, which includes other modalities of treatment of potentially debilitating physical disorders.

The therapeutic nihilism associated with the aged psychiatric patients is unwarranted. A broad array of individual and group therapies, learning strategies, and environmental manipulations, as well as pharmacotherapies, are effective with this population. In some settings, psychotropic medications may be used unwisely, especially in attempts to control recalcitrant individuals with excessive sedation. Such abuses are more likely to occur in the "hopeless and helpless" atmosphere of custodial rather than therapeutically oriented environments.

Psychopharmacologic agents alone, or in conjunction with other forms of treatment, can, in many instances, produce gratifying therapeutic success among the aged. Results will be far more satisfactory, however, when more is known about the psychologic, social, and physiologic bases for age-related changes, and when the avenues of intervention are defined with greater clarity.

References

Altman H, Mehta D, Evenson R, Sletten IW: Behavioral effects of drug therapy on psychogeriatric inpatients: 1. Chlorpromazine and thioridazine. J Am Geriatr Soc 21:241–248, 1973

American Psychiatric Association: Diagnostic and Statistical Manual II. Washington, DC, 1968

Ball JAC, Taylor AR: Effect of cyclandelate on mental function and cerebral blood flow in elderly patients. Br Med J 3:525–528, 1967

Baltes PB, Labouvie GV: Adult development of intellectual performance: description, explanation and modification. In Eisdorfer C, Lawton MP (eds): The Psychology of Adult Development and Aging. Washington DC, American Psychiatric Association, 1973

Bellville JW, Forrest WH, Miller E: Influence of age on pain relief from analgesics. JAMA 217:1835, 1971

Bender AD: Pharmacodynamic principles of drug therapy in the aged. J Am Geriatr Soc 22:296–303, 1974

Cameron DE, Sued S, Solyom L, Wainrib B, Barik H: Effects of ribonucleic acid on memory defect in the aged. Am J Psychiatry 120:320–324, 1963

Chien CP: Psychiatric treatment for geriatric patients "pub" or drug? Am J Psychiatry 127:1070–1075, 1971

———, Stotsky BA, Cole JO: Psychiatric treatment for nursing home patients: drug, alcohol and milieu. Am J Psychiatry 130:543–558, 1973

Davis JM: Use of psychotropic drugs in geriatric patients. J Geriatr Psychiatry 7:145–164, 1974

Dawson-Butterworth K: The chemopsychotherapeutics of geriatric sedation. J Am Geriatr Soc 18:97–114, 1970

DeAlarcon R: Hypochondriasis and depression in the aged. Gerontol Clin 6:266–277, 1964

Eisdorfer C, Nowlin J, Wilkie F: Improvement of learning in the aged by modification of autonomic nervous system activity. Science 170:1327–1329, 1970

———, Raskind MA: Aging, hormones and human behavior. In Sprott RL, Eleftheriou BE (eds): Hormonal Correlates of Behavior. New York, Plenum, 1975

———, Wilkie F: Intellectual changes with advancing age. In Jarvik LF, Eisdorfer C, Blum JE (eds): Intellectual Functioning in Adults. New York, Springer, 1973

Emmengger H, Meier-Ruge W: The actions of hydergine on the brain. A histochemical circulatory and neurophysiological study. Pharmacology 1:65, 1968

Frolkis VV, Bezrukov VV, Duplenko YK, Genis ED: The hypothalamus in aging. Exp Gerontol 7:169–184, 1972

Garattine S, Marcucci F, Morselli PL, Mussini E: The significance of measuring blood levels of benzodiazepines. In Davies DS, Prichard BNC (eds):

Biological Effects of Drugs in Relation to Their Plasma Concentrations. Baltimore, University Park Press, 1973, p 211

Gilbert J, Donnelly KJ, Zimmer LE, Kubis JF: Effect of magnesium pemoline and methylphenidate on memory improvement and mood in normal aging subjects. Aging Hum Dev 4:35–51, 1973

Goldfarb AI, Hochstadt NJ, Jacobson JH, Weinstein E: Hyperbaric oxygen treatment of organic mental syndrome in aged persons. J Gerontol 27:212–217, 1972

Gregerman RI, Bierman EL: Aging and hormones. In Williams RH (ed): Textbook of Endocrinology. Philadelphia, Saunders, 1974

Honigfeld G, Rosenblum MP, Blumenthal IF, Lambert HL, Roberts AJ: Behavioral improvement in the older schizophrenic patient: drug and social therapies. J Am Geriatr Soc 13:57–71, 1965

Hurwitz N: Predisposing factors in adverse reactions to drugs. Br Med J 1:536–539, 1969

Jacobs EA, Winter PM, Alvis HJ, Small SM: Hyperoxygenation effect on cognitive functioning in the aged. N Engl J Med 281:753–757, 1969

Jarvik LF, Cohen D: A biobehavioral approach to intellectual changes with aging. In Eisdorfer C, Lawton MP (eds): The Psychology of Adult Development and Aging. Washington DC, American Psychiatric Association, 1973

Kay DW: Epidemiology of brain deficit in the aged: Issues in patient identification. 10th International Congress of Gerontology, Jerusalem, Israel, 1975

Kral VA, Cahn C, Deutsch M: Procaine (Novocain) treatment of patients with senile and arteriosclerotic brain disease. Can Med Assoc J 87:1109–1113, 1962

————, Solyom L, Enesco HE: Effect of short-term oral RNA therapy on the serum uric acid level and memory function in senile versus senescent subjects. J Am Geriatr Soc 15:364–372, 1967

Learoyd BM: Psychotropic drugs and the elderly patient. Med J Aust 1:1131–1133, 1972

Lehmann HE, Bann TA: Chemotherapy in aged psychiatric patients. Can Psychiatr Assoc J 14:8361–8369, 1969

Lifshitz K, Kline NS: Use of an estrogen in the treatment of psychosis with cerebral arteriosclerosis. JAMA 176:501–504, 1961

Lu LM, Stotsky BA, Cole JO: A controlled study of drugs in long-term geriatric psychiatric patients. Arch Gen Psychiatry 25:284–288, 1971

Lukas ER, Hambacher WD, Fullica AJ: A note on the use of anticoagulant therapy in chronic brain syndrome. J Am Geriatr Soc 21:224–225, 1973

MacFarlane DM, Besbris H: Procaine (Gerovital H3) therapy: mechanism of inhibition of monoamine oxidase. J Am Geriatr Soc 22:365–371, 1974

Michael CM: Further psychometric evaluation of older women—the effect of estrogen administration. J Gerontol 25:337, 1970

Mishara BL, Kastenbaum R: Wine in the treatment of long-term geriatric patients in mental institutions. J Am Geriatr Soc 22:88–94, 1974

Nies A, Robinson DS, Davis JM, Ravaris CL: Changes in monoamine oxidase with aging. In Eisdorfer C, Fann WE (eds): Psychopharmacology and Aging. New York, Plenum, 1973

Nursing Home Care in the United States: Supporting paper No. 2. Drugs in nursing homes, misuse, high costs and kickbacks. Washington, DC, U.S. Government Printing Office, 1974

Office of the Secretary for Health, Education and Welfare: Interim report on nursing home survey. Washington, DC, U.S. Government Printing Office, 1975

Pacha W, Salzman R: Inhibition of the reuptake of neuronally liberated noradrenaline and receptor blocking action of some ergot alkaloids. Br J Pharmacol 38:439–443, 1970

Post F: The Clinical Psychiatry of Late Life. Oxford, Pergamon, 1965

Prien RF, Caffey EM, Klett J: Factors associated with treatment success in lithium carbonate prophylaxis. Arch Gen Psychiatry 31:189–192, 1974

Ratner J, Rosenberg G, Vojtech AK, Engelsmann F: Anticoagulant therapy for senile dementia. J Am Geriatr Soc 21:556–559, 1972

Roubicek J, Geiger SC, Abt K: An ergot alkaloid preparation, hydergine, in geriatric therapy. J Am Geriatr Soc 20:222–229, 1972

Sakalis G, Oh D, Gershon S, Shopsin B: A trial of Gerovital H3 in depression during senility. Curr Ther Res 16:59–63, 1974

Smith WL, Lowrey JB, Davis JA: The effects of cyclandelate on psychological test performance in patients with cerebral vascular insufficiency. Curr Ther Res 10:613–618, 1968

Terry RD, Wisniewski HM: Ultrastructure of senile dementia and of experimental analogs. In Gaitz CM (ed): Aging and the Brain. New York, Plenum, 1972

Van Der Velde CD: Toxicity of lithium carbonate in elderly patients. Am J Psychiatry 127:1075–1077, 1971

Walsh AC, Walsh BH: Senile and presenile dementia: further observations on the benefits of dicumarol—psychotherapy regimen. J Am Geriatr Soc 20:127–131, 1972

Yousef MK, Janowsky DS, Davis JM, Sekerke HJ: Reversal of antiparkinsonian drug toxicity by physostigmine: a controlled study. Am J Psychiatry 130:2, 1973

psychotherapeutic drugs in childhood and adolescence

commentary

The use of psychoactive drugs to treat psychiatric disorders in children is fairly common. The treatment of the hyperactive child with stimulants and other drugs is discussed in another chapter (see p 291). Some of the common childhood disorders that may be treated with drugs are enuresis, school phobia, affective disorders, night terrors, and anxiety states. Enuresis is a self-limiting disorder that disappears with advancing age. If it threatens to persist into adolescence, it may be a source of extreme embarrassment and inconvenience to both the child and the parents. Tricyclic antidepressant medication sometimes helps, perhaps by providing enhanced adrenergic inhibitory input upon micturition. By contrast, cholinergic stimulation has the opposite effect.

The use of tricyclic drugs to treat school phobia is an heroic measure that may be necessary in severe cases in which desensitization and persuasion do not work. Childhood depression and mania do occur and are treated with the same drugs as are used in adults, namely, tricyclics and lithium. The diagnosis should be carefully established before treatment is started. Persistent night terror or somnambulism can be extremely disturbing to both parents and child. Sedative hypnotics and antidepressant drugs appear to be useful but much more research is needed. Anxiety in children is treated with sedative hypnotic drugs, particularly benzodiazepines, just as in adults. Diphenhydramine (Benadryl) is also quite useful, although it may not be as acceptable as a benzodiazepine. Parental reassurance and psychotherapy may be very useful in all mental disturbances in children.

psychotherapeutic drugs in childhood and adolescence

Robert O. Friedel, M.D.
Carl Eisdorfer, Ph.D., M.D.

In this chapter the use of psychotherapeutic agents is discussed for the treatment of most common childhood behavioral disorders presented to the practicing physician—hyperactive child syndrome (minimal brain dysfunction), enuresis, school phobia, affective disorders, night terrors, and anxiety states. Most physicians will recognize the need for other forms of therapeutic interventions, such as parental and teacher counseling, for all children manifesting symptoms of these disorders. However, since it is beyond the scope of this article to deal with these additional treatment modalities comprehensively, the reader will be referred to other sources for this information, when appropriate.

The effective use of psychotherapeutic agents in children presents the practicing physician with at least four problems in addition to those commonly encountered in treating adults with these medications. (a) Criteria for the diagnosis of psychiatric disorders in children are not as clearly defined as in adults; children present with a vast variety of physical symptoms, some of which are thought of mask underlying emotional conditions. (b) Due to pharmacokinetic effects, only one of which is a function of body size, therapeutic dose ranges are more variable in children than in adults. (c) Even when the diagnostic picture is fairly clear, some of the drugs commonly used in adolescents and adults are not approved for use in children by the Food and Drug Administration. (d) There is concern that drug use in children will increase subsequent drug-abuse tendencies and will act to produce a population of adolescents and adults who use medications far too liberally to solve ordinary life problems (Lennard et al 1971). Although there are no data substantiating these fears and there are some refuting them (Beck et al 1975), they are still most likely a major determinant in the development of treatment plans for behaviorally disturbed children. Hopefully, additional information and a realistic and supportive approach to parents with these concerns will reduce the impact of these latter factors.

Prevalence of Psychotherapeutic Drug Use in Children and Adolescents

Parish (1971) surveyed the records of 13,259 patients aged 15 to 92 years seen by general practitioners in England and Wales from May 1967 to April 1968. Of those aged 15 to 20 years, 8 percent of the males and 34 percent of the females received psychotropic medications, the most commonly prescribed being antidepressants and tranquilizers. Rowe (1973a, b) reviewed more than one million prescriptions for antidepressant drugs written by general practitioners in Australia during a 9-month period in 1971 and found that 4.1 percent of the prescriptions were written for males and 3.3 percent were written for females 14 years and younger. In a cross-national study (excluding the United States) Balter et al (1974) found that between 4.0 percent and 13.5 percent of the males between 5.3 percent and 17.2 percent of the females between 15 and 24 used antianxiety/sedative drugs during the years prior to their study. Rowe (1973a, b) also found that these medications were prescribed for the treatment of mental disorders in 2.8 percent and 2.2 percent of the male and female patients under 14 years of age by 796 general practitioners surveyed in Australia. In general, then, the data indicated that psychotherapeutic agents are prescribed by general practitioners for children and adolescents in significant amounts in other parts of the world and that it is relatively safe to assume that a similar pattern exists in the United States (Parry et al 1973).

Hyperactive Child Syndrome

The subject of drug effects on minimal brain damage or the hyperactive child syndrome has been covered elsewhere in this book (p 291).

Enuresis

The frequent occurrence of enuresis in children makes this a common problem in general practice. Meadow (1970) estimated that between 10 and 15 percent of 5-year-olds, 5 percent of 10-year-olds, and 1 percent of 15-year-olds wet their bed at night. A recent survey (WHO, unpublished data) revealed similar findings with 13 percent of 6- and 7-year-olds and 3 percent of 13- and 14-year-olds still reported to be wetting their beds more than once a month. Thorne (1944) reported that 1 in 50 Army draftees in World War II were still enuretic at age 18. Boys are more likely to have this problem than girls, the ratio being about 3:2 to 2:1. Approximately two-thirds of enuretic children have never achieved a dry period and are called "primary" enuretics. The remaining one-third, having experienced a dry period at some point prior to the onset of recurrent wetting, are designated "secondary" enuretics. Andersen and Petersen (1974) proposed that these two subtypes be further divided into those without and those with behavioral disturbances. Their data suggest that boys are more likely to present with primary enuresis without behavioral disturbances, whereas girls predominate in the other three subtypes. Girls more commonly present with enuresis of a diurnal nature and with symptoms of urinary tract infection. The associated symptom of encopresis was found to be twice as common in boys as in girls by these authors. Ritvo and co-workers (1969) describe two subgroups of children with enuresis on the basis of sleep electroencephalogram derived events, terming them arousal and nonarousal enuretics. Subjects with arousal enuresis showed increased evidence of neuroticism, a history of sporadic wetting, and no family history of enuresis. Subjects with nonarousal enuresis had minimal evidence of maladjustment, a history of regular wetting, family history of enuresis, and a better response to imipramine.

Feldman (1973) lists eight theories of the etiology of enuresis that have been proposed at one time or another. Among these are: small bladder capacity, failure of conditioning, nocturnal epilepsy, obstructive uropathy, spina bifida occulta, food allergy, and psychologic factors. The relative prevalence of these different proposed causes of enuresis has not been clearly determined, but relatively few are attributable to organic lesions.

Treatment

As one might surmise, no single treatment program has gained universal acceptance. Some authors recommend a complete history, physical examination, laboratory studies, including urinalysis, urine culture, and urologic investigation consisting of intravenous pyelograms and voiding cystourethrograms. Others consider this approach too heroic to be employed routinely and opt for a more conservative program relying on radiologic procedures only in those cases refractory to the more commonly used therapeutic approaches.

In addition to counseling and psychotherapy, the two interventions that have received the most attention have been the electric alarm system and drug treatment with a tricyclic antidepressant, most commonly imipramine. The proponents of the alarm system (Young and Morgan 1973) feel that with the full cooperation of parents this system is highly effective, although it does not lend itself readily to controlled studies. In spite of reported high success rates, it is suggested (Fraser 1972) that buzzer training not be undertaken until a urinary tract infection has been excluded (psychiatric assessment has been reqeested when several symptoms of emotional disturbance are present in addition to the symptom of enuresis), until waking the child in the late evening or early morning has been tried; and a course of extended treatment with tricyclic antidepressants and chlordiazepoxide has been attempted. When all of these approaches have failed and the alarm system has been unsuccessful, many practitioners feel that more extensive urologic and psychiatric evaluation should then be pursued.

Prior to treatment with imipramine, children with organic heart disease, hyperthyroidism, glaucoma, diabetes, kidney or liver disease should be excluded by careful history, physical examination, and routine laboratory tests. Patients receiving treatment with monoamine oxidase inhibitors should also be excluded. Imipramine is approved for use in children of 6 and over suffering from enuresis. An oral dose of 25 mg given 1 hour before bedtime is the recommended starting dose. If improvement has not been noted after 1 week, the dose is increased to 50 mg nightly. In children over 12 years of age an additional increase of 25 mg to a total of 75 mg per night may be attempted in those who do not respond after the second week of treatment. Improvement frequently takes 1 to 2 weeks to occur, and both patients and parents should be alerted to this response pattern. Once a successful response has occurred, it is recommended that the child be maintained on the medication for a 3- to 6-month period, since it appears that exacerbation of symptoms frequently occurs when shorter time periods are employed. The evidence is not clar that rapid cessation of medication after the treatment program is complete results in a greater rate of exacerbation of symptoms than a gradual tapering of medications. However, the latter course is to be preferred until conclusive data are available.

Adverse Reactions

Side effects do not appear to be common in children treated with imipramine for enuresis. When reported, they include anticholinergic effects, tremors, anorexia, and diarrhea.

There is a growing concern about the increasing incidence of sublethal and lethal poisoning in children with tricyclic compounds (Brown et al 1971). Such medications now rank second to salicylates as a cause of childhood death due to self-poisoning (Bain 1973). Goel and Shanks (1974) report that 60 percent of 60 children admitted over a 7-year period were receiving treatment for enuresis. The most prevalent symptoms are convulsions, coma, cardiac arrythmias, and vascular collapse. Treatment is difficult. In addition to supportive measures, intravenous physostigmine (Rumack 1973), potassium chloride (Schneider 1972), glucagon (Ruddy et al 1972), and sodium bicarbonate (Brown et al 1973) are reported to be beneficial. Careful counseling of parents in the proper use and care of this medication is a prerequisite to prescribing it for a disease that itself is not life threatening.

At the very least, enuresis has a significant emotional overlay associated with it, even when it is not primarily psychogenic. Therefore, it is recommended that ample time be taken to discuss the problem and management with both parents and child, provoking as little guilt as possible, in an effort to determine what these factors may be and to reduce them when possible.

School Phobia

School phobia, like enuresis, presents more frequently to the primary medical practitioner than to the mental health specialist. The presenting symptom is typically marked anxiety associated with the thought of going to school or being at school, which is reduced significantly by staying home. The symptoms often include malaise, nausea, stomach pains, and pallor, which are associated with the anxiety. "School phobia" is to be differentiated from school truancy primarily by the observation that separation anxiety from mother or from home is the central issue among school phobic children and absent among truant children. Thus *separation phobia* may be a more apt term for many such children. Gittelman-Klein and Klein (1973) report that in addition to the primary anxiety occasioned by separation, the child also demonstrates a marked anticipatory anxiety and refuses to go to school. It is clear that in children who have completely refused to attend school for a 1- to 2-week period that a crisis situation exists and that medical help is urgently needed. Unfortunately, there have been few studies directed at defining the epidemiology, typology, and controlled evaluation of a variety of therapeutic approaches to this problem. Some authors recommend that children be immediately separated from parents (Eisenberg

1958), while others feel it imperative that the therapist must be employed by, and only responsible to, the communities, since the therapist paid by and under the control of the family is often left when he fails to meet their manipulative demands (Skynner 1974). School phobias often occur following illness of the child, a parent or loss of some loved object, and may occur at the initiation or at some later point in one's school history. School phobias associated with traumatic events may be more responsive to measures involving the cooperation of the parents and school in forcing the child into the classroom situation. School problems associated with a history of disturbed parent-child relationships and that build up over longer periods require different strategies.

There have been only two reports of controlled studies evaluating the effects of drug therapy on the treatment of severe school phobia. Frommer (1967) treated 32 depressed children, 15 with phobia, with phenelzine-chlordiazepoxide combination and phenobarbital for 2 weeks each, finding the antidepressant and minor tranquilizer combination superior to the sedative. Gittelman-Klein and Klein (1973) treated 35 school-phobic children in a double-blind, placebo controlled study design with imipramine or placebo. Both groups were treated the same regarding counseling of parents in the use of persuasive and desensitization techniques and supportive efforts by social workers. The reader is recommended to this paper for more details on the combination of the counseling approach and the use of active medications.

Since the tricyclic antidepressants are safer to use than the monoamine oxidase inhibitors, the authors suggest that if attempts at returning the child to school using more conservative techniques are not successful, imipramine should be tried. Patients are given 25 mg per day fdor the first 3 days, then 50 mg for the next 4 days, followed by 75 mg per day during the second week. Thereafter, the dose is adjusted weekly by increments of 25 mg. Parents and patient are told to expect a reduction of fear and parents are instructed to maintain a firm attitude toward promoting school attendance, with a family member accompanying the child to school and remaining there until the anticipatory anxiety has been reduced significantly. In the Gittelman-Klein and Klein (1973) study, doses below 100 mg per day were indistinguishable from placebo and no child was found to respond to doses of less than 75 mg per day. In some children doses had to be increased to 200 mg per day and in one instance to 300 mg per day. Children were found to vary widely in their response to imipramine dosage, and since blood levels were not determined it can only be speculated that this is a function of interpatient differences in drug absorption, metabolism, distribution, elimination, or tissue sensitivity. Treatment should be continued for a minimum of 6 weeks in order to evaluate the effectiveness of the medication. Since no long-term follow-up of the children is reported in the above study, it is not clear at this point how long medication must be continued to maintain any progress noted. Once improvement has been observed, it is recommended that the child be maintained on the lowest possible dose for a period of several months, since this appears to be the minimal amount of time necessary for the successful management of other problems with this medication.

Side effects at the dosage of imipramine recommended were reported by Gittelman-Klein and Klein (1973) to consist predominantly of dry mouth, constipation, dizziness, and tremor. These authors conclude that on the whole there was remarkably little difficulty due to side effects in their study group.

It should be emphasized that the successful return to school of children who suffer from school phobia depends on a number of independent factors, including parental and school cooperation, the quality of the support given parents, school, and patient, as well as the skillful use of medication as an adjunctive treatment.

Affective Disorders

It is apparent that children, and to a greater degree, adolescents, experience symptoms of both depression and mania. Criteria for the diagnosis of affective disorders in children and in adolescents have not been clearly defined, however, primarily because the presenting symptomatology often differs significantly from that seen in adults. While some children present with the classic symptoms of these disorders, most have a considerable amount of difficulty in expressing feelings of helplessness, hopelessness, rejection, emptiness, loneliness, or worthlessness. It is also suggested that such feelings frequently underlie or accompany acting-out, delinquent behavior, poor school performance, temper tantrums, truancy, running away, excessive alcohol intake, promiscuous behavior, boredom, restlessness, and poor communication. The classic biologic symptoms of depression, such as sleep disturbance, anorexia, and psychomotor retardation, are also absent frequently, and mild hyperactivity is much more common than psychomotor retardation. The acting-out behaviors are thought to serve as a defense against depression and regression, chronic feelings of low self-esteem, and as a deterrent to realistically confronting the sources of grief.

Prevalence and incidence figures for affective disorders in children and adolescents have been showing an increase since 1961 when Annesley (1961) found affective disorders in only 4 percent of 362 adolscents admitted to the St. Ebba's Hospital. Using conventional, (ie, adult-derived) diagnostic criteria with adolescents, King and Pittman (1970) examined the psychiatric workup of 65 patients less than age 19 admitted during 1 year to Renard Hospital, Washington University. Twenty-six patients (40 percent) met the criteria of Woodruff et al (1974) for depression. Cytryn and McKnew (1972) define three categories of depressive reaction of midchildhood ages 6 to 12: masked depressive reaction, acute depressive reaction, and chronic depressive reaction. These authors find that the masked depressive type is the most frequent but unfortunately give no data as to the frequency of these subtypes of depression. Weinburg et al (1973) reported that 45 of 72 children (63 percent), referred to an educational diagnostic clinic for poor school performance or behavioral problems, were felt to be depressed. The diagnosis of depression was made by clearly stated criteria. Suicide among adolescents is also an increasing phenomenon.

Although there are statements in the literature that medications are not effective in the treatment of affective disorders in children and adolescents, these statements are typically not substantiated by data. On the other hand, in one of the two controlled studies reported to date, Lucas et al (1965) found amitriptyline effective in the treatment of 14 children and adolescents presenting with symptoms of depression, while Frommer (1967) found a phenlzine-chlordiazepoxide combination superior to phenobarbital in a mixed group of 32 children, half of whom were described as suffering from mood disorder. In addition Rifkin et al (1972), in a controlled study, found lithium efficacious in the treatment of adolescent girls presenting with a syndrome they describe as "emotionally unstable character disorder."

What may be said with some degree of assurance at present is that children and adolescents do suffer from affective disorders and that the general practitioner should maintain a high "index of suspicion" for this problem before affixing the diagnosis of antisocial personality disorder to young people with a variety of acting-out disorders. Attempts should be made to elicit feelings of hopelessness, helplessness, inability to experience pleasure, and worthlessness from the child. A positive family history for affective disorders or alcoholism also supports the diagnosis of an underlying affective disorder. Since many of these children frequently have problems of such severity that educational and social growth are severely impeded, and since there is no demonstrated effective treatment for moderate to severe behavior disorders, it is the author's contention that in the presence of the above symptoms and family history, pharmacologic management should be considered. For children presenting with predominantly hyperactive or maniclike behavior, a trial on lithium carbonate is recommended. Since this medication is not approved for this particular use, parental consent, after full discussion with them, is advisable. To minimize side effects, it is recommended that initial doses be low and increased gradually until a blood level of approximately 1.0 mEq per liter is achieved. Lower levels than this are probably therapeutic in many instances. For those children presenting with symptoms more consistent with depression and manifested by lower levels of activity, we have found that doxepin and amitriptyline are very effective in this population, especially when given in single doses at bedtime, thus minimizing side effects such as drowsiness during the day with concomitant impairment of school performance. Dosage should be adjusted at weekly intervals until the therapeutic effect is obtained or dose limits are achieved. These tricyclic antidepressants are not approved for use in children under 12 years of age and, therefore, consent should be obtained from parents before doing so.

Pavor Nocturnis (Night Terrors) and Somnambulism

Symptoms of night terror in children are quite readily diagnosed. The child wakes up screaming, usually in the first hour or two of sleep, perspiring, terrified and in a state of panic, and typically unconsolable. The child then goes back to sleep in a few minutes to one half hour and has no recollection of the attack in the morning. Somnambulism also usually occurs during the first several hours of sleep. The child quietly arises and walks around his room or other parts of the house in a confused manner. Episodes may last from a few minutes to a half an hour and, as in the case of pavor nocturnis, the child does not recall any of his behavior in the morning. Although there are no controlled studies evaluating the efficacy of medications in the treatment of pavor nocturnis and somnambulism, several open studies report favorable results with diazepam and imipramine. Pesikoff and Davis (1971) treated 7 children with either pavor nocturnis or somnambulism or both, with imipramine at bedtime for a minimum of 8 weeks, with a complete cessation of symptoms in all patients. Glick et al (1971) treated 7 children with sleep disorders, three with night terrors and somnambulism, with diazepam 2 to 5 mg at bedtime, with a successful response in all cases. Tec (1974) reports the successful treatment of 12 children with somnambulism and night terrors with 25 to 50 mg of imi-

pramine at bedtime. The latter author found that in his series 2 weeks
of medication was sufficient. This author also reports that in one
case in which imipramine was unsuccessful, nortriptyline therapy
was successful. It is recommended that when the symptoms of these
disorders present significant problems, diazepam be tried initially,
since the toxicity and side effects of this medication are less than
those of the tricyclic antidepressants. Controlled studies are clearly
indicated in this area.

Anxiety States

Most prescriptions for antianxiety agents in this country are written
by general practitioners (Parry et al 1973). At the present time indications for the use of these agents in children and in adolescents are
not clearly defined. Anxiety is a symptom most individuals have
experienced at one point or another, and the decision to use medications for its relief in these age groups is certainly open to debate. The
authors recommend that only anxiety of a moderate to severe degree
and clearly of an acute nature be treated by the practitioner, and that,
pharmaceutical advertisements to the contrary, prophylactic doses
of antianxiety medication to help one over the anticipated problems
of adjustment to a new school, a new neighborhood, separation from
parents, a hard day at school, or one's first date are medically unwarranted indications.

Since benzodiazepine derivatives are the least toxic, are not addictive antianxiety agents, and result in the fewest number of adverse interactions with other drugs (Greenblatt and Shader 1974),
these are currently the drugs of choice in this area. Prescriptions
should be written so that the drug is taken only when needed rather
than on a fixed schedule. Long-term use of the medication should be
avoided. Patients needing more than a few weeks treatment should
be referred to a psychiatrist when possible. If symptoms are not
relieved by a benzodiazepine compound, diphenhydramine (Benadryl) has been found to be effective in prepubertal children. Young
children appear to require higher doses of this medication by body
weight than do adults, and the drug reduces symptoms before producing drowsiness or lethargy in the prepubertal child (Fish 1968).

Summary

Psychopharmacologic agents are powerful tools, each with specific
indications for use and most with anticipated side effects. As such,

they represent a quite significant and valuable adjunct to the practitioners armamentarium, but one requiring careful judgment of the options. In most cases these medications should be seen as part of a therapeutic package, much as the treatment of a diabetic with insulin should be accompanied by a program of diet and exercise management. In some instances the long-term consequences of drug use is not known, and this should be a factor in treatment decisions. Occasionally psychotherapeutic drugs are taken lightly, since they have (as a rule) a very low index of lethality. This is not warranted. In other cases moral rudgments concerning an overmedicated society clouds an appropriate clinical decision with regards to a specific patient.

It seems clear that blanket condemnation or praise of such medication is naive. What is important is that well-informed, sound clinical decisions be based upon careful evaluation, efforts at alternative or conjoint strategies (where helpful), consultation and discussions with parents or guardians (as well as the patient, where appropriate), careful follow-up and reevaluations with periodic trials off drugs, and careful attention to side effects, including growth changes. These are the hallmarks of effective use of psychopharmacology in the patient's best interests.

References

Andersen OO, Petersen KE: Enuresis: an attempt at classification by genesis. Acta Paediatr Scand 63:512, 1974

Annesley PT: Psychiatric illness in adolescence: presentation and prognosis. J Ment Sci 107:268, 1961

Bain DJG: A criticism of the use of tricyclic antidepressant drugs in the treatment of childhood enuresis. J R Coll Gen Practit 23:222, 1973

Balter MB, Levine J, Manheimer DI: Cross-national study of the extent of antianxiety/sedative drug use. N Engl J Med 290:769, 1974

Beck L, Langford WS, MacKay M, Sum G: Childhood chemotherapy and later drug abuse and growth curve: a follow-up study of thirty adolescents. Am J Psychiatry 132:436, 1975

Brown TCK, Barker GA, Dunlop ME, Loughnan PM: The use of sodium bicarbonate in the treatment of tricyclic antidepressant-induced arrhythmias. Anaesth Intensive Care 1:203, 1973

———, Dwyer ME, Stocks JG: Antidepressant overdosage in children—a new menace. Med J Aust 2:848, 1971

Campbell M: Pharmacotherapy in early infantile autism. Biol Psychol 10:399, 1975

Cytryn L, McKnew DH Jr: Proposed classification of childhood depression. Am J Psychiatry 129:149, 1972

Eisenberg L: School phobia: a study in the communication of anxiety. Am J Psychiatry 114:712, 1958

Feldman W: Enuresis. CMA Journal 109:218, 1973

Fish B: Drug use in psychiatric disorders in children. Am J Psychiatry 124:(Suppl 1)31, 1968

Fraser MS: Nocturnal enuresis. Practitioner 208:203, 1972

Frommer EA: Treatment of childhood depression with antidepressant drugs. Br Med J 1:729, 1967

Gittelman-Klein R, Klein DF: School phobia: diagnostic considerations in the light of imipramine effects. J Nerv Ment Dis 156:199, 1973

Glick BS, Schulman D, Turecki S: Diazepam (Valium) treatment in childhood sleep disorders. Dis Nerv Syst 32:565, 1971

Goel KM, Shanks RA: Amitriptyline and imipramine poisoning in children. Br Med J 1:261, 1974

Greenblatt DJ, Shader RI: Benzodiazepines in Clinical Practice. New York, Raven, 1974

King LJ, Pittman GD: A six year follow-up study of sixty-five adolescent patients: natural history of affective disorders in adolescence. Arch Gen Psychiatry 22:230, 1970

Lennard HC, Epstein LJ, Bernstein A, Ransom DC: Mystification and Drug Misuse. New York, Harper, 1971

Lucas RC, Lockett HJ, Grimm F: Amitriptyline in childhood depressions. Dis Nerv Syst 26:105, 1965

Meadow R: Childhood enuresis. Br Med J 4:787, 1970

Parish PA: The prescribing of psychotropic drugs in general practice. J R Coll Gen Practit 21:(Suppl 4)1, 1971

Parry HJ, Balter MB, Mellinger GD, Cisin IH, Manheimer DI: National patterns of psychotherapeutic drug use. Arch Gen Psychiatry 28:769, 1973

Pesikoff RB, Davis PC: Treatment of pavor nocturnis and somnambulism in children. Am J Psychiatry 128:778, 1971

Rifkin A, Quitkin F, Carrillo C, Blumberg AG, Klein DF: Lithium carbonate in emotionally unstable character disorder. Arch Gen Psychiatry 27:519, 1972

Ritvo ER, Orvitz EM, Gottlieb F, Poussaint AF, Maron BJ, Ditman KS, Blinn KA: Arousal and non-arousal enuretic events. Am J Psychiatry 126:77, 1969

Rowe IL: Prescription of psychotropic drugs by general practitioners: 2. General. Med J Aust 1:589, 1973a

————: Prescription of psychotropic drugs by general practitioners. 2. Antidepressants. Med J Aust 1:642, 1973b

Ruddy JM, Seymour JL, Anderson NG: Management of tricyclic antidepressant ingestion in children with special reference to the use of glucagon. Med J Aust 1:630, 1972

Rumack BH: Anticholinergic poisoning: treatment with physostigmine. Pediatrics 52:449, 1973

Schneider S: Imipramine poisoning: successful treatment. Pediatrics 49:787, 1972

Skynner ACR: School phobia: a reappraisal. Br J Med Psychol 47:1, 1974

Tec L: Imipramine for nightmares. JAMA 228:978, 1974

Thorne F: The incidence of nocturnal enuresis after age five. Am J Psychiatry 100:686, 1944

Weinburg WA, Rutman J, Sullivan L, Penick EC, Dietz SG: Depression in children referred to an educational diagnostic center: diagnosis and treatment. J Pediatr 83:1065, 1973

WHO-International Collaborative Project of Medical Care Utilization. Baltimore Supplementary Questionnaire. Unpublished data

Woodruff RA Jr, Goodwin DW, Guze SB: Psychiatric Diagnosis. New York, Oxford Univ Press, 1974

Young GC, Morgan RTT: Rapidity of response to the treatment of enuresis. Dev Med Child Neurol 15:488, 1973

rational and irrational use of narcotic analgesics

commentary

For a long time the opioids have been known to have a serious potential for inducing addiction in their users. However, fear of drug dependence may sometimes be so exaggerated that many physicians fail to provide adequate relief of pain and suffering for patients who need it. Dr. Sachar discusses this very important problem and suggests that physicians should be more intrepid and place greater reliance upon patient reports. Above all, no patient should be allowed to suffer when adequate doses of pain relieving drugs are available.

rational and irrational use of narcotic analgesics

Edward J. Sachar, M.D.

Amid the national concern about narcotic drug abuse in the United States, another type of misuse of narcotic drugs has received relatively little attention. Ironically, the latter problem may have been aggravated by efforts to deal with the former. I am referring to the widespread undertreatment with narcotic analgesics of medical patients in pain. It appears that a significant percentage of medical inpatients suffer needless agony because physicians and nurses fail to administer narcotic analgesics in an adequate dose regimen.

Our systematic data on this point comes from a study conducted in 1970 on the inpatient service of a major New York City teaching hospital (Marks and Sachar 1973). The study was prompted by numerous instances in which psychiatric consultation was requested because of patient behavior judged inappropriate by medical house staff, and which turned out to be partly iatrogenic, that is, the "inappropriate" behavior was occasioned by severe distress due to pain inadequately treated by the physician.

We then administered structured interviews to 37 consecutively admitted medical inpatients who were receiving parenteral narcotic analgesics (mostly meperidine) for pain arising from a wide variety of medical conditions. The interviewers made quantitative assessments of the degree of distress from pain that patients reported experiencing, despite the analgesic medication. The interviewers scored not only the patient's response to a global question about pain relief and residual distress, but also the degree of distress expressed in specific difficulties with sleep, concentration, eating, anxiety, depression, irritability, and crying spells. We found that 32 percent of the patients reported they were still experiencing severe distress, while 41 percent were in moderate distress. Only 27 percent of the patients reported adequate pain relief. Forty-three percent of the patients also reported severe return of pain well before their next dose.

Interestingly the response of patients to the global question correlated poorly with their subsequent responses to detailed questions about specific areas of distress. This suggests that if physicians really want to find out how their patients are responding to analgesics, it is important not to stop with a general question but to pursue the matter with specific, focused questions in the same way physicians are accustomed to doing when assessing clinical responses to drugs for peptic ulcers, congestive heart failure, and so forth. It appears, however, that physicians rarely do this.

The average dose of meperidine prescribed for the total group of 37 patients was 66 mg intramuscularly every 4 hours (usually as required), a dose judged by pharmacologists to be insufficient to relieve severe pain in a substantial percentage of subjects. The amounts of drug *actually received* by the patients was much less than this. Only one patient was given a meperidine dosage regimen above 75 mg every 4 hours, even though the optimum dose range for meperidine, for effective relief of severe pain, for the maximum number of patients with the minimum amount of side effects, is 80 to 100 mg, and the average duration of action is only 3 hours (Beecher 1966, Buchsbaum 1975, Evans 1974, Glassman and Perel 1975).

A chart review revealed that a third of the patients were suffering from acute myocardial infarctions or coronary ischemia, conditions for which relief of pain is considered vital, while others in severe distress included some suffering from advanced cancer. Only 1 of the 37 patients had a medical contraindication to larger doses.

While these data were drawn from a single hospital, our strong impression is that the findings reflect a widespread phenomenon, based on communication we have received from many medical centers and our experiences in lecturing and consulting at other hospitals.

What underlies this significant undertreatment? One possibility is that physicians have inadequate or incorrect information about narcotic drugs. In order to clarify this point, in 1971 we gathered questionnaire data from 102 medical interns and residents at two major New York City teaching hospitals (Marks and Sachar 1973). The 25 multiple choice questions were designed mainly to assess their information and attitudes about the clinical administration of intramuscular meperidine (the most commonly used narcotic analgesic in inpatients). We should emphasize that our results pertain to house staff in 1971. It may be that older, more experienced clinicians would have responded differently and that beliefs and practices may have changed during the past several years. On the other hand, the house staff were closely supervised by attending physicians, and our impression is that most of the misunderstandings noted in 1971 still persist.

It was still interesting (and ironic) that 100 percent of respondents claimed that the desirable end-point of an analgesic regimen was either complete relief of pain or enough relief so that the pain is noticed but is not distressing. Yet, in general, their choice of drug dosage in a variety of hypothetical clinical situations would not have achieved these goals for a great percentage of cases.

The points of information most commonly misunderstood by many of the residents and students were the following:

Therapeutic Dose Range of Intramuscular Meperidine

Ten milligrams of morphine are equivalent to 80 to 100 mg of meperidine (but meperidine is shorter acting), and this dose will relieve severe pain in the great majority of subjects, although not all. Lesser doses, equivalent to 62 to 72 mg, will leave one-third of subjects experiencing severe pain or significant distress. Doses of 125 to 150 mg may be required by a small percentage of subjects, but above 100 mg the incidence of side effects (eg, decreased tidal volume, hypotension) is greater (Lasagna and Beecher 1954, Beecher 1966, Lasagna 1964, Jaffe 1966).

Many physicians underestimated the optimum doses of meperidine and evidently did not realize that there is a distribution curve among patients in terms of their dosage requirements of narcotic analgesics. In all likelihood, part of this variation is due to differences in blood levels attained after a standard dose, since genetic differences in the rate of metabolism by the liver of a variety of medical and psychiatric drugs have been well demonstrated in recent years (Glassman and Perel 1975). Furthermore, while we did not address this point in our questionnaire, we have since learned that many physicians do not realize that an oral dose of meperidine is only one-third to one-half as effective as the same dose administered intramuscularly.

In clinical practice it is quite reasonable in many situations to begin with a dose that statistically has a 66 percent chance of being adequate—say, 75 mg intramuscularly. It is imperative, however, for the doctor then to assess the patient's response to that dose and to be prepared to increase it if it is inadequate. On the other hand, in cases such as acute myocardial infarction, where the doctor wants to be relatively certain he will relieve pain immediately, a starting dose of 100 mg would seem to be indicated; the dose could then be reduced

later, if necessary, after the patient's response is clinically reasses-
ed.

Duration of Action

Intramuscular meperidine is shorter acting than morphine, with a
range of 2 to 4 hours, and an average duration of 3 hours (Jaffe 1975).
This means that many patients receiving a standard 4-hour regimen
will be suffering for an hour, and some for 2 hours, before they get
their next injection. Nearly half of the patients we interviewed reported this phenomenon as being severe. We don't know how often
doctors ask patients how long the analgesic effect lasts, but in response to a questionnaire item describing a patient on a 4-hour regimen, who reported significant pain return after 3 hours, a third of
the respondents rejected the alternative of switching to a 3-hour
regimen, stating they would make no change.

Addiction Liability and Tolerance Phenomena

Addiction and tolerance are two separate pharmacologic issues.
Tolerance is a very common concomitant of repeated narcotic administration. Probably there are changes over time in the opiate
receptor, altering its sensitivity. Clinically, tolerance is manifested
in an increase in the dose required to achieve the same pharmacologic effect, and, usually, in some symptoms associated with
drug withdrawal (physical dependence). By the end of 2 weeks of
around-the-clock administration of narcotic analgesics in the
therapeutic range, some increase in dosage will probably be required
in most patients if the severity of the underlying pain remains the
same. However, since tolerance also usually develops to side effects,
no increase in incidence of these side effects would be anticipated. If
the drug is abruptly discontinued at the end of 2 weeks, some mild
withdrawal symptoms will be detectable in nearly all patients, with
transient sleep disturbance and rhinorrhea being the most common
(Jaffe 1975).
    Addiction, on the other hand, is a behavioral pattern of compul-
sive drug use characterized by overwhelming preoccupation with
the use of the drug and securing its supply, and a tendency to relapse after withdrawal (Jaffe 1968). In the process of becoming addicted, tolerance and physical dependence are frequent and important elements, but not absolutely necessary. A more important contribution to the etiology of addiction is social involvement in a
drug-abuse culture (Jaffe 1975).

The point is that the probability is virtually nil of making a mentally healthy person an addict after 1 to 3 weeks of rational narcotic therapy for a time-limited pain problem in the controlled environment of a hospital, where the emphasis is on the drug's specific medicinal properties. What is more, the percentage of narcotic addicts in the United States who began their addictive career after hospital narcotic treatment for pain is quite negligible (Marks and Sachar 1973, Jaffe 1975).

There was much confusion about these issues among house staff in 1971, and this confusion appeared to influence their prescribing patterns. Thus, 22 percent of physicians thought the likelihood of a patient becoming addicted after 10 days of 100 mg of meperidine every 4 hours was greater than 6 percent (!), and these respondents were also less likely to prescribe adequate doses of meperidine for acute myocardial infarction. Fifteen percent of the doctors thought that the percentage of American narcotic addicts who had first become addicted after a course of in-hospital narcotic therapy for pain was greater than 5 percent; these physicians were much less likely to increase the dose of medication for a terminal cancer patient whose severe pain was no longer being relieved—indeed many recommended substituting placebos.

This raises one of the most troubling aspects of the inappropriate concern about addiction—the failure to treat with adequate narcotic analgesics patients with terminal malignancies. To quote Jaffe's comment (1975) in Goodman and Gilman's textbook of pharmacology.

> Some degree of physical dependence and tolerance develops whenever a narcotic is given in therapeutic dosage over a prolonged period, but in patients with painful terminal illnesses such considerations should not in any way prevent the physician from fulfilling his primary obligation to ease the patient's discomfort. The physician should not wait until the pain becomes agonizing; no patient should ever wish for death because of his physician's reluctance to use adequate amounts of potent narcotics.

Indeed, in Cecily Saunder's hospice for fatally ill patients in England, those narcotic drugs with greater euphoric properties are deliberately chosen, regardless of their addictive risk.

We have emphasized the negligible likelihood that addiction will occur in the controlled setting of the hospital. For outpatients with chronic pain, who are given the responsibility of regulating their own narcotic medication, the probability of addiction is significantly higher, and the physician should not abdicate his responsibility for supervising the medication regimen in the context of a supportive relationship.

Euphoria

The incidence of euphoria associated with therapeutic doses of meperidine has been reported as between 10 and 25 percent. A clear relationship to dose has not been established. A euphoric response should not be seen as a contraindication to meperidine or as a reason for reducing a dose previously established as effective and not excessive.

Half of the physicians in our sample, however, said they would reduce the dose for a patient who reported mild euphoria, and, in another clinical situation involving a herniated lumbar disc, almost half of the doctors would reduce the dose if the patient merely reported he felt relief not only of the pain but also of the depression associated with pain.

It is remarkable that so many physicians responded in this way. Possibly some have puritanical attitudes about a medicine that makes people feel good, but more likely there is concern that a euphoric reaction might lead the patient to seek the drug later for purposes of abuse. Once again, there is no evidence to support such a concern.

The observations drawn from our questionnaire study have since been supplemented by further impressions of areas of significant misunderstanding, which may interfere with the rational use of narcotic analgesics.

Placebo Response

There seems to be a widespread view among physicians and nurses that relief of pain following administration of a placebo proves that the patient is malingering or neurotic or that the pain is functional rather than organic in origin. Nothing is further from the truth.

Much is still mysterious about the placebo response in pain reduction, but certain facts have been established. (a) In severe clinical pain, numerous studies have shown that about a third of the patients achieve at least 50 percent relief after placebos (Evans 1974). There is no relationship between suggestibility or hypnotizability and responsiveness to placebo (Orne 1974, see also p 47). (b) The potency of the placebo is closely related to the potency ascribed by the patient to the analgesic it has replaced. This relationship is remarkably constant at a figure of about 50 percent. Thus, for the placebo-responder, a placebo-morphine is 50 percent as effective as morphine, placebo-aspirin is 50 percent as potent as aspirin, and so on (Evans 1974). (c) The mechanism of the placebo response is not by its relief of anxiety, although there are differences between anxious and nonanxious subjects in their response to placebo (Evans 1974). These facts should make it clear that the derogation of the placebo responder is entirely inappropriate.

Virtually all studies on the placebo response deal with responses to the first dose. The potency of chronic placebo administration is unclear, but the general impression is that effectiveness declines rapidly with repeated doses.

Individual Differences in Response to Pain

Just as there is a range of individual responses to drugs, so there is a range of response to pain itself. All too frequently, the physician, based on his personal experience, has a mental image of what an appropriate pain response to a particular clinical situation should be and may make inappropriate moralistic and pharmacologic judgments regarding the patient whose response falls outside the physician's conception.

The factors related to the individual experience of pain are exceedingly complex, and some appear to be constitutional. Thus, there is wide variation among subjects in both their threshhold of pain and their upper limit of tolerance to pain. Some of these differences are correlated to whether the subjects are "augmenters" or "reducers" in their electroencephalographic responses to stimuli of increasing intensity (Buchsbaum 1975).

Ethnic factors also alter the response to pain: patients from different ethnic groups tend to differ in their attitudes toward pain, in their expression of pain, and even in their autonomic responses to experimentally induced painful stimuli (Zborowski 1952, Sternbach and Tursky 1965).

For individual patients, the psychologic context of the pain alters the perception of it and tolerance for it. In Beecher's classic study, he noted that war wounds that warranted evacuation of soldiers from combat and to safety were experienced as much less painful than similar wounds sustained by civilians (Beecher 1956). One might expect then, that pain following a successful operation, and which the patient knows will be self-limiting, could be tolerated much more easily than pain from a life-threatening condition for which the outlook is clouded.

Summary

There is a wide variation among subjects in their response to narcotic medication and in their experience of pain. There certainly are neurotic patients whose inappropriate responses and demands must be dealt with primarily psychologically rather than pharmacologically, as well as patients whose severe anxiety intensifies their experience of pain and who require combined psychologic and pharmacologic care. Nevertheless, in the great majority of instances, the most common difficulties can be avoided by an appreciation and application of the known pharmacology of narcotic analgesics. The physician has no laboratory measure of pain and must rely heavily on the patient's reports of his subjective experience. If he comes to distrust the patient's reports, or interposes a moralistic or ethnocentric attitude toward pain tolerance, or confuses the medical analgesic role of the narcotic with its use in the drug culture, the outcome is likely to be a bad one, involving needless suffering for the patient and frustration for the doctor. If, on the other hand, he can trust the patient and adjusts the dose of medication to an end point of relief he and the patient mutually agree upon, drawing upon appropriate understanding of the pharmacology of the drug, the outcome can be a good one in which the doctor can realize one of his traditional responsibilities—the relief of suffering.

References

Beecher HK: Relationship of significance of wound to pain experienced. JAMA 161:1609–1613, 1956

————: The use of clinical agents in the control of pain. In Knighton RS, Dumke P (eds): Pain. Boston, Little, Brown, 1966

Buchsbaum M: Average evoked response augmenting 'reducing' in schizophrenia and affective disorders. Freedman DX (ed): Biology of the Major Psychoses. New York, Raven, 1975, pp 129–142

Evans FJ: Placebo response in pain reduction. Adv Neurol 4:289–296, 1974

Glassman AH, Perel JM: Clinical pharmacology of imipramine. Arch Gen Psychiatry 28:649–653, 1975

Jaffe J: Narcotics in the treatment of pain. Med Clin North Am 52:33–45, 1968

————: Narcotic analgesics. In Goodman L, Gilman A (eds): The Pharmacological Basis of Therapeutics, 5th ed. New York, Macmillan, 1975, pp 237–275

Lasagna L: The clinical evaluation of morphine and its substituting as analgesics. Pharmacol Rev 16:47–83, 1964

————, Beecher HK: The optimal dose of morphine. JAMA 156:230–239, 1954

Marks R, Sachar E: Undertreatment of medical inpatients with narcotic analgesics. Ann Intern Med 78:173–181, 1973

Orne M: Pain suppression by hypnosis and related phenomena. Adv Neurol 4:563–572, 1974

Sternbach RA, Tursky B: Ethnic differences among housewives in psychophysiological and skin potential responses to electric shock. Psychophysiology 1:241–246, 1965

Zborowski M: Cultural components in responses to pain. J Soc Issues 8:16–30, 1952

part IV
drugs of
dependence

Introduction

Drugs of dependence may be used by patients as nonprescription self-medication. They relieve anxiety and alleviate depression; or else they enable the patient to escape from the tedium or suffering of his unsatisfying everyday life. Sometimes highly successful and artistic individuals may take drugs for novel experiences and inspirations. Some of the more commonly used non-drugs, such as caffeine and nicotine, provide people with a welcome lift during the day. All of these drugs have dangers when used in large doses and these are discussed in each of the chapters. There are strong feelings and much controversy as to how strongly these drugs should be regulated by the government. Today, regulation ranges from complete prohibition (opioids such as heroin) to complete accessibility (caffeine, alcohol, and nicotine).

Some of these drugs are also used as therapeutic agents on occasion. Under such circumstances, care must be taken not to habituate the user. There was a period of time from 25 to 10 years ago when therapeutic uses were actively being sought for the hallucinogenic drugs. Now it is very difficult to obtain or do human research with these agents. However, more research under carefully guarded conditions would be very desirable.

alcohol

commentary

Alcohol is the most venerable of all psychopharmaceutical agents. Dr. Goodwin gives us a compact summary of its pharmacology and toxicology. Alcoholism is a disease characterized by an overwhelming compulsion to drink alcoholic beverages. The social and physiologic factors responsible for the habit are not well understood, but genetic susceptibility plays a role and there is cross-dependence to other sedative-hypnotic drugs. As with all drug dependencies (pp 327, 419, and 467) the positively reinforcing effect of the drug must be countered by competing reinforcers, such as fear of consequences, social pressure, self-help groups, psychotherapy, and pharmacologic aids, such as disulfiram (Antabuse), in treating this habit. It is important for the primary care physician to know the physiologic and psychologic effects of alcohol outlined in this chapter.

alcohol

Donald W. Goodwin, M.D.

When yeast grows in sugar solutions without air, most of the sugar is converted (fermented) into carbon dioxide and alcohol. When the alcohol concentration reaches about 12 or 13 percent, the process stops. This is why unfortified wines have alcohol concentrations of no more than 12 or 13 percent.

As a rule, people do not drink just alcohol. They drink alcoholic beverages. Alcoholic beverages are mostly water and ethyl alcohol. Tiny amounts of other chemicals are present, providing most of the taste and smell and all of the color, if any. Called congeners, these chemicals include amino acids, minerals, vitamins, methanol, and the "higher" alcohols, known as fusel oil (Leake and Silverman 1966).

Beverages differ according to the sugar source: from grapes, wine; from grain and hops, beer; from grain and corn, whiskey; from sugarcane, rum; from the potato, vodka.

Man discovered distillation about 800 AD in Arabia (alcohol comes from the Arabic alkuhl, meaning essence). Distillation boils away alcohol from its sugar bath and recollects it as virtually pure alcohol. The water is then put back, so that instead of 100 percent alcohol, the result is, perhaps, 50 percent alcohol or 100 proof alcohol (percent being one-half of proof).

Alcohol's Fate in the Body

What happens to alcohol when you drink it? Essentially the same thing that happens if you don't drink it. It turns to vinegar. When

alcohol sours in open air, bacteria are responsible. To become vinegar (acetic acid) in the body, two enzymes are required: alcohol
dehydrogenase (Adh) and aldehyde dehydrogenase (AldDH).

The first is located in the liver in surprisingly large supply. Surprisingly because, as far as we know, alcohol dehydrogenase does
nothing except metabolize alcohol. A minute amount of ethyl alcohol is produced in the gastrointestinal tract by bacteria, and
perhaps this accounts for alcohol dehydrogenase in the liver.
Infinitesimal amounts of alcohol may also be produced by normal
metabolic processes in the body. If these sources are the reason the
alcohol enzyme is present in such large quantity, it is clearly a case
of biologic overkill. It disposes of 86 proof distilled spirits at about
the rate of one ounce per hour. Fed into the body's normal metabolic
machinery, acetic acid becomes carbon dioxide and water, burning
or storing 7 cal/g of alcohol.

Between alcohol and acetic acid, there is an intermediate step,
which is why a second enzyme is required. The intermediate chemical is an aldehyde and very toxic. The enzyme that destroys the
aldehyde is found not just in the liver but throughout the body. It
quickly turns the aldehyde into harmless acetic acid. This enzyme,
aldehyde dehydrogenase, is inhibited by disulfiram (Antabuse). This
results in an accumulation of acetaldehyde and a toxic reaction
characterized mainly by vasodilation and hypotension.

Alcohol is almost entirely oxidized in the liver. A small amount is
expired in the breath and excreted in urine and sweat. In the oxidation of alcohol, two molecules of diphosphopyridine nucleotide
(DPN) are changed to reduced diphosphopyridine nucleotide
(DPNH).

ADH

C_1H_5OH + DPN ———————— CH_3CHO + DPNH

AldDH

CH_3CHO + DPN ———————— CH_3COOH + DPNH

Vinegar may be harmless, but how it is produced may not be. In
being oxidized, alcohol is stripped of hydrogen atoms, which must
go somewhere. Where they go results in some interesting biochemical changes that may or may not be harmless (the evidence is not in
yet; Lieber and Davidson 1962). Here are some:

1. There is an increase in lactic acid. This is interesting because

increased lactic acid has been associated with anxiety attacks, and heavy drinking is also associated with anxiety attacks.

2. There is an increase in uric acid. This is interesting because increased uric acid is associated with gout, and gout, for centuries, with alcohol.

3. There is an increase in fat—not the slow increase that comes from calories (those 7 cal /g) but a rapid increase from the oxidation of alcohol. The fat is seen mainly in the liver or blood. One night of serious drinking—say, six or seven highballs—discernibly increases the fat content of the liver. The liver will be fattier still if fatty food is eaten (Wallgren and Barry 1970).

Is a fatty liver bad? Admittedly it doesn't sound good, but on the other hand, the connection between fatty liver and liver diseases, such as hepatitis and cirrhosis, is undetermined. For one thing, the fat goes away soon after the drinker stops drinking. Also, most people drink but most do not develop liver disease. Among those very heavy drinkers called alcoholics, perhaps only 5 or 10 percent develop liver disease. On the other hand most people who develop aparticular type of liver disease, Laennec's cirrhosis, are heavy drinkers.

Many disorders connected with heavy drinking are believed to be due to malnutrition, but this may not be true of cirrhosis. Laennec's cirrhosis has been produced in well-nourished baboons after 4 years of drunkenness (Lieber and Rubin 1974). Most of the drunk baboons, however, only developed a fatty liver, and controversy still thrives about whether alcohol alone causes cirrhosis. Obviously it doesn't in everybody.

Intoxicating amounts of alcohol also increase fat in the bloodstream. In high enough dose, particularly combined with a fatty meal, alcohol may even produce *visible* fat in the blood (chylomicrons).

It is possible, of course, that the so-called medical complications of alcoholism are not due to alcohol at all. Alcoholics are almost universally heavy smokers and many are malnourished. Even alcoholics who have a normal dietary intake may have nutritional deficiencies, because alcohol in large quantities inhibits the absorption of amino acids, vitamins, and other nutrients. Damage to the nervous system associated with alcoholism—eg, peripheral neuropathy, Wernicke-Korsakoff encephalopathy, cerebellar degeneration—is almost definitely related to vitamin deficiency, particularly vitamins of the B group (Victor et al 1971). There is no direct evidence that alcohol alone, in the amounts consumed by even alcoholic individuals, damages the brain.

Many things have been tried—insulin, caffeine, exercise—to speed up the elimination of alcohol. Fructose in large doses does this, but the dose is so large it is sickening, and most people prefer to stay drunk (Pawan 1967).

Alcohol behaves similarly to water, travels everywhere that water travels, and, because of its waterlike properties, can be accommodated by the body in vastly greater amounts than any other drug. A person's blood can consist of one-half of one percent alcohol without producing death or even unconsciousness.

The Effects of Alcohol

The effects of alcohol do not depend on how much a person drinks, but on how much gets into the bloodstream. This in turn depends on many things.

1. Some alcohol is absorbed through the stomach wall but most reaches the bloodstream through the small intestine.
2. For rapid absorption, it is important that alcohol reach the small intestine in the highest possible concentration in the shortest possible time. People who have had their pyloric valve removed surgically, as for ulcers, find they get drunk faster than previously.
3. Other factors affecting absorption include the presence of food in the stomach and the type of beverage. With the same amount of alcohol consumed over the same length of time, the blood alcohol concentration may vary greatly. Gin on an empty stomach has a far different effect from beer combined with a meal.

In addition to how much alcohol is in the blood, it matters how quickly the alcohol is absorbed. In general, the faster the rate of absorption, the more striking the effect. Also, as alcohol remains in the blood over longer periods, its effects become less. In practical terms, if you make five errors per minute while typing sober, you may make 15 errors per minute while typing with X blood alcohol concentration after one hour of drinking, but only seven errors at the same X concentration after five hours of drinking.

In general, people feel better getting drunk than they do sobering up. That is, as the blood alcohol level climbs from A to B to C, a person may feel euphoric at B and C, but as the blood level falls from C to B to A, not only is there no euphoria at B, but the person feels discomfort, presaging the hangover to come at A. This "slope" effect is closely related to and hard to separate from the duration effect. As people drink more over days, months, and years, they gradually need to drink more to obtain the same effect. The importance of "tolerance," however, is often exaggerated. A seasoned alcoholic at the prime of his drinking capacity may be able to drink, at most, twice more than a teetotaler of similar age and health. Compared to tolerance for morphine, which may be manifold, tolerance for alcohol is modest.

More striking than "acquired" tolerance may be inborn tolerance. Individuals vary widely in the amount of alcohol they can tolerate, independent of drinking experience. Some people cannot drink more than a small amount of alcohol without developing a headache, sick stomach, or dizziness. They rarely become alcoholic but deserve no credit: they can't drink much.

Differences in tolerance for alcohol apply not only to individuals, but to racial groups. For example, some Oriental groups develop flushing of the skin, sometimes with nausea, after drinking a little alcohol (Wolff 1972). Alcoholism is rare in these groups.

Tolerance is reversible. People who have had encephalitis, brain tumors, or other damage to the brain commonly experience at least a temporary decrease in tolerance for alcohol. Alcoholics, after many years of heavy drinking, also may lose tolerance as they grow older. Older people, in general, have less tolerance for alcohol than do younger people.

Any drug response that involves thinking and mood is bound to be influenced by expectation (set). If a person believes alcohol will improve his mood, diminish fatigue, or make him feel sexy, the chances of these occurring may be improved. If he believes alcohol will make him sleepy or produce a headache, these also may occur.

Set is linked to setting. Where is the person drinking? With whom? If he enjoys the people he is with, he may also enjoy the alcohol more. If the occasion is a celebration, a drink may have a livelier effect than would the same amount taken routinely before dinner.

Alcohol is said to make people talk louder, and it often seems true. On the other hand, two men in a duck blind, having a little bourbon to warm up, may talk more softly than usual.

The "Four Stages" of Intoxication

There is an old saying that alcohol affects a person in four ways. First, he becomes jocose, then bellicose, then lachrymose, and finally comatose.

Comatose he does indeed become, if he drinks enough, but the other three stages are not all that inevitable. Some people hardly feel jocose at all. Many become argumentative and some combative, but these responses are strongly influenced by social circumstances. The legendary barroom fight usually occurs in lower class bars. Countless parties are held nightly in middle class surburbia, and although drinking is common, fighting is not.

One of the paradoxes about alcohol is that people do cry sometimes when they drink. They become anxious and depressed. This challenges the assumption that people drink mainly to feel less anxious and depressed. The motives for drinking are complex, with no single explanation sufficing.

Alcohol is often described as a "depressant" drug that depresses first the "higher" centers in the brain and then downwardly anesthetizes the "lower" centers until finally, in lethal dosage, it snuffs out life itself by depressing the respiratory center at the base of the brain. This is an oversimplification.

What is alcohol "depressing"? Many people get a lift from alcohol and become animated and energetic. Nerve fibers fire about as readily in an alcohol solution as they do otherwise, unless the concentration is far above what most people can drink. It is sometimes said that by depressing the "higher" centers of the brain, alcohol releases the "lower," and this is why people are more animated or uninhibited when they drink. The problem is that studies do not support the top-to-bottom action of alcohol. Coordination, a "lower" function, often is impaired at lower doses of alcohol than is memory, a "higher" function (Goodwin et al 1969).

Dosage is crucial. Alcohol in rather small doses improves certain types of performance, perhaps because it reduces anxiety. Apparently this is most likely to occur in activities where the person is not very proficient. If he does poorly hitting the target on a firing range, he may improve somewhat after several drinks of alcohol. On the other hand, if he does well normally, his performance may fall off after small amounts of alcohol. Nevertheless, in moderate-to-high amounts, alcohol generally diminishes function across the board. Alcohol has been shown (in cats, at any rate) to dampen activity of the reticular formation before it does other areas of the brain, and this may be the reason.

An interesting exception to the above has emerged in several recent studies. If a person learns certain things while intoxicated —even severely intoxicated—he will remember them better when reintoxicated than when sober, a phenomenon that has been well demonstrated in man as well as animals (Goodwin 1974). Called state-dependent learning (p 73), this is one of the few exceptions to the overall impairing effect of alcohol at moderate and high doses.

Alcohol does something else almost unique among drugs. It produces a classic amnesia called *blackout*. While drinking, the drinker does highly memorable things and cannot remember them the next day. Many social drinkers have had this experience, but it occurs most frequently in alcoholics (Goodwin et al 1969).

These are mental effects. There are also physical effects which should be mentioned, if only because there are misconceptions about them.

1. It is known that alcohol increases urination by inhibiting antidiuretic hormone. It is generally not known that the increase is temporary, and that after a fairly short period of drinking, the need to urinate decreases.
2. It is commonly believed that alcohol causes dehydration. It does not. When a person has a dry mouth and thirst after an evening of drinking, it may be due partly to the astringent effect of alcohol on the mucous membranes of the mouth. If anything, heavy drinkers may be slightly overhydrated because of the large volume of fluid they consume.
3. It is generally known that alcohol produces a feeling of bodily warmth and, therefore, is just the thing for St. Bernard's to carry around their necks in caskets and to have at a frosty football game. Alcohol produces a feeling of warmth because it dilates blood vessels in the skin, which is why some drinkers have red noses. However the warmth is subjective and can be harmfully illusionary. A person's resistance to the effects of severe cold, such as frostbite, in no way is increased by alcohol, although the victim may temporarily think it is.

When Alcohol is Contraindicated

Alcohol is contraindicated in alcoholism. Follow-up studies indicate that a small proportion of individuals diagnosed as alcoholic return to "normal" drinking for extended periods, but the consensus is that this occurs rarely and that total abstinence is the best policy for most alcoholics. Temporary abstinence is well-nigh obligatory, if only because it is almost impossible to diagnose other psychiatric and sometimes medical conditions when a person is intoxicated or during withdrawal.

Epileptics probably should not drink, or if they do so, with caution and moderation. Drinking is related to an increased frequency of seizures in epileptics (Lennox 1941). There is no evidence that alcohol *causes* epilepsy, although grand mal seizures (rum fits) may occur during withdrawal.

Since antiquity, alcohol has been associated with gout. There is evidence that alcohol does indeed increase blood levels of uric acid but only at high blood alcohol levels, and even then the increase is slight. Patients with gout can probably drink moderately with no ill effects. It may be well to avoid large amounts of beer, since beer is rich in purines.

Ever since Beaumont gave alcohol to his gastrostomized patient, Alexis St. Martin, a century and a half ago, it has been recognized that alcohol produces inflammation of the gastric mucosa. However, more recent studies indicate that the inflammation disappears after continued use of alcohol (Wolff 1970). Nevertheless, there is general agreement that patients with gastritis, gastric cancer, and bleeding in the upper digestive tract should not drink.

There is less agreement about whether a patient with gastric and duodenal ulcers should drink. There seems no question that alcohol stimulates acid secretion in the same manner as that produced by histamine, the secretion being rich in acid and low in pepsin. There is also evidence that alcohol produces changes in the mucosal barrier of the stomach that *might* predispose to ulcers. On the other hand, there is no convincing evidence that ingestion of alcohol alone causes gastric mucosal hemorrhage in man. One investigator found that peptic ulcer was diagnosed in only 5 percent of 430 consecutive alcoholics surveyed for symptoms of peptic ulcer (Bingham 1960). This incidence is comparable to the 5 to 10 percent lifetime incidence of peptic ulcer in the general population. Therefore, whether an ulcer patient is discouraged from drinking depends on the patient and his physician. If alcohol produces local irritation, then he will probably abstain without any advice. Some physicians *encourage* modest use of alcohol on the grounds that it has a tranquilizing effect. In addition alcohol reduces hunger contractions, at least in dogs. In view of these factors, no definitive advice can be given.

With regard to alcohol and coronary artery disease, a "fact" accepted by physicians since Heberden's days—namely, that alcohol was good for heart patients and relieved angina pectoris—has recently been challenged by studies in man and animals indicating that alcohol reduces cardiac contractility and may indeed be contraindicated in patients with heart disease. This may occur for a number of reasons, one being that ethanol increases osmolarity of the serum and extracellular fluid, which, in turn, leads to a loss of electrolytes from cardiac muscle cells. On the other hand alcohol in modest amounts has been prescribed to cardiac patients for a long time, and there is no direct evidence that it increases the incidence of myocardial infarction or cardiac failure. The effect of alcohol on the heart is probably dose related, as it usually is. There is certainly no absolute contraindication against heart patients using alcohol in small amounts.

During withdrawal from heavy drinking, the blood pressure is commonly elevated. However, alcohol apparently does not produce chronic hypertension and because of the tranquilizing effects from alcohol, it may indeed have a kind of phenobarbital effect on blood pressure and lower it slightly.

Alcohol is definitely contraindicated in pancreatitis.

The role of alcohol in liver disease, even with respect to the three liver diseases associated with alcoholism (fatty liver, alcoholic hepatitis, and portal cirrhosis), remains controversial. No one questions that patients with acute hepatitis should abstain from alcohol. The disagreement arises from the question, "How long should they abstain after laboratory tests and other indicators of the disease have returnedto normal?" Some clinicians believe they should abstain practically forever, particularly if alcohol appears to be the prime offender. Others believe it makes little difference. One investigator reported that patients consuming large amounts of alcohol during convalescence after acute hepatitis showed no more evidence of posthepatitic liver damage than did those who drank little or no alcohol (Gardner 1949). Since recurring bouts of alcoholic hepatitis may result in irreversible cirrhosis, the question is hardly trivial, but the clinician must base his advice on evidence that is less than conclusive.

Patients with acute kidney disease should not drink. Those with chronic nephritis can probably drink in moderation but should avoid beer, since beer contains considerable sodium.

Nobody knows why, but apparently alcohol worsens prostatitis. At the very least, where prostatic hypertrophy is present, the diuretic effect of alcohol may result in urgency and urinary retention.

Alcohol has additive or synergistic effects with other drugs. Relatively modest amounts of alcohol in combination with halogenated compounds (such as dry-cleaning agents, insecticides, and pesticides) can have devastating effects on the liver. The "accidental" suicides resulting from mixing alcohol with barbiturate and barbituratelike hypnotics have been well publicized. The minor tranquilizers, particularly the benzodiazepine group, apparently have less damaging effects in combination with alcohol, but caution naturally should be exercised, if only because these drugs make people sleepy and so does alcohol. Other drugs may interact with alcohol to produce distressing, if not disastrous, effects. Among these are the oral antidiabetic agents, such as tolbutamide and chlorpropamide. Metronidazole may also produce mildly unpleasant effects in people drinking alcohol, although this is less well documented.

References

Bingham JR: Precipitating factors in peptic ulcer. Can Med Assoc J 83:205–208, 1960

Gardner HT: Hepatitis among American occupation troops in Germany: follow-up study with particular reference to interim alcohol and physical activity. Ann Intern Med 30:1009–1019, 1949

Goodwin DW: Alcoholic blackouts and state-dependent learning. Fed Proc 33:1833–1835, 1974

———, Crane JB, Guze SB: Alcoholic blackout: a review and clinical study of 100 alcoholics. Am J Psychiatry 126:77–85, 1969

———, Powell BE, Bremer D, Hoine H, Stern J: Alcohol and recall: state-dependent effects in man. Science 163:1358–1361, 1969

Leake CD, Silverman M: Alcoholic Beverages in Clinical Medicine. Chicago, Year Book, 1966

Lennox WG: Alcohol and epilepsy. Q J Stud Alcohol 2:1–11, 1941

Lieber C, Rubin E: Fatty liver, alcoholic hepatitis and cirrhosis produced by alcohol in primates. N Engl J Med 209:128–135, 1974

———, Davidson CS: Some metabolic effects of ethyl alcohol. Am J Med 33:319–327, 1962

Pawan GLS: Alcohol metabolism in man: acute effects of physical exercise, caffeine, fructose and glucose on the rate of ethanol metabolism. Biochem J 109:19, 1967

Victor M, Adams RD, Collins GH: The Wernicke-Korsakoff Syndrome. Philadelphia, Davis, 1971

Wallgren H, Barry H: Actions of Alcohol, New York, Elsevier, 1970, (Chap 9)

Wolff G: Does alcohol cause chronic gastritis? Scand J Gastroenterol 5:289–298, 1970

Wolff PH: Ethnic differences in alcohol sensitivity. Science 175:449–450, 1972

characteristics
of opioid
addiction
commentary

Heroin addiction is considered a major public health and sociologic problem in our country today. The roots of this dependence are complex, involving economic, social, psychologic, and pharmacologic factors. Dr. Wikler, who has had a lifelong acquaintance with various aspects of the problem, discusses the characteristics of opioid addiction in this chapter. The primary care practitioner may encounter addicts from time to time and should be able to make a diagnosis, with guidance, from this chapter. By contrast, medical addiction is very rare, but it does occur and Dr. Wikler describes it. The various parameters of opioid addiction on an acute and chronic basis are discussed in some detail. Such phenomena as tolerance, physical dependence, and abstinence are described. Signs to watch out for in diagnosing opioid addiction are described. Opioid poisoning is also mentioned. Similarities and differences between the various opioids may sometimes present problems in diagnosis, and these are also described.

characteristics of opioid addiction

Abraham Wikler, M.D.

The term *opioids* refers to any drug, regardless of chemical structure, with actions similar to those of morphine. Morphine itself constitutes about 10 percent of opium, prepared from the sap of the poppy, *Papaver somniferum*. Opium also contains codeine (3-methoxymorphine), about 0.5 percent by weight. Morphine and codeine have analgesic activity, and chemically they possess a phenanthrene nucleus. Another alkaloid with a phenanthrene nucleus present in opium is thebaine, which, however, has strong stimulant (eg, convulsive) and minimal analgesic properties. Opium also contains compounds, such as papaverine and noscapine, which possess a benzylisoquinoline nucleus and are devoid of analgesic action.

Morphine and heroin are classed as opioids, whereas thebaine, papaverine, and noscapine are not. Compounds synthetically derived from morphine, which are classed as opioids, include heroin (diacetylmorphine), hydromorphone (Dilaudid), oxymorphone (Numorphan), and oxycodone (Percodan). Purely synthetic compounds include methadone (Dolophine), meperidine (Demerol), phenazocine (Prinadol), and D-propoxyphene (Darvon). On a milligram-per-milligram basis, the analgesic potencies of these opioids relative to morphine (all drugs given subcutaneously) are: codeine, 1/12; heroin, 2 to 3; hydromorphone, 6 to 8; oxymorphone, 7 to 10; oxycodone, 2/3 to 1; methadone, 1; meperidine, 1/8 to 1/10; and phenazocine, 3. By the oral route 65 mg of D-propoxyphene is equivalent to 32 to 45 mg of codeine for analgesia, but 32 mg of D-propoxyphene may be no more effective than a placebo.

Though differing in potency as well as in degree of tolerance and physical dependence produced by repeated administration, the pattern of effects of equivalent single doses of these opioids in a nontolerant person is similar to those of morphine. The analgesia produced by these drugs is part of a general antiprotective action (Schaumann 1954). Not only pain but also cough, dyspnea, bowel and bladder urgency, and hunger pangs are reduced or abolished. Experimental studies in man have indicated that morphine has no effect on the ability to discriminate the intensities of brief, painful electric shocks but does reduce the effects of anxiety on such discriminatory ability (Hill et al 1952a, Hill et al 1952b). Also, morphine reduces the disruption of performance caused by anticipation of punitive, self-administered electric shocks (Hill et al 1955, Hill et al 1952c), and reduces the effects of experimentally manipulated incentive levels upon performance (Hill et al 1957). Because of such general antiprotective actions, single doses of opioids produce in nontolerant persons who are distressed (by pain, pain-anticipatory anxiety, dyspnea, and others) a sense of unusual well-being termed *euphoria* by their observers and a "high" by themselves. However, many normal persons, presumably not so distressed, do not feel unusually well after a dose of morphine (Smith et al 1959, Smith et al 1962) and may react negatively to it because the antiprotective actions may interfere with their activities and because of unpleasant side effects (nausea, vomiting, giddiness, or fainting).

However, the occurrence of opioid-type euphoria alone cannot be a sufficient reason for the production of habitual, compulsive, opioid-seeking behavior (addiction or opioid dependence). Countless numbers of people are given opioids for relief of pain, and probably very many of them experience an unusual sense of well-being in consequence. If the pain is continuous, they may be given opioids repeatedly, at frequencies and in amounts sufficient to produce physical dependence; when the pain has disappeared, opioids are discontinued and they go through the discomfort of the opioid-abstinence syndrome. Yet few such persons continue to seek opioids compulsively after the pain is gone and the opioid-abstinence syndrome has subsided.

In the cases of the vast majority of habitual opioid addicts, the circumstances of their initial experiences with the drug are quite different. Generally, they are young (in their teens), they are not in pain, they associate with other young people among whom are heroin or other opioid users, and they *self-administer* the drug because of curiosity and /or a need to establish an identity as a member of an exclusive peer group. Often their first experience with heroin is unpleasant (nausea, vomiting, giddiness, faintness), but after several repetitions of self-administration of the drug and under tutelage by their peers, they learn to recognize the heroin "high" despite the recurrence of nausea, faintness, and so on, which they now call "a good sick."

From this point on the typical addict "hustles" for the drug, again under peer group tutelage. He is constantly busy establishing "connections," outwitting the law, and, if necessary, committing crimes (usually against property) to obtain money for "a fix," which may or may not be forthcoming. Sooner or later this drug-seeking activity is interrupted by arrest and jail sentences, admission to a hospital, or temporary disappearance of heroin (or other opioids) from the illicit market. The addict "kicks his habit" (undergoes opiod withdrawal or detoxification), but regardless of the duration of jail sentence or of hospitalization, he relapses to opioids and "hustles" for them when he returns to the environment in which his previous addiction developed.

As emphasized by Bejerot (1972), this pattern of opioid dependence is an *epidemic addiction* in that it is contagious—ie, one addict induces another person or persons into addiction, and the newly recruited addicts do likewise. As such, epidemic addiction is to be distinguished from drug abuse, from single addictions, and from endemic addiction. In this context drug abuse is considered to be the occasional use of nonmedically indicated chemical agents. Single addictions are those consciously accepted during medical treatment for relief of pain in patients with incurable illnesses or in dying patients, those inadvertently but rarely caused by medical treatment, and the self-established addictions in persons whose professions give them easy access to opioids. Endemic addictions are socially accepted addictions, such as alcoholism in the United States and Europe, opium smoking in ancient China, hashish smoking in North Africa, and coca chewing among South American Indians. This chapter is concerned with the "epidemic" type of opioid dependence in the United States.

Epidemiology

Ball and Chambers (1967) estimated that in 1967 there were 108,424 opioid addicts in the United States; in 1972, the number was conservatively estimated at about 300,000 (City Almanac 1972). The majority of opioid addicts reside in the metropolitan slum districts, about half of them in New York City, while the rest are found mainly in Washington, DC, Chicago, and Los Angeles. A smaller but substantial number come from rural areas in Southern states. In 1936 only

16 percent of addicts were nonwhite, but by 1966, 57 percent were
black, Puerto Rican, or Mexican residents of Northern metropolitan
ghetto areas; in the Southern states the majority are predominantly
white. The ratio of male to female addicts is about 5 to 1. Stated age
at first use of opioids was given at less than 20 years by 16 percent of
addicts in 1936, while age of onset was given at less than 19 years by
53 percent in 1966. In 1936, morphine was used by 51 percent of the
addicts; heroin by 43 percent; opium by 4 percent; and 2 percent
used all other opioids. In 1966, heroin was used by 70 percent;
morphine by 7 percent; hydromorphone (Dilaudid), 6 percent;
codeine, 6 percent; meperidine (Demerol), 4 percent; methadone, 1
percent; and all other opioids, 2 percent. The route of self-
administration has also changed from smoking of opium, sniffing of
heroin, and subcutaneous injections of morphine or heroin in the
nineteenth and early part of the twentieth century to intravenous
self-injection, which is by far the predominant route today.

Etiology

The personalities of addicts of the "epidemic" type have been
studied intensively at the federal hospital in Lexington, Kentucky.
In the early 1960s the great majority were found to have significant
elevations on the Psychopathic and Neurotic Scales of the Minnesota Multiphasic Personality Inventory (MMPI) (Hill et al 1960). In
1971, Monroe et al published the results of studies with the Lexington Personality Inventory on 837 opioid addicts at the Clinical Research Centers in Lexington, Kentucky, and Fort Worth, Texas.
Characterologic disorder (psychopathy or sociopathy) was found in
42 percent; emotional disturbance in 29 percent, and thinking disorder in 22 percent; while only 7 percent were asymptomatic. However, control studies (Hill et al 1962) have revealed similar elevations of the Psychopathic Scale on the MMPIs of chronic, institutionalized alcoholics and of institutionalized juvenile delin-
quents who were neither opioid addicts nor alcoholics. Gerard and
Kornetsky (1955) found that half of a control (nonaddict) sample
from a New York slum area showed evidence of psychiatric disorder,
although the addict sample was more severely disturbed. In favor of
a relationship between psychopathy (or other psychiatric disorder)
and opioid dependence is the finding of Hill et al (1968) that addict
physicians showed moderate elevations on the Psychopathic and
Neurotic Scales of the MMPI, whereas the MMPIs of nonaddict
physicians were within the normal range. The issue of personality
deviation and opioid addiction can be resolved only by additional

control studies, such as on the personalities of nonaddict siblings reared in the same metropolitan slum environment in which "psychopathic" attitudes toward conventional middle-class norms are prevalent.

Regardless of this issue, the development of habitual, compulsive opioid-seeking behavior may be ascribed, in part at least, to the process of reinforcement. The future addict, particularly of the "epidemic" variety, self-administers the drug, and the recurrence of this operant (drug self-administration) becomes increasingly more probable in consequence of the rewarding effects (subjectively interpreted as a "high") of each dose. In time, the initial rewarding effects of opioids, ascribable to the reduction of antecedent needs or sources of reinforcement (eg, hypophoria, anxiety, and /or the need to belong) decrease because tolerance develops. Concomitantly, physical dependence develops. With narcotic antagonists, it has been possible to precipitate morphine-abstinence phenomena in subjects who had received only nine doses of 15 mg each, or equivalent doses of heroin or methadone, over a period of 3 days (Wikler et al 1953).

Thus, very early, a new pharmacogenically induced need is developed, which is reduced by each dose of the drug. Because of tolerance, the prevailing mood of the addict is now dysphoric (Haertzen and Hooks 1969, Wikler 1952), and he tends to increase the dose. This, however, results in further development of tolerance and intensifies physical dependence. As long as opioids are in adequate supply, the addict is unable to distinguish his pharmacogenically induced need from his antecedent needs. Hence, reduction of the pharmacogenically induced need by each dose of opioid is likewise interpreted by him as a "high," albeit of diminished magnitude.

Along with these changes in needs, the addict of the "epidemic" variety also develops techniques of "hustling" and elaborate rituals of opioid self-administration, which are likewise reinforced by the need-suppressing effects of the opioid, as well as by other rewards, such as elevation of esteem in the eyes of the "drug culture." Sometimes hustling results in the acquisition of opioids and sometimes not (variable interval reinforcement). When opioids are not obtained, a frank opioid-abstinence syndrome emerges. Inasmuch as hustling involves other people (pushers and other sources of drug supply) in specific neighborhoods, these eventually acquire the properties of classically conditioned stimuli that can evoke the cycle of opioid abstinence and its termination as classically conditioned responses. In response to such stimuli, transient signs of opioid abstinence may appear long after detoxification, when the presumably cured addict returns to the neighborhood frequented by active addicts and pushers.

Concomitantly with the occurrence of such conditioned abstinence (narcotic hunger or craving), renewed hustling for opioids occurs and, if successful, the former addict is said to have relapsed (Wikler 1973). Augmenting this process is the long persistence, up to 30 weeks following morphine withdrawal (Martin and Jasinski 1969), of low-grade physiologic changes (the protracted abstinence syndrome) that are generally opposite in direction to those of the well-known early or acute opioid-abstinence syndrome that reaches peak intensity about 48 hours after abrupt morphine withdrawal and subsides over the next few weeks (see below). The protracted opioid-abstinence syndrome constitutes another pharmacogenically induced need, which likewise acts as a source of reinforcement for opioid-seeking behavior in the detoxified opioid addict.

Regardless of whether or not an abnormal personality predisposes certain individuals to opioid dependence, the development of new, pharmacogenically induced needs, together with classical conditioning of opioid-abstinence phenomena and operant conditioning of opioid-seeking behavior, constitute a disease sui generis, which must be treated as such after detoxification (see below), before or concomitantly with therapies directed toward the presumed personality disturbance. As Bejerot (1972) has stated, addiction is "an artificially induced drive," and "the reason why people start taking drugs is quite different from the reason they continue."

Clinical Syndromes

Effects of Single Doses in Nontolerant Individuals

Although heroin is most widely used by opioid addicts, neither they nor their observers can distinguish heroin from morphine when the drugs are given in equipotent doses subcutaneously (Frazer et al 1961). On the other hand, when given intravenously, opioid addicts distinguish heroin from morphine readily (Martin and Fraser 1961), possibly because morphine produces a more intense "pins and needles" sensation in the skin (histamine release?). Shortly after intravenous injection of either drug, many addicts report a transient rush or thrill, which they describe as an orgasmic sensation in the abdomen. Later the state of unusual well-being already described supervenes. The subject may "go on the nod," sitting in a chair or lying in bed, gazing at a newspaper, dozing and rousing suddenly in alternation, and frequently scratching his nose. Others may "drive," talking volubly and boastfully and displaying unwanted energy in discharging assigned or unassigned tasks. A given subject may nod or drive alternatively, depending on the social situation. Concomitantly, the pupils are markedly constricted (miosis), the eyelids are droopy (pseudoptosis), respiratory rate is slowed, body temperature is slightly lowered, there may be slight slowing of dominant frequencies in the electroencephalogram, diuresis is inhibited (by release of antidiuretic hormone), and constipation is produced by a general spasmogenic action on smooth muscle. Addicts also report that in the nontolerant state, libido is decreased but sexual potency (in the male) may be increased because of delay in sexual orgasm (Wikler 1952).

The duration of these effects is positively correlated with the dose but by 4 hours the subjective effects of 10 mg of morphine or 4 mg of heroin, intravenously, have declined to less than half of their peak intensity (which is reached within one-half hour after intravenous injection); however, the decline of pupillary constriction is slower (Martin and Fraser 1961).

Tolerance

When the same dose of morphine or heroin is repeated, the subjective effects of the drug decrease in duration and intensity (except for the pins and needles sensation, and perhaps the thrill). On the other hand, there is little attenuation of the miotic or constipating effects. If the size of the dose is increased, there is some temporary increment in the subjective effects, but these likewise decline eventually. In this "tolerant" state, the addict is not "normal" either physiologically or behaviorally. In fact, a new homeostatic state appears to have developed, characterized by elevation of blood pressure, pulse rate, and rectal temperature, with smaller pupillary diameter and slower respiratory rate compared to preaddiction control values (Martin and Jasinski 1969). Behaviorally, the addict exhibits increased irritability and hypochondriasis, with decreased motivation for activity and decreased social involvement (Haertzen and Hooks 1969).

Physical Dependence and the Abstinence Syndrome

As already mentioned, opioid abstinence syndromes (evidence of physical dependence) have been precipitated by subcutaneous injection of an opioid antagonist (nalorphine) after 3 days of administration of morphine, heroin, or methadone (Wikler et al 1953). Very recently Nutt and Jasinski (1974) reported that they were able to precipitate abstinence phenomena by injection of another opioid antagonist (naloxone) 24 hours after administration of a single 30-mg dose of morphine or a week after a single 40-mg dose of methadone. However, without the use of such narcotic antagonists, the earliest sign of opioid abstinence after abrupt withdrawal of morphine or heroin is restlessness, detectable about 4 hours following the last dose of the drug. Gross abstinence phenomena appear about 8 hours later and consist, roughly in order of their appearance, of anxiety, chills, rhinorrhea, lacrimation, yawning, perspiration, waves of piloerection, pupillary dilatation (mydriasis), anorexia, muscular aches and pains, nausea, craving for sweets (but aversion to tobacco), abdominal cramps, tremors, elevation of rectal temperature, blood pressure, pulse and respiratory rates, insomnia, repeated vomiting, and loss of weight. Ejaculations may occur in men and menorrhagia in women. The signs and symptoms of this early or acute opioid-withdrawal syndrome reach peak intensity between the thirty-sixth and forty-eighth hour of abstinence, then decline until about the tenth day of abstinence when physiologic changes are within normal ranges, although asymptotic values are not reached for up to 6 months (Himmelsbach 1942), or 30 weeks (Martin and Jasinski 1969). During this period, morphine addicts display a protracted abstinence syndrome, physiologic changes generally being in a direction opposite to those of the early abstinence syndrome: decreased blood pressure, pulse rate, rectal temperature, pupillary diameter, and sensitivity of the respiratory center to carbon dioxide, compared with preaddiction control values (Martin and Jasinski 1969, Martin et al 1968).

Diagnosis of Opioid Addiction

Habitual use of opioid drugs may be suspected if blue or black pinhead-sized needle marks or pigmented streaks are noted in the skin, particularly in the antecubital regions, arms, volar surfaces of the forearms, and dorsum of the hands and feet; in women, needle marks may be found on the abdomen and thighs. Current opioid use may be suspected if the pupils are markedly constricted, the patient goes on the nod, and'or if a urine sample is positive for morphine (after taking morphine or heroin), methadone, meperidine, or other opioid. It should be noted that after experimental intravenous injections of heroin in a dose of 5 mg /70 kg in nontolerant human subjects, morphine can be detected in urine only for 16 to 24 hours with thin-layer chromatography (iodoplatinate spray) preceded by hydrolysis and extraction or by the free radical assay technique, and up to 48 to 56 hours by radioimmunoassay. For smaller doses of heroin, the time span for detectability of morphine in the urine will be correspondingly shorter.

Proof of physical dependence on opioids can be made only by the demonstration of typical signs of opioid abstinence. This can be accomplished either by isolating the patient without medication of any kind for at least 48 hours and observing closely for pupillary dilatation; lacrimation; rhinorrhea; piloerection; frequent yawning; increased sweating; rise in rectal temperature, pulse, and respiratory rates; or by administering a narcotic antagonist, which, in a patient who is physically dependent, will precipitate all of the above-mentioned signs within minutes. Two narcotic antagonists, nalorphine (Nalline) and naloxone (Narcan), are commonly used for this purpose, naloxone being 10 times as potent as nalorphine. An experienced physician may give the narcotic antagonist *slowly* by the intravenous route, observing the patient carefully for abstinence signs, especially pupillary dilatation, lacrimation, rhinorrhea, sweating, and an increase in respiratory rate. Generally, these signs appear after intravenous injection of 1 to 4 mg of nalorphine or 0.1 to 0.4 mg of naloxone. If these abstinence signs do appear, the injection of narcotic antagonist should be stopped, as further injection could precipitate a more violent and potentially dangerous abstinence syndrome. For less experienced physicians, the subcutaneous route is safer. The initial dose of narcotic antagonist, given subcutaneously, should be 3 mg of nalorphine or 0.4 mg of naloxone. If the cardinal signs of opioid abstinence do not appear within 15 minutes, another dose of 5 mg of nalorphine or 0.7 mg of naloxone should be given subcutaneously and if abstinence signs fail to appear within 15 minutes, a final dose of 7 mg of nalorphine or 1 mg of naloxone is injected subcutaneously. If no signs of abstinence appear after this last dose of narcotic antagonist, it is concluded that the patient is not physically dependent.

Opioid Poisoning

Typical signs of opioid poisoning include stupor or coma, miosis, and slowed or periodic respiration. However, in very severe opioid poisoning the pupils may be dilated because of hypoxia, and frequently the clinical picture is obscured by the effects of other drugs, such as barbiturates, alcohol, or amphetamines, that are often abused by addicts. If the patient can be aroused by mild sensory stimulation, this should be continued, the airways should be cleared and an airway inserted, and adequate respirations should be maintained artificially (do not use 100 percent oxygen). Hypotension should be combated with intravenous infusions of 5 percent glucose in water and by vasopressor amines, such as methoxamine (Vasoxyl), 10 to 20 mg intramuscularly. If the opioid poisoning is more severe, or if the patient does not respond to the above-mentioned procedures, a narcotic antagonist should be given. Naloxone is preferred to nalorphine for this purpose as it has no agonistic actions (see above) and therefore, unlike nalorphine (a partial agonist), it will not further depress the patient, should the presumed signs of opioid poisoning actually be due to some other cause (eg, sedative drug poisoning, increased intracranial pressure, or other neurologic condition). The initial dose of nalozone should be 0.01 mg/kg (0.7 mg/70) given intravenously. This dose may be repeated once or twice at intervals of 5 minutes to obtain an adequate respiratory response. If the patient does not respond, the diagnosis of opioid poisoning should be questioned. If the patient does respond, he should be watched carefully for the next 24 hours or more, as the antagonistic actions of naloxone last only 2 to 3 hours or so while the depressant actions of large doses of heroin last much longer, and in the case of methadone, as long as 24 to 48 hours. If, after the initial narcotic antagonistic actions of naloxone have subsided, the respiratory rate falls to unacceptable levels, naloxone may be given again by the intramuscular routes as often as necessary, in doses 50 percent larger than that found to be adequate by the intravenous route initially (Dole et al 1971). Alternatively, in methadone overdosage, naloxone may be given continuously by intravenous drip, 0.4 mg/30 min, until the respiratory rate remains adequate after the drip has been interrupted (Waldron et al 1973).

Addictions to Other Opioids

In general, the features of addiction to hydromorphone (Dilaudid), oxymorphone (Numorphan), phenazocine (Prinadol), levorphanol (Levo-Dromoran), and oxycodone (Percodan) are similar to addiction to morphine or heroin. However, there are special features of addictions to other opioids, viz:

1. Codeine is rarely self-administered intravenously by addicts because it often produces intense flushing of the skin, edema of the face, and sometimes severe hypotensive reactions. Taken subcutaneously or orally in adequate amounts, codeine does produce

physical dependence. In clinical practice, codeine-abstinence phenomena are generally mild. Codeine may be abused by the oral route in the form of elixirs (eg, of terpin hydrate), and the patient may become physically dependent on both codeine and the alcohol content of the elixir.

2. Meperidine (Demerol) addicts often exhibit cutaneous disklike scars and multiple subcutaneous indurated areas in the arms and forearms due to the local irritating effects of meperidine injected subcutaneously or to extravasations from intravenous injections. The duration of action of meperidine is relatively short and becomes even shorter as tolerance develops; consequently, abstinence phenomena, consisting of extreme restlessness, muscle twitches, sweating, and anxiety, become manifest if the interval between doses is more than 4 hours. When the daily dose of meperidine reaches 2000 mg, generalized convulsions (with characteristic changes in the electroencephalogram) may appear as a toxic effect. After recovery from postseizure stupor, the patient may exhibit meperidine abstinence phenomena. The problem is best handled by reducing the daily dose of meperidine but increasing its frequency of administration (eg, to every 2 or 3 hours) and carrying out subsequent withdrawal by the rapid-reduction method.

3. The physical dependence-producing potency of D-propoxyphene (Darvon) is somewhat less than that of codeine, but overdoses of D-propoxyphene can produce coma (reversible by nalorphine or naloxone), and chronic overdosage can produce toxic psychoses and /or convulsions, sometimes with a fatal termination (Karliner 1967).

4. Pentazocine (Talwin) is a weak opioid antagonist with analgesic properties, 40 to 60 mg being equivalent to 10 mg of morphine when given parenterally; the analgesic action of the oral preparation is about one-third that of the parenteral. Overdosage with pentazocine can produce stupor or coma, which is reversible by naloxone but not by nalorphine or other partial agonists. In some patients pentazocine produces psychotomimetic effects, principally visual hallucinations, also reversible by naloxone but not by nalorphine. Tolerance develops to pentazocine and on its abrupt withdrawal, a mild, atypical abstinence syndrome ensues (abdominal cramps, nausea, vomiting, restlessness, dizziness, chills, and fever). In patients physically dependent on pentazocine, an abstinence syndrome can be precipitated by naloxone but not by nalorphine (Fraser and Rosenberg 1964). Withdrawal of pentazocine can be accomplished by the rapid-reduction method.

Polydrug Addiction

Frequently, opioid addicts give histories, or a urinary drug screen reveals that they have been using quantities of other classes of drugs as well, such as alcohol, barbiturates and nonbarbiturate sedatives, minor tranquilizers, amphetamines and other stimulants, marihuana, LSD, and other psychotomimetic agents.

The prevalence of polydrug abusers has increased over the past two decades probably because of "progress" in developing new nonbarbiturate sedatives for therapeutic purposes and new psychotomimetic agents for research. Often the polydrug user himself does not know the identity of the drugs he is using. However, the diagnosis of polydrug abuse has been facilitated by the development of new analytic techniques such as gas chromatography, mass spectrometry, and radioimmunoassay by which one can detect these drugs in body fluids such as blood or urine.

References

Ball JC, Chambers CD (eds): The Epidemiology of Opiate Addiction in the United States. Springfield, Ill., Thomas, 1970

Bejerot N: Addiction. An Artificially Induced Drive. Springfield, Ill., Thomas, 1972

City Almanac, Center for New York City Affairs of the New School for Social Research 6:2, 1972

Dole VP, Foldes FF, Trigg H, Robinson JW, Blatman S: Methadone poisoning—diagnosis and treatment. NY State J Med 71:541–543, 1971

Fraser HF, Rosenberg DE: Studies on the human addiction liability of 2'hydroxy-5, 9-dimethyl-2-(3,3-dimethylallyl)-6, 7-benzomorphan (Win 20, 228): a weak narcotic antagonist. J Pharmacol Exp Ther 143:149–156, 1964

————, Van Horn GD, Martin WR, Wolbach AB, Isbell H: Methods for evaluating addiction liability. (A) "attitude" of opiate eddicts toward opiate-like drugs (B) a short-term "direct" addiction test. J Pharmacol Exp Ther 133:371–387, 1961

Gerard DL, Kornetsky C: Adolescent opiate addiction: a study of control and addict subjects. Psychiatr Q 29:457–489, 1955

Haertzen CA, Hooks NT: Changes in personality and subjective experience associated with the chronic administration and withdrawal of opiates. J Nerv Ment Dis 148:606–614, 1969

Hill HE, Belleville RE, Wikler A: Studies on anxiety associated with anticipation of pain. II. Comparative effects of pentobarbital and morphine. Arch Neurol Psychiatry 73:602–608, 1955

————: Motivational determinants in the modification of behavior by morphine and pentobarbital. Arch Neurol Psychiatry 77:28–35, 1957

————, Haertzen CA, Davis H: An MMPI factor analytic study of alcoholics, narcotic addicts and criminals. Q J Stud Alcohol 23:411–431, 1962

————, Haertzen CA, Glaser R: Personality characteristics of narcotic addicts as indicated by the MMPI. J Gen Psychol 62:127–139, 1960

————, Haertzen CA, Hamahiro RS: The addict physician: a Minnesota Multiphasic Personality Inventory of the interaction of personality characteristics and availability of narcotics. In Wikler A (ed) The Addictive States. 46:321–332, 1968 Res Publ Assoc Nerv Ment Dis

————, Kornetsky CH, Flanary HG, Wikler A: Relationship of electrically induced pain to the amperage and wattage of shock stimuli. J Clin Invest 31:464–472, 1952a

————: Effects of anxiety and morphine on discrimination of intensities of painful stimuli. J Clin Invest 31:473–480, 1952b

————: Studies on anxiety associated with anticipation of pain. I. Effects of morphine. Arch Neurol Psychiatry 67:612–619, 1952c

Himmelsbach CK: Clinical studies of drug addiction: physical dependence, withdrawal and recovery. Arch Intern Med 69:766–772, 1942

Karliner JS: Propoxyphene hydrochloride poisoning: report of a case treated with peritoneal dialysis. JAMA 199:152–155, 1967

Martin WR, Fraser HF: A comparative study of physiological and subjective effects of heroin and morphine administered intravenously in post-addicts. J Pharmacol Exp Ther 133:388–399, 1961

————, Jasinski DR: Physiological parameters of morphine dependence in man—tolerance, early abstinence, protracted abstinence. J Psychiatr Res 7:9–17, 1969

————, Jasinski DR, Sapira JD, Flanary HG, Kelly OA, Thompson AK, Logan CR: The respiratory effects of morphine during a cycle of dependence. J Pharmacol Exp Ther 62:182–189, 1968

Monroe JJ, Ross WR, Berzins JI: The decline of the addict as "psychopath": Implications for community care. Int J Addict 6:601–608, 1971

Nutt JG, Jasinski DR: Methadone-Naloxone mixtures for use in methadone maintenance programs. I. An evaluation in man of their pharmacological feasibility. II. Demonstration of acute physical dependence. Clin Pharmacol Ther 15:156–166, 1974

Schaumann O: Analgetika und protektives system. Dtsch Med Wochenschr 79:1571–1573, 1954

Smith GM, Beecher HK: Measurement of "mental clouding" and other subjective effects of morphine. J Pharmacol Exp Ther 126:50–62, 1959

———, Semke CW, Beecher HK: Objective evidence of mental effects of heroin, morphine and placebo in normal subjects. J Pharmacol Exp Ther 136:53–58, 1962

Waldron VD, Klimt CR, Seibel JE: Methadone overdose treated with naloxone infusion. JAMA 225:53, 1973

Wikler A: A psychodynamic study of a patient during self-regulated re-addiction to morphine. Psychiatr Q 26:279–293, 1952

———: Sources of reinforcement for drug using behavior—a theoretical formulation. In Pharmacology and the Future of Man, Vol 1. Proceedings of the 5th International Congress of Pharmacology, San Francisco, Basel, Karger, 1973, pp 18–30

———, Fraser HF, Isbell H: N-allylnormorphine: effects of single doses and precipitation of acute "abstinence syndromes" during addiction to morphine, methadone, or heroin in man (postaddicts). J Pharmacol Exp Ther 109:8–20, 1953

treatment of
opioid
addiction

commentary

Heroin addiction, as well as dependence upon other opioids, remains a problem of paramount importance in our country. Although no treatment has been totally successful, many have achieved partial success. Dr. Wikler discusses detoxification, maintenance on narcotic antagonists, methadone, or heroin itself as treatment modalities. Arguments pro and con are considered. Since heroin addicts tend to be polydrug users, other drugs they tend to use are discussed.

treatment of opioid addiction

Abraham Wikler, M.D.

A variety of treatments for opioid addiction have been advocated and tried during the past century. None has been unequivocally successful, and the ideal treatment remains to be investigated. In general therapeutic approaches involve detoxification and the use of antagonists or agonists, such as methadone or heroin itself. Arguments for and against these approaches will be considered.

Detoxification of Opioid Addicts

Rapid Withdrawal Technique

In patients with low degrees of physical dependence the opioid, whatever its nature, may be withdrawn by first administering the drug subcutaneously or intramusculary (or orally in the cases of methadone or D-propoxyphene) in daily amounts just sufficient to suppress all abstinence phenomena and then reducing the daily dose each day over a period of 5 to 10 days. In the case of heroin addiction, morphine may be substituted, since in the United States heroin is a Schedule I drug (available for research purposes only, to specially licensed physicians). When morphine has been used in the reduction schedule, codeine (30 mg) may be combined with morphine on the last day of the reduction schedule and the patient may be continued on codeine alone for an additional day or two. Subsequently, one or two "pick-up" doses of small doses of morphine (6 to 10 mg) may be given if there are persistent complaints of muscular

aches and pains, anorexia, nausea, and vomiting. During the reduction period, intravenous infusions of 5 percent glucose in saline
should be given to combat dehydration due to excessive sweating,
vomiting, or diarrhea. Warm flow baths for 2 or 3 hours, once or
twice daily, are of value in the treatment of restlessness and complaints of muscular pains. Aspirin may be given for muscular pains,
and hypnotics may be prescribed at bedtime to promote sleep.

Methadone Substitution and Withdrawal

Methadone is an opioid that, unlike morphine, is effective by mouth
(probably because of more complete absorption), has a long duration
of action, and while it does produce physical dependence, the abstinence syndrome is of lesser intensity though complaints of muscular
and bony aching and insomnia may be prolonged (Isbell et al 1948).
Substitution of 1 mg of methadone for 3 to 4 mg of morphine or 1 mg
of heroin or 0.5 mg of hydromorphone or 20 mg of meperidine will
suppress the corresponding abstinence syndromes. In practice 10 to
20 mg of methadone by mouth, two or three times daily, has been
found sufficient to achieve this end. After the patient is stabilized on
an abstinence-suppressing daily oral dose of methadone for 3 to 5
days, the daily dose of methadone can be reduced to zero over a
period of 7 to 10 days with minimal discomfort for the patient,
although he may complain of vague anxiety, anorexia, poor sleep,
weakness, and muscular and bony aching for weeks. Because of its
convenience for physicians and nurses, methadone substitution and
withdrawal have been preferred to rapid reduction techniques in the
management of patients with moderate to high degrees of physical
dependence on opioids.

Detoxification should be carried out in a hospital, with due
safeguards against smuggling of drugs, including opioids, either by
the patient (concealed in his clothing and other personal effects or in
the case of females, in containers inserted into the vagina) or by
visitors. For the use of methadone in detoxification, new FDA regulations (Federal Register 1972) require that the hospital pharmacy be
approved for this purpose by the FDA and state authorities, and that
the procedures for methadone substitution and withdrawal be completed within 21 days. Methadone administered for longer than 21
days constitutes "methadone maintenance," for which special authority and facilities are required.

Relapse

More than 90 percent of 1881 (of a total of 1912) opioid addicts who
had been detoxified and institutionalized for variable periods of time

at the Federal hospital in Lexington, Kentucky, between 1952 and 1955, relapsed to heroin addiction within 2 years, and more than 90 percent of those who became readdicted did so within 6 months after discharge from the hospital (Hunt and Odoroff 1962). On longer follow-up, the percentage of readdictions decreases. Thus, Duvall et al (1963) found that of a sample of 453 addicts in the previously mentioned study, only an estimated 46 percent were readdicted by the fifth year after discharge from the hospital. In other studies, Vaillant (1966, 1973) found that 46 percent were abstinent from heroin 12 years after discharge from the Lexington hospital, and 35 percent after 20 years. Similar results were obtained by O'Donnell (1969) in a long-term (2 to 18 years) follow-up of addicts residing in rural areas of Kentucky who had been detoxified in the Lexington hospital. Winnick (1962) noted a sharp increase in the rate at which names of "active addicts" are dropped from the File of Active Addicts of the former Bureau of Narcotics between the ages of 35 and 40 years and has suggested that in some cases maturation may lead to permanent abstention from opioids with or without previous treatment and despite relapses.

Provision of aftercare (individual or group psychotherapy, vocational training, education, job counseling) following detoxification and release from hospital or jail seems not to have altered the prognosis for relapse significantly. Therapeutic communities, such as Synanon in California, in which ex-addicts live permanently, and Daytop Village in New York, where residents may live for months or years and then graduate into the general society, have claimed great success in decreasing relapse rates, but for various reasons their data, if made public at all, have been extremely difficult to evaluate (Glasscote et al 1972).

Pharmacologic Prevention of Relapse—Temporary Maintenance on Narcotic Antagonists (Currently Under Restricted Investigation)

Narcotic antagonists are synthetically derived from certain opioids by substituting an allyl or cyclopropylmethyl radical for the methyl radical on the tertiary nitrogen. Some, like naloxone (N-allylnoroxymorphone) and naltrexone (N-cyclopropyl-methylnoroxymorphone) are relatively "pure" antagonists, exert-virtually no actions of their own other than competitively antagonizing agonistic effects of opioids (euphoria, miosis, respiratory depression, and so on). Others, like nalorphine (N-allylnormorphine) and cyclazocine (N-cyclopropylmethylbenzomorphan), are classed as partial agonists (of the nalorphine type) because, in addition to their competitive antagonism of opioid agonistic actions, they exert agonistic actions of their own (morphinelike and psychotomimetic) and on repeated administration produce a peculiar state of physical dependence.

When pure antagonists like naloxone or naltrexone are administered in adequate doses to a nontolerant person after a single dose of an opioid, the effects of the latter are antagonized promptly. When partial agonists, like nalorphine or cyclazocine, are given after a small dose of an opioid, certain effects of the latter (miosis, sedation) may be augmented, but if the dose of opioid was large, the effects of the opioid will be antagonized. In persons tolerant to and physically dependent on opioids, administration of either pure antagonists or partial agonists precipitates an opioid-abstinence syndrome promptly.

On the other hand, if narcotic antagonists are given in adequate single doses to a nontolerant person before an opioid is administered, the agonistic actions of the opioid will be prevented. On repeated administration of narcotic antagonists to an otherwise untreated person, no tolerance develops to this opioid-blocking action, and no physical dependence develops if the person takes or is given repeated doses of opioids in amounts insufficient to overcome the blockade produced by the narcotic antagonist. In contrast to the absence of tolerance to the opioid-antagonistic actions of narcotic antagonists, tolerance does develop to the agonistic effects of the partial agonists. Thus, by beginning with very small doses and increasing the dose gradually, previously detoxified opioid addicts can be made tolerant to the frequently unpleasant agonistic actions of nalorphine or cyclazocine, without attenuating the opioid-antagonistic actions of these narcotic antagonists.

In 1966 Martin and his collaborators proposed that detoxified opioid addicts be placed on daily doses of a long-lasting, orally effective narcotic antagonist that would block the effects of heroin and other opioids in amounts usually obtainable "on the street." During the action of narcotic antagonists, such amounts of heroin will not produce euphoria, and even repeated self-injections of heroin will not result in physical dependence. Hence, provided that the narcotic antagonist-maintained patient *does* attempt to overcome the opioid blockade by opioid self-administration, both conditioned opioid-seeking behavior and conditioned abstinence should undergo extinction. (Extinction should be differentiated from suppression as in the case of alcoholics maintained on disulfiram who become violently ill if they drink alcohol.) It has been proposed (Wikler 1974) that maintenance on narcotic antagonists in outpatient status be maintained for about 10 months after detoxification, not only to ensure extinction of the conditioned responses but also to permit recovery from protracted abstinence. During this period of narcotic antagonist maintenance, efforts should be at rehabilitation, including psychotherapy, vocational retraining, education, and counseling.

For temporary maintenance, the narcotic antagonist should be effective when administered by mouth, and a single dose should block opioid effects for at least 24 hours. The duration of the opioid-antagonistic actions of nalorphine is too short (4 to 5 hours) for this purpose, and naloxone is both too short acting and relatively ineffective by the oral route. (Single doses of 2000 to 3000 mg per day of naloxone are required to block opioid effects for 24 hours [Zaks et al 1973].) In their 1966 paper, Martin et al presented experimental data indicating that by starting with very small oral doses, which were increased gradually, detoxified addicts could be made tolerant to the agonistic actions of 2 mg of cyclazocine given orally twice daily (4 mg per day), and that when maintained on this daily dose, they showed marked degrees of tolerance to 60 mg of heroin given parenterally and developed only mild degrees of physical dependence on morphine when this opioid was given subcutaneously in ascending doses up to 240 mg per day and then abruptly withdrawn. Eventually, when cyclazocine was abruptly discontinued, a mild, atypical abstinence syndrome (including complaints of "electric shocks" in the head and neck) ensued, which was not accompanied by opioid-seeking behavior. In clinical trials it has been found that slightly higher single oral doses of cyclazocine (eg, 5 mg per day) are required to block 25 mg of heroin intravenously for 24 hours, whereas the blockade can last 48 hours after single oral doses of 10 mg of cyclazocine (Resnick et al 1974). A number of preliminary reports of clinical results with cyclazocine have appeared (Wikler 1975), some of which indicate that in addicts who choose a cyclazocine program rather than methadone maintenance a high rate of abstention from heroin and other opioids can be expected (Fink 1973, Kissin et al 1973).

Very recently Martin et al (1973) reported the results of experimental studies on naltrexone. This long-lasting, orally effective narcotic antagonist has few, if any, agonistic actions and does not produce physical dependence on chronic oral administration. In daily oral doses of 25 mg twice daily (50 mg per day), naltrexone markedly attenuates the effects of 100 mg of morphine (subcutaneously) and the abstinence syndrome that ensues when such subjects are given increasing doses of morphine up to 240 mg per day followed by abrupt withdrawal of morphine. In clinical trials a single daily oral dose of naltrexone, 50 mg, has been found to block the effects of heroin, 25 mg intravenously, for 24 hours, while 100 to 150 mg per day of naltrexone will exert the same blocking action for 48 hours (Resnick et al 1974). Clinical trials of naltrexone in the treatment of addicts are currently under way.

This pharmacologic approach to the management of detoxified opioid addicts, particularly if it can be combined with programmed self-administration of heroin or other opioids while under narcotic antagonist blockade (experimental extinction), represents an attempt to deal with opioid addiction as a disease *sui generis*. However, one investigator (Altman et al 1974) reports that when placed on daily oral doses of naloxone or naltrexone, detoxified addicts refuse to challenge the opioid blockade by self-administration of heroin, or do so in desultory fashion. Whether this is due to a cognitive awareness that opioids would have no effect, or to a hitherto unknown satiating action of the narcotic antagonist on opioid-deprived receptors remains to be determined. If addicts do not challenge the opioid blockade by self-administration of heroin, then theoretically extinction will not take place and the patient is likely to relapse again when the narcotic antagonist is discontinued. Nevertheless, even without programmed self-administration of heroin, a high proportion of addicts maintained on cyclazocine are reported to have remained abstinent from heroin for as long as 6 months (to date) after cyclazocine has been discontinued (Fink 1973, Kissin et al 1973). At the present time clinical therapeutic trials with narcotic antagonists are restricted to investigators whose IND (Investigational New Drug) application has been approved by the FDA.

Methadone Maintenance

In contrast to methods of treatment that aim at total and permanent abstention from all opioids, Dole and Nyswander (1965) proposed that opioid addicts be maintained indefinitely on single, daily oral doses of methadone dispensed legally in amounts sufficient to establish a high degree of tolerance to it and cross-tolerance (blockade) to heroin and other opioids. The rationale for such methadone maintenance is as follows: (a) For a long time after detoxification from heroin, addicts have a metabolic defect experienced as "drug hunger," which, they have learned, can be reduced by opioids——hence the addict's notorious propensity to relapse. (b) By the oral route, methadone is said not to produce euphoria, but it does reduce "drug hunger." (c) Even after a high degree of tolerance has developed to others of its actions, methadone (in daily oral doses of about 40 mg or more) continues to reduce "drug hunger"; hence the addict maintained on high doses of methadone does not seek to increase the dose (achievement of euphoria is not the addict's primary goal). (d) Because cross-tolerance develops to heroin, the addict maintained on large daily doses of methadone will not experience heroin effects (including euphoria) if he tries to administer heroin intravenously to himself. As a consequence, he will soon desist from such attempts. (Heroin-seeking behavior will become extinguished.) (e) Tolerance to the performance-impairing actions of methadone having been established, "drug hunger" having been suppressed, and heroin hustling (with its attendant criminalism) having been given up, the addict can now be rehabilitated in society—he can, with some assistance, find a place to live and a job, or go back to school and refrain from criminal activities. (f) Maintenance on methadone for long periods of time does not produce serious impairment of health (Kreek 1973).

Criticisms of methadone maintenance include the following:

1. Methadone is a drug that produces physical dependence and causes withdrawal. Especially after the prolonged administration of the high daily doses used in methadone maintenance, withdrawal is followed by a prolonged, distressing abstinence syndrome. (The protracted abstinence syndrome lasted from 6 to 8 weeks and up to 24 weeks after abrupt withdrawal of methadone from experimental subjects who had received methadone orally for 15 weeks, attaining a daily dose of 100 mg by the seventh week [Martin et al 1973a and b]). If the postulated metabolic defect and "drug hunger" are consequences of long-term heroin use, then they should be aggravated by prolonged maintenance on another opioid, like methadone, which produces physical dependence with protracted abstinence.

2. Although some well-rehabilitated, selected methadone maintenance patients can be withdrawn from methadone without relapsing to heroin ". . . there is no evidence in the medical literature to support the assumption that detoxification can be achieved in most cases without compromising the patient's rehabilitation" (Dole 1973).

3. Although reduction of criminal activity and increase in gainful (legal) employment of addicts are salutary social achievements, methadone maintenance constitutes a method of social control through pharmacologic reinforcement—a method that conceivably could be abused by unscrupulous reinforcers (those who control the dispensing of methadone).

4. Patients maintained on methadone are, physiologically at least, not normal. Electroencephalograms of subjects experimentally stabilized on methadone 100 mg per day, orally, show increased

delta bursts and rapid eye movement (REM) sleep as well as more vocalization during REM periods, decreased blood pressure, pulse rate, respiratory rate, and pupillary diameter, and increased body temperature; sexual activity is markedly decreased initially but returns to almost the control level later (Martin et al 1973). In methadone-maintenance treatment populations, about half of the patients complain of excessive sweating, and lesser but substantial numbers report constipation, decreased libido, sleep disturbances, and pain in the bones and joints. About one-third of babies born to mothers maintained on methadone are underweight at birth and are considered premature (Wilmarth and Goldstein 1974). Roughly 80 percent of babies born to mothers maintained on 60 mg per day or more of methadone display methadone-withdrawal phenomena, such as irritability, hypertonicity, tremors, excessive sucking needs, and excessive crying (Davis et al 1973).

5. Like heroin or morphine, methadone given *intravenously* does produce euphoria (Isbell et al 1948) as well as physical dependence. For these reasons, diversion of the drug from methadone maintenance programs could give rise to a serious problem of methadone addiction (and overdose) "on the street." Indeed, a black market for methadone already exists, and in some cities the number of methadone-related deaths exceeds those attributable to heroin (Bourne 1973).

When a patient is admitted to a methadone maintenance program, the initial dose of methadone is 10 or 20 mg per day in divided doses, given orally. This dose is gradually increased, as tolerance develops, until a stabilization level is reached, after which the patient is maintained on a single daily oral dose of methadone at the stabilization level, without a further increase in dose. Stabilization on methadone may take as long as 6 weeks and preferably should be carried out in a hospital. After the patient is stabilized, he is discharged to the outpatient department where he reports daily for his dose of methadone for supportive therapy and at random intervals to submit a urine specimen for the detection of morphine (heroin), other opioids, barbiturates, amphetamines, cocaine as well as quinine, which is commonly mixed with illicit heroin. According to Dole and Nyswander (1968), the stabilization dose of methadone should be between 80 and 120 mg per day, but Wilmarth and Goldstein (1974) note that blind studies failed to reveal important differences in the use of heroin or in other program criteria at doses as widely different as 40 mg or 160 mg. They feel that daily oral doses of 50 to 80 mg are generally sufficient, provided there is no evidence of an unusually low plasma level. Comparing the outcomes of these different methadone maintenance programs, Wilmarth and Goldstein (1974) found that heroin use was markedly reduced, employment rates were increased, and arrest rates were decreased. They emphasize the roles of rehabilitative efforts and of outreaching, nonpunitive, and nonjudgmental attitudes on the part of the staff in achieving these results.

Effective June 17, 1973, the FDA has issued new regulations intended to (a) prevent the diversion of methadone into the illicit market, (b) ensure that methadone maintenance is offered only to physically dependent opioid addicts who are otherwise unlikely to abstain from using heroin or other opioids, and (c) facilitate the acquisition of data on the long-term effects of methadone. Shipments of methadone by manufacturers are restricted to approved methadone maintenance programs, approved hospital pharmacies, and approved community pharmacies. A private licensed physician may prescribe methadone for oral administration to alleviate severe pain (only) in outpatients, but the prescription can be filled only by approved hospital or community pharmacies. For inpatients, a private licensed physician may prescribe methadone orally or parenterally for severe pain in patients hospitalized for treatment of medical or surgical disorders and for detoxification of opioid addicts, provided that the latter does not exceed 21 days. A methadone treatment program is defined as a person or organization, approved by the state authorities and by the FDA, that furnishes a comprehensive range of services, using methadone for the detoxification and /or maintenance of opioid addicts, and provides counseling, rehabilitative, and other services, including vocational and educational guidance and employment placement.

Admission to methadone treatment programs must be voluntary (with written consent); the patient must be over 16 years of age, dependent on opioids for at least 2 years, and show evidence of physical dependence at time of admission (except for eddicts within 1 week of discharge from a prison or other institution where he had spent 1 month or longer). All methadone must be dispensed in liquid form for oral administration. During the first 3 months methadone must be administered under close supervision, daily, at least 6 days a week; after 3 months, three times weekly (with no more than a 2-day take-home supply). These rules may be relaxed in cases of acute illness, family crises, or necessary travel. The maximal daily dose of methadone is generally 100 mg; higher doses, up to 120 mg per day, must be justified in the medical record and approval must be obtained from state authorities and the FDA for doses over 120 mg per day (or over 100 mg per day for take-home methadone).

Urine tests for morphine (heroin) should be made randomly, at least
once a week, and tests for methadone, barbiturates, amphetamine,
and other drugs, randomly, at least once a month (Methadone
Treatment Manual 1973).

The British System

What is presently called the *British System* evolved out of a number
of ad hoc measures taken to deal with an alarming increase in the
number of opioid addicts in Great Britain, noted by the Interdepart-
mental Committee on Drug Addiction (the *Brain Committee*) in
1965. Prior to 1968 physicians were urged but not required to report
addicts they were maintaining (usually on morphine) to the Home
Office. Up to 1961 the number of addicts known to the Home Office
in any given year was less than 500, mostly middle-aged, largely
from medical or paramedical professions, and their addiction was
usually of therapeutic origin. In 1959 a few London physicians
began to prescribe heroin (a legal drug in England) for addicts in
amounts far in excess of their requirements. These addicts gave or
sold their excess heroin to others, many of whom had not used
heroin. By 1965 the number of heroin addicts known to the Home
Office doubled. The rapid increase in the number of known addicts
continued until, in 1968, their number rose to 2782 (Bewley 1974).
These new addicts differed from those known to the Home Office
before 1961 in that they were younger (the majority being 20 to 34
years old), had a history of arrests prior to using heroin, and were of
lower social class.

In 1968 legislation in the Dangerous Drugs Act of 1967, recommended by the Brain Committee in 1965, was implemented. This
provided that notification of addiction to dangerous drugs (including heroin) be required and that prescribing heroin (or cocaine) for
an addict be restricted only to specially licensed physicians, working mainly in special clinics, most of which were in the London
area. At these clinics attempts are made at detoxification, and it is
believed that some 20 percent become abstinent. For the majority,
however, maintenance on opioids is practiced. During the year 1971,
the number of addicts reported to the Home Office was 2769, but as
of December 31, 1971, only 1555 addicts were receiving prescriptions for daily self-administration of opioids (Bewley 1974). Of these
addicts, 1161 were receiving methadone (mostly for intravenous
use) either alone or, in 229 cases, with heroin as well; 156 addicts
were receiving heroin either alone or in combination with drugs
other than methadone; and 238 addicts, whose addiction was mostly

of therapeutic origin, were receiving other opioids (mainly morphine or meperidine).

Some of the advantages claimed for this system are that the rate at which new cases of addiction have appeared has been much lower than before the clinics were set up; the rate of increase in the overall death rate of opioid addicts has declined since the 1960s; and some patients have been helped to abstain entirely from drug use, while others have been able to lead more stable lives despite their continuing use of opioids. Also, "there are advantages in using a medical model for addiction, as sickness is generally less attractive than sin" (Bewley 1974).

In principle the arguments for and against the British System are the same as those for and against methadone maintenance in the United States. Whether or not the British System will prevent the development of a black market in opioid drugs in Great Britain and the concomitant accelerated rate at which new addicts are recruited in the future, remain to be seen.

Treatment of Polydrug Addiction

As treatment for intoxication due to amphetamines and other stimulants—marihuana, LSD, and other psychotomimetic agents—consists of abrupt withdrawal of these drugs, they present no immediate problem. However, repeated use of alcohol, barbiturates, nonbarbiturate sedatives, and minor tranquilizers can produce a type of physical dependence, and abrupt withdrawal may result in convulsions and delirium, which may be dangerous to life. In patients who have used these drugs as well as opioids, it is best to stabilize them on pentobarbital in doses and frequency of administration (by the oral route, if possible, or by intramuscular injection) just sufficient to prevent all signs of barbiturate-type abstinence (tremulousness, weakness, postural hypotension, anxiety, sweating, anorexia, convulsions, and later delirium) and to produce minimal signs of barbiturate intoxication (slight nystagmus and ataxia, mild drowsiness). Or, chlordiazepoxide (Librium) may be used for the same purpose with less danger of overdosage. At the same time, the patient may be stabilized on his opioid of "choice" or on methadone. Stabilization on pentobarbital or chlordiazepoxide is then maintained, while the opioid is withdrawn by the rapid reduction or the methadone substitution and withdrawal method. After this has been accomplished, the dose of pentobarbital (or of chlordiazepoxide) may be progressively reduced at a rate of not more than 100 mg per day of pentobarbital, or 25 mg per day of chlordiazepoxide. The postwithdrawal treatment of polydrug addicts, insofar as their opioid addiction is concerned, is the same as for "pure" opioid addicts. Unfortunately, neither narcotic antagonists nor methadone maintenance appears to affect abuse of drugs other than opioids, but in the case of alcoholism, disulfiram (Antabuse) may be tried.

References

Altman JL, Meyer RE, Mirin SM, Mcnamee HB: The effects on narcotic antagonists upon heroin self-administration behavior. In National Academy of Sciences-National Research Council: Proceedings, Committee on Problems of Drug Dependence, 1974 p 752–763

Bewley TH: Treatment of opiate addiction in Great Britain. In Fisher S, Freedman VH (eds): Opiate Addiction: Origins and Treatment. Washington, DC, Winston, 1974

Bourne PG: Methadone diversion. In National Association for the Prevention of Addiction to Narcotics. Fifth National Conference on Methadone Treatment. New York, 1973, pp 839–841

Davis MM, Brown BS, Glendinning ST: Neonatal effects of heroin addiction and methadone-treated pregnancies. Preliminary report of 70 live births. In National Association for the Prevention of Addiction to Narcotics. Proceedings of the Fifth National Conference on Methadone Treatment. New York, 1973, pp 1153–1162

Dole VP: Detoxification of methadone patients and public policy. JAMA 226:780–781, 1973

————, Nyswander M: A medical treatment for diacetylmorphine (heroin) addiction. JAMA 193:646–650, 1965

————, Nyswander ME: Methadone maintenance and its implications for theories of narcotic addiction. In Wikler A (ed): The Addictive States, Vol 46. Research Publication of the association of nervous and mental Diseases, 1968, pp 359–366

Duvall HJ, Locke BZ, Brill L: Follow-up study of narcotic drug addicts five years after hospitalization. Pub Health Rep 78:185–196, 1963

FDA regulations governing methadone. In Federal Register, Vol 37, Section 130.44, Conditions for the Use of Methadone, Dec 15, 1972

Fink M: Questions in cyclazocine therapy of opiate dependence. In Fisher S, Freedman AM (eds): Opiate Addiction: Origins and Treatment, Washington, DC, Winston, 1973, pp 203–209

Glasscote RM, Sussex JN, Jaffe JH, Ball J, Brill L: The Treatment of Drug Abuse. Programs, Problems, Prospects. Washington, DC, American Psychiatric Association, 1972

Hunt GH, Odoroff ME: Follow-up study of narcotic drug addicts after hospitalization. Pub Health Rep 77:41–54, 1962

Isbell H, Eisenman AJ, Wikler A, Frank K: The effects of single doses of 6-dimethylamine-4, 4-diphenyl-3-heptanone (Amidone, methadon or "10820") on human subjects. J Pharmacol Exp Ther 92:83–89, 1948

———, Wikler A, Eisenman A, Daingerfield M, Frank K: Liability of addiction to 6-dimethylamine-4, 4-diphenyl-3-heptanone (methadon, "amidone" or "10820") in man. Arch Intern Med 82:362–396, 1948

Kissin B, Ottomanelli G, Sang E, Halloran G: Cyclazocine treatment for heroin addicts. In National Association for the Prevention of Addiction to Narcotics. Proceedings of the Fifth National Conference on Methadone Treatment. New York, 1973, pp 658–666

Kreek MJ: Medical safety and side effects of methadone in tolerant individuals. JAMA 223:665–668, 1973

Martin WR, Gorodetzky CW, McClane TK: An experimental study in the treatment of narcotic addicts with cyclazocine. Clin Pharmacol Ther 7:455–465, 1966

———, Jasinski DR, Haertzen CA, et al: Methadone—a re-evaluation. Arch Gen Psychiatry 28:286–295, 1973a

———, Jasinski DR, Mansky PA: Naltrexone, an antagonist for the treatment of heroin dependence: effects in man. Arch Gen Psychiatry 28:782–791, 1973b

Methadone Treatment Manual. Prescriptive Package. Washington, DC, U.S. Department of Justice, 1973, p 104

O'Donnell JA: Narcotic addicts in Kentucky. Public Health Publication 1881, Washington, DC, Supt of Documents, 1969, p 297

Resnick R, Fink M, Freedman AM: High-dose cyclazocine therapy of opiate dependence. Am J Psychiatry, 131:595–597, 1974

———, Volavka J, Freedman AM, Thomas M: Studies of EN-1639A (Naltrexone): a new narcotic antagonist. Am J Psychiatry, 131:646–650, 1974

Vaillant GE: A twelve year follow-up of New York narcotic addicts. I. The relation of treatment to outcome. Am J Psychiatry, 122:727–736, 1966

———, A twenty year follow-up of New York narcotic addicts. Arch Gen Psychiatry 29:237–241, 1973

Wikler A: Requirements for extinction of relapse-facilitating variables and for rehabilitation in a narcotic-antagonist treatment program. In Braude MC, Harris LS, May EL, Smith JP, Villareal JE (eds): Narcotic Antagonists, Advances in Biochemical Psychopharmacology, Vol 8. New York, Raven, 1974, pp 399–414

————: Opioid antagonists and deconditioning in addiction treatment. In Drug Dependence—Treatment and Treatment Evaluation. Skandia International Symposium, 15-17 Oct 1974, Boström H, Larsson T, Ljunqstedt (eds), Stockholm, Almaquist and Wiksell Internat, 1975, pp 159–182

Wilmarth SS, Goldstein A: Therapeutic Effectiveness of Methadone Maintenance Programs in the Management of Drug Dependence of Morphine-Type in the USA. Geneva, World Health Organization, 1974, p 53

Winick C: Maturing out of narcotic addiction. UN Bull Narcotics 14:1–7, 1962

Zaks A, Jones T, Fink M, Freedman AM: Naloxone treatment of opiate dependence. JAMA 215:2108–2110, 1973

psychopharmacology of caffeine

commentary

Caffeine is one of the most widely used psychoactive agents. Even though, as a component of coffee or tea, it is generally considered a nondrug, its pharmacologic properties are just as real as those of other drugs. Caffeine is occasionally prescribed alone or in drug mixtures, as in caffeine sodium benzoate, a mild stimulant, or with aspirin and phenacetin as a headache remedy. Two related methylated xanthines are theophylline, which is used as a cardiac stimulant, and theobromine, which has no medical application today. Some of the safety in caffeine resides in the fact that it is obtainable only in diluted form in beverages. Furthermore, stimulation may result from the possible ability of caffeine to inhibit the enzyme, phosphodiesterase. However, more research is needed to demonstrate whether the effects of caffeine are mediated through cyclic AMP or some other mechanism.

It is fascinating to speculate that the purine structure of caffeine may explain its influence on the adenosine moiety of cyclic AMP. Whether it influences purines and pyrimidines in nucleic acids is still a moot point.

psychopharmacology of caffeine

Harold S. Levenson, Ph.D.
Erin Charles Bick

Caffeine, as a constituent of the social beverages and as an ingredient in popular cola soft drinks and countless nonprescription pharmaceutical combinations, is the most widely used stimulant in the world. Caffeine, nicotine, and ethanol are the only naturally occurring psychoactive substances accepted by our culture for recreational use. Each of these three nonmedical, mind-affecting drugs has had a great influence on human civilization, undoubtedly greater than that of all other psychopharmacologic agents combined. This is true by any measure chosen: the number of people using them regularly, number of hours spent "under the influence," the quantities of each produced and consumed, as well as the amount of money spent to obtain them.

Caffeine's sought-after psychopharmacologic actions generally consist of a mild and agreeable central stimulation, which may be manifested, under the right circumstances, as enhanced alertness, wakefulness, increased energy, and elevated mood.

Background Information on the Caffeine Beverages

Caffeine occurs naturally in six distinct botanical families: in coffee, tea, kola nuts, guarana paste, in maté and cassina leaves, and in smaller amounts in cacao and chocolate.

Of the three major natural caffeine-containing beverages, coffee is the most important commercially. The United States imported 2.86 billion pounds of green coffee in 1973 to satisfy a per capita con-

451

TABLE 1.
CAFFEINE-CONTAINING PLANTS AND PREPARATIONS

Beverage (and other names)	Natural Sources and Botanic Distribution	Type of Preparation	Caffeine Content of Beverage (Per Average Serving)	% Caffeine/Other Xanthine Alkaloids in Plant Sources	Other Constituents in the Plant Source or Beverage	Green Beans %	Roasted Beans %	Comments
COFFEE (Cafe, Mocha, Java)	Seeds ("beans"), berries of *Coffea arabica* or *Coffea canephora* (*robusta*) (Rubiaceae). Original habitat Ethiopia; now widely cultivated in tropical zones surrounding the equator; Brazil, Africa, Colombia, South and Central America, Indonesia.	Roast and ground brewed coffee	85 mg/cup (aver.) 65–125 mg/cup (range)	Caffeine 1.2–2.3%	Trigonelline	1.2	0.7	
		Brewed instant or freeze-dried coffee	60 mg/cup (aver.) 40–100 mg/cup (range)	Adenine 0.02%	Acids (mostly chlorogenic)	7.0	3.5	
		Decaffeinated roast and ground brewed coffee	3 mg/cup (aver.) 2–8 mg/cup (range)	Theophylline	Carbohydrates	22.0	24.0	
		Decaffeinated instant coffee	3 mg/cup (aver.) 2–8 mg/cup (range)	Theobromine	Protein	12.0	13.0	
				Xanthine (traces)	Oils	11.0	13.0	
				Guanosure	Ash	3.0	4.0	
					Volatiles	trace	trace	
					Cellulose — nonhydrophy.	18.0	17.0	
					Cellulose — hydrolysible	13.0	14.0	
					H_2O	12.0	2.0	
					CO_2	0	2.0	
TEA (Chai, Te)	Leaves of *Thea sinensis* or *Camellia sinensis* (Theaceae) Original home in central Asia but now grown in wide range	Leaf tea (bags)	40 mg/cup (aver.) 30–50 mg/cup (range)	Caffeine 1.5–5.0% Theobromine 0.2%	>25% tannins or polyphenols (flavenols, gallocanthocyanins), amino acids, simple carbohydrates, polysaccharides, acids and depsides (theagallin), ash (flourine), vitamins (niacin, C, riboflavin, thiamin),			Essential oils present in black or fermented tea only.
		Instant tea	30 mg/cup (aver.) 25–35 mg/cup (range)	Theophylline 0.1% Adenine 0.01% Xanthine Hypoxanthine				

of latitudes; India, China, Burma, Ceylon, Japan, Brazil, Rhodesia, Russia, East Africa.			3,4-Dimeth- (traces) Oxyphenyl- Ethylamine	lignin, cellulose, volatiles.	
COCOA (Chocolatl) Seeds (shells and husks) of *Theobroma cacao* (Sterculiaceae) Original habitat Mexico; now cultivated widely in the tropics; West Africa, Brazil, Central America, Madagascar.	Cocoa beverage (African) Cocoa beverage (S. American) Sweet chocolate	7 mg /cup (aver.) 40 mg /cup (aver.) 20 mg /oz	Caffeine 0.3–1.8% Theophylline 0.05%	Fats (cocoa butter or theobroma oil), starches, pentosans, pectins, proteins, cacao red, tannins, (6%). Chocolate (plain)—crushed & shelled cacao "nibs"; sweet chocolate contains 50% + sugar, vanillin, and flavorings; milk chocolate has added milk solids.	Theobromine also occurs in plants of the Cascarilla family. Much of the theobromine extracted from cocoa is chemically converted to caffeine.
COLA (Kola nut, Guru nut, Sudan coffee) Seeds ("nuts" or dried cotyledons) of *Cola vera* or *C. nitida* or *Sterculia acuminata* (Sterculiaceae) Original habitat West Africa; grown in E & W Indies, Ceylon.	Cola (nut infusion) Cola (soft drinks)	— 20–36 mg /6 oz. bottle beverage	"Pods" contain caffeine 1.5–3.0% Theobromine 0.1%	Tannins (4.0%), glucose, resins, "kola red," kolantin, other unknown constituents. Cola-type soft drinks *may* contain cola nut extractives and decoccainized coca leaves; sugar, phos. acid, flavoring	Cola drinks must contain added caffeine (Standards of Identity); cola flavor is blended from lime and orange oils, cinnamon bark, ginger, and methyl salicylate (oil of wintergreen).

sumption of 136 pounds. Total world production exceeds 4 million
tons of green coffee annually. This annual coffee crop, valued at 4
billion dollars, provides a livelihood for some 20 million people in
60 countries.

The genus *Coffea* is a large one, numbering between 40 and 70
species. Only two of these species have attained commercial importance: *C. arabica* (accounting for about 75 percent of the coffee crop),
and *C. canephora* (Robusta coffee, mainly produced in Africa and
accounting for about 25 percent of the crop).

About 2 million pounds of caffeine were synthesized or extracted
in the United States in 1970. In addition, the United States imported
1,616,264 pounds of caffeine that year, mostly from West Germany
and the Netherlands, at a cost of more than 2 billion dollars. Over
two-thirds of this caffeine was used in cola-type beverages, with the
remainder going into headache and cold remedies and nonprescription stimulant tablets. For a summary of sources and preparations,
see Table 1.

Chemistry

Caffeine, or 1,3,7-trimethylxanthine, theophylline, and theobromine
are structurally related methylated xanthines, differing only in the
number and position of methyl groups substituted on the xanthine
parent ring.

Purine derivatives are widely distributed in nature and include
such vitally important endogenous substances as uric acid and the
nucleotide constituents of nucleic acid, adenine and guanine.

Guanine (2-amino-6-oxypurine) and adenine (6-aminopurine)
occur both in the free state and in complex combinations, such as the
nucleic acids, which serve as hereditary determinants in all living
creatures.

Structure-activity relationships involving methylation distinguish the three xanthine compounds. For instance, methyl substitution on the 1 position is associated with central nervous system
stimulation, diuresis is linked to the 3-methyl group, and cardiac
stimulation with the methyl group on the 7 position. Thus caffeine,
1,3,7-trimethylxanthine, shows all three effects, theobromine,
3,7-dimethylxanthine possesses relatively weak central nervous system activity, and theophylline, 1,3-dimethylxanthine, has increased
cardiac stimulant properties. All three compounds possess the
3-methyl group and all produce diuresis.

Cyclic adenosine-3,5-monophosphate (cyclic-AMP or c-AMP) is
an adenine nucleotide of vital importance in regulating metabolic
and cellular processes. Caffeine and theophylline bear a close family

resemblance to adenine and this similarity is now thought to underlie their pharmacologic actions.

Caffeine is often described as being tasteless; there may be curious
genetic implications in this oddity. It has recently been reported
(Hall et al 1975) that a substantial part of the population is insensitive to the bitter taste of caffeine. Caffeine taste blindness is correlated with taste deficiencies for the bitter substance phenylthiocarbamide and related compounds containing "CSNH" groups. Though
caffeine lacks this group, its threshold shows a similar bimodal distribution between bitter-sensitive people and nontasters. Genetic
studies on phenylthiocarbamide insensitivity indicate that this
Mendelian hereditary trait exists in about 30 percent of the population.

Since it is physiologically active, contains nitrogen, and is of botanical origin, caffeine is considered an alkaloid. It is not easy to give
an exact definition of the word *alkaloid*, however, and since there is
some question about their inclusion in this category, the methyl
xanthines are occasionally designated *pseudo alkaloids*.

Caffeine differs from most other alkaloids in being somewhat
water soluble, lacking a center of asymmetry, being biosynthetically
unrelated to amino acids, and showing scarcely any basic properties.
Caffeine is a very weak monoacidic base. A saturated aqueous solution is neutral to litmus and, similarly, almost neutral by other more
accurate methods of testing pH. The usual salts are formed with
mineral acids, but they are unstable in water or on prolonged exposure to air.

Pharmacology

Caffeine acts mainly as a stimulant to the central nervous system
(CNS), especially the higher centers, but its complex pharmacologic
actions extend to most physiologic systems. These include: contraction of striated muscle (including the cardiac muscle); relaxation of
smooth muscle (notably the coronary arteries, the uterus, and the
bronchi); a diuretic effect on the kidneys; a stimulatory effect on
respiration (at high doses); elevation of basal metabolism; and various endocrine and enzymatic effects.

In toxic and lethal quantities, caffeine produces convulsions. This
action can be elicited in decerebrate animals, indicating a direct
effect on the spinal cord. Caffeine produces an increase in the electrical activity of the cortex, evoking a shift in frequency comparable
to that shown with attention. It lowers reflex thresholds and increases the amplitude of synaptic potentials.

Single doses of caffeine, by various routes, cause an increase in the spontaneous motor activity of animals. Actually, caffeine exerts a biphasic psychomotor effect, depressing activity with larger doses. Chronic ingestion elicits a tolerance to this stimulation, which is dose dependent. Sufficient intake completely obliterates the response.

The psychologic effects of therapeutic doses of caffeine depend to some extent on the subject's initial state and can include enhanced alertness, relief from drowsiness and boredom, a delayed onset of fatigue, a sense of well-being and increased self-confidence, improved powers of concentration, brightening intellect, and an increased desire and capacity for work.

These subjective effects, like those of all centrally active drugs, depend on the expectations and personality of the individual user, on the environment, and on the dose and mode of administration. Caffeine is capable of elevating mood without altering perception of reality. The mild arousal resulting from social doses of caffeine is not followed by a marked compensating depression. These effects are considered pleasant by most people, and they represent valued attributes in an achievement-oriented society.

Caffeine's undesirable central effects are best understood as dose-related extensions of its characteristic pharmacologic actions. Within the central nervous system, toxic symptoms (usually referred to as *side effects* but actually dose-related consequences of over-stimulation) may include: delayed onset of (and motor disturbance during) sleep, and headache, restlessness, palpitation, tremulousness, unsteadiness, vertigo, reflex hyperexcitability, irritability, agitation, anxiety, and general discomfort. This syndrome has been popularly described as "coffee nerves," and is for the most part, preventable simply by rationing caffeine intake.

Caffeine, theophylline, and theobromine are essentially similar in qualitative action, but differ markedly in the intensity of their effects on various organs. Caffeine has the most potent psychomotor stimulatory and behavioral effects. Theophylline causes less central nervous system and respiratory stimulation, while it has stronger cardiac and diuretic effects. Theobromine is almost devoid of stimulating properties. It has a stronger inotropic action on striated muscles than caffeine, however, and more lasting effect on the renal system than theophylline.

Pharmacokinetics

Absorption of caffeine after intramuscular injection has been shown to take twice as long as absorption of the same dose by mouth. After absorption, caffeine is rapidly and quite uniformly distributed throughout the body. The levels reached in various tissues are in proportion to their water content. This applies not only to somatic cells but also to germ cells. Most of the caffeine administered is stored in muscle tissue, since these tissues hold the greatest deposits of body water. Furthermore, caffeine has been found to penetrate cells of the fetus and reaches the same concentration there as in tissues of the mother.

The tissue concentration is significant in relation to allegations of genetic risks involved in the consumption of caffeine-containing beverages. Kihlman (1974) after an extensive survey of the effects of caffeine on genetic material, concluded: "In my opinion, these risks, if any, are exceedingly small. The concentrations needed to produce chromosomal aberrations are at least 40 times higher than those we are likely to be exposed to as a result of consumption of caffeine-containing beverages."

After absorption, the blood plasma concentration declines very rapidly in man and most other mammals. The human half-life is 3.5 hours (ie, 15 percent is metabolized per hour). There is some indication of a saturation level for caffeine because plasma half-life shows a relationship to the quantity of caffeine administered, though dramatic differences are not observed. Studies have shown that when two cups of coffee were ingested at four equal intervals over a 12-hour period, considerable amounts of caffeine were stored in the body; specifically 180 mg of the alkaloid were present 1 hour after the last cup. However, Axelrod and Reichenthal (1953) found no caffeine in plasma the following morning, indicating that there was no day-to-day accumulation.

Caffeine is not a substrate for xanthine oxidase, but several of the monomethylxanthines are. Uric acid is produced in the body from guanine via xanthine or from adenine via hypoxanthine and xanthine. The xanthine is then oxidized by the enzyme xanthine oxidase to the rather insoluble acid, which produces gout by precipitating in joints and soft tissues. Basically, the metabolism of caffeine in man and animals involves a series of dimethylation steps and oxidation in the reactive 8-position, forming dimethyl and monomethylxanthines with uric acid derivatives as end-products. However, uric acid, per se, is not formed as a caffeine metabolite. Thus caffeine intake need not be restricted in gout sufferers.

Toxicity

Acute

Caffeine is considered a relatively safe and nontoxic compound, both acutely and when moderately large amounts are ingested chronically for long periods of time.

In the rat, rabbit, guinea pig, cat, and dog, the lethal dose of the alkaloid is reported to be in the range of 140 to 250 mg/kg body weight. A 70-kg human who drinks one cup of coffee containing 100 mg of caffeine has an initial level, before metabolic activity, of about 1.4 mg/kg of body weight of caffeine in his tissues.

The nature of caffeine's acute toxicity is an extension of its characteristic pharmacologic actions to a harmful degree and involves the central nervous system, cardiovascular, gastrointestinal, renal, and respiratory systems.

Fatal poisonings due to caffeine are extremely rare. There were none reported in the medical literature until 1959. Only six deaths, worldwide, have been reported since then, and the lowest toxic dose was 3.2 g (57 mg/kg) intravenously. The oral lethal dose in humans has been estimated to be 10 g.

Chronic

The clear-cut existence of chronic toxic effects from caffeine, coffee, tea, or cola drinking in moderate or even in large quantities is quite debatable in man, though the chronic administration of very large doses of caffeine to animals has been shown to produce a variety of adverse effects, including weight loss (transient) and reduced reproductive capacity.

Cyclic AMP and Hormone Action

The methylxanthines are competitive inhibitors of cyclic nucleotide phosphodiesterase (PDE), the enzyme catalyzing the conversion (and inactivation) of cyclic adenosine $3'5'$-monophosphate (c-AMP) to adenosine 5-monophosphate (AMP).

This action of caffeine and theophylline was first reported by Butcher and Sutherland in 1962 (Robison 1971) who suggested this was the mechanism underlying the methylxanthine's physiologic and metabolic effects. Whether or not this eventually proves to be the case, caffeine's inhibition of PDE has secured for it a leading role in the most significant and potentially useful biochemical developments of recent years.

Cyclic AMP is now recognized to be a key regulating agent in most mammalian tissues. It modulates the rate of a broad spectrum of cellular activities and vital metabolic processes. Cyclic AMP mediates the actions of large numbers of hormones and regulates the release of most, if not all, other hormones.

Abnormal levels of cyclic AMP are also associated with a variety of disease states. Deficiencies or excesses of the cyclic nucleotide and the enzymes affecting it may be important in the etiology of diabetes, hypertension, obesity, hepatomas, asthma, and psoriasis.

Caffeine's Effects on Human Performance

One of the most valuable investigations of caffeine's effects on the human mind was conducted over 60 years ago by H. L. Hollingworth (1912) who studied the influence of caffeine on mental and motor efficiency and found that in appropriate doses it improved both. Weiss and Laties (1962) summarized and critically evaluated the earlier psychophysiologic studies on caffeine's effects on human performance. They list their conclusions as follows:

1. Caffeine has little or no effect on reaction time, whereas amphetamine seems to lower it, especially in fatigued subjects.
2. Caffeine impairs hand steadiness, whereas amphetamine seems to improve it.
3. Caffeine has equivocal effects on coordination, while amphetamines improve such performance, especially the more complex.
4. Both caffeine and amphetamine can to some extent counteract the decrement of motor performance produced by alcohol.
5. Both caffeine and amphetamine counteract fatigue produced by exhausting physical activity.

Neuropharmacology

It is generally agreed that caffeine, like other psychostimulants, shifts the electroencephalogram and frequency distribution toward the fast side, with a slight rise in voltage level. These electroencephalographic effects are very similar to those seen with increased "alertness."

Gibbs and Maltby (1943) tested epinephrine, amphetamine, and caffeine and found all three caused a frequency shift toward the faster end of the spectrum. Epinephrine's effect was strongest and caffeine's least (despite its ability to penetrate the blood-brain barrier). The depressant drugs, thiopental, morphine, and phenobarbital, produced a shift in the opposite direction.

Sulc and Broyek (1974) gave 8 young volunteers 200 mg of caffeine and sodium benzoate and measured the electroencephalogram, critical flicker fusion threshold, and efficiency in "pursuit" tests, 2 and 4 hours later. Caffeine improved the test results, had no effect on critical flicker fusion, and caused a spectral redistribution (a shift to faster frequencies in the electroencephalogram). The authors were puzzled by the fact that electroencephalographic changes were progressively greater at 4 hours than at 2, although plasma caffeine levels were decreasing.

Klein and Salzman (1975) have reported paradoxic effects of caffeine on averaged evoked responses to sound stimuli of low intensity (1000 cps, 60 db). Seven of 10 male subjects showed statistically significant lowering of evoked response amplitude 2 hours after ingesting 300 mg of caffeine. Only 2 of 10 females tested showed a similar paradoxic effect. Other researchers have observed this same sort of transient depression in electrical brain activity (usually accompanied by drowsiness) in a high percentage of normal subjects receiving 10 mg amphetamine.

This study seems to emphasize the need for caution in applying the term *stimulant* uncritically to characterize drug action. Electroencephalographic effects of psychopharmacologic drugs vary in their actions in time, and apparently the predominant or typical actions of many stimulant drugs include a phase of transiently depressed brain activity over the course of time.

There have been several other electroencephalographic studies with caffeine, but like those described so far, they seem to add little to direct behavioral analysis or to a basic understanding of caffeine's mechanism or locus of action in the central nervous system.

Psychologic Effects

The power of suggestion is illustrated by an interesting experiment performed by Goodfellow in 1946. Regular or decaffeinated coffee was administered to subjects on different occasions and auditory thresholds measured. When the coffee with and without caffeine was administered "blind," both depressed the thresholds in an almost identical fashion. After subjects were informed that only decaffeinated coffee was being used, all thresholds returned to normal.

A similarly strong effect from suggestion was observed by Goldstein et al (1964 a,b) in his experiment on caffeine-induced wakefulness. "A most interesting phenomenon was revealed when a known caffeine sample was given on the first night, followed by blind administration of caffeine or lactose on the succeeding four nights. The wakefulness produced by known caffeine was minimized in subjects' reports, so that effects appeared to be hardly greater than on lactose nights; yet the identical caffeine dose given to the same subjects in a blind experiment produced definite wakefulness. We are confronted with a 'reverse placebo effect' of striking magnitude."

An experiment by Mitchell and Ross (1974) was specifically designed to control placebo effects and assess caffeine's effects on cognitive performance in "isolation." Sixty subjects were given a difficult recall test (Paced Sequential Memory Task) after receiving either 300 mg caffeine in capsules or the same dose in orange juice. A quarter received placebo capsules, while another quarter received only orange juice. No statistically reliable caffeine effects were found. When the raw test data were subjected to analysis of variance, however, a significant interaction between "drug" and "pill" factors was observed. The "drug plus pill" combination produced facilitation. The investigators conclude that caffeine served as an "active placebo" with which "enhanced suggestive power" was effective, while the normal inert placebo was not.

Goldstein, Kaiser, and Whitby (1969) made a survey showing that heavy and light coffee drinkers differed in a number of significant ways. Caffeine's predominant effects on those who were nondrinkers were to cause upset stomach and a feeling of anxiety and jitteriness, without any stimulation of alertness or sense of well-being. In contrast, the habitual drinkers displayed no anxiety or jitteriness in response to caffeine; quite the contrary, jitteriness was noted on placebo administration and was relieved by caffeine. The habitual drinkers also reacted positively with feelings of improved alertness, awakeness, and well-being. All the effects observed were dose-related.

The findings related to morning coffee are of particular interest since morning coffee has a special place in the habits of most people. Those who drank coffee regularly at breakfast and again after breakfast did so because they were convinced it helped wake them and made them more efficient for the day's tasks. For the heaviest drinkers, caffeine played the role of a drug required to ward off a mild abstinence syndrome consisting of anxiety, dysphoria, feeling of sluggishness, and (sometimes) headache. In greater or lesser degree, most people who drink coffee in the morning take advantage of the mood-elevating effect of caffeine at this time of day, even though they may drink little coffee later and none at all in the evening. Those who are sensitive to caffeine, it seems, take advantage of the wakening effect in the morning, but for the same reason shun coffee at night; while the insensitive can drink in the morning and throughout the day without disturbing their sleep. Generally those drinking coffee habitually tended to be less sensitive to its effects than light users. This could be taken to indicate the development of tolerance, but it is also possible that such nonreactors drink more coffee because they are intrinsically less sensitive to all stimulants. (Goldstein et al 1965a)

Caffeine Addiction—A Question of Semantics

Drug dependence, typically encompassing psychologic craving, a tendency toward increasing dose, the phenomenon of acquired tolerance, and physical dependence accompanied by an abstinence syndrome upon abrupt withdrawal, has always been most clearly represented by addiction to opiates and other narcotics. Indeed, it has been only relatively recent that pharmacologists have become aware that many drugs and substances other than opiates may have some or all of the characteristics mentioned above as characterizing addiction.

Caffeine withdrawal symptoms are relatively mild and variable, however. They are characterized by irritability, inability to concentrate, nervousness, lethargy, and, in some people, by a characteristic headache. We have referred to the survey by Goldstein and Kaiser (1969) in which the heavy coffee drinkers described these typical dysphoric symptoms.

When heavy users abstained from morning coffee (ie, were given decaffeinated coffee in a blind experiment), in some cases they developed a characteristic headache that could be relieved promptly by taking about 150 mg of caffeine.

Therapeutic Uses

Caffeine, theophylline particularly, and to a lesser extent theobromine, do, however, have several important medical indications supported by extensive clinical experience. Theophylline is an active ingredient in aminophylline, used in the treatment of asthma, both cardiac and bronchial. Caffeine is a constituent of headache remedies (such as APC—aspirin, phenacetin, and caffeine) and of mild stimulants (caffeine sodium benzoate). In many instances their value in conditions for which they have been traditionally recommended has stood up very well in the light of current research.

References

Axelrod J, Reichenthal J: The fate of caffeine in man and a method for its estimation in biological material. J Pharmacol Exp Ther 107:519–523, 1953

Burg A: Effects of caffeine on the human system. Tea Coffee Trade J 40:40–43, 1974

Gibbs F, Maltby G: Effect on the electrical activity of the cortex of certain depressant and stimulant drugs—barbiturates, morphine, caffeine, benzedrine, and adrenaline. J Pharmacol Exp Ther 78:1–10, 1943

Goldstein A, Warren R, Kaiser S: Psychotropic effects of caffeine in man. Part 1: Individual differences in sensitivity to caffeine-induced wakefulness. J Pharmacol Exp Ther 49:156–159, 1965a

———, Warren R, Kaiser S: Psychotropic effects of caffeine in man. Part II: Alertness, psychomotor coordination and mood. J Pharmacol Exp Ther 150:146–151, 1965b

———, Kaiser S: Psychotropic effects of caffeine in man. Part III. A questionnaire survey of coffee drinking and its effects in a group of housewives. Clin Pharmacol Ther 10:477–487, 1969

———, Kaiser S, Whitby O: Psychotropic effects of caffeine in man: Part IV: Quantitative and qualitative differences associated with habituation to caffeine. Clin Pharmacol Ther 10:489–497, 1969

Goodfellow LD: Significant incidental factors in the measurement of auditory sensitivity. J Gen Psychol 35:31–41, 1946

Hall MJ, Bartashuk LM: PTC taste blindness and the taste of caffeine. Nature 253:442–43, 1975

Hollingworth H: The influence of caffeine on mental and motor efficiency. Arch Psychol 20:1–166, 1912

Kihlman BA: Effects of caffeine on the genetic material. Mutat Res 26:53–71, 1974

Klein RH, Salzman LF: Paradoxical effects of caffeine. Percept Mot Skills 40:126, 1975

Mitchell VE, Ross S: Drugs and placebos: effect of caffeine on cognitive performance. Psychiatr Rep 35:875–883, 1974

Robison GA, Butcher RW, Sutherland EW: Cyclic AMP. New York, Academic, 1971

Sulc J, Broyek G: Neurophysiological effects of small doses of caffeine in man. Act Nerv 16:217, 1974

Weiss B, Laties VG: Enhancement of human performance by caffeine and the amphetamines. Pharmacol Rev 14:1–36, 1962

amphetamine and cocaine
commentary

The stimulant drugs, particularly the amphetamines, their molecular relatives, and cocaine, which is pharmacologically related, are quite effective in relieving fatigue, reducing appetite, improving mood, and maintaining wakefulness. Unfortunately for their medical usefulness, tolerance gradually develops, and there is a significant abuse potential, probably related to their euphoric subjective effects. Amphetamines have specific use in the treatment of narcolepsy and hyperactivity in children. Although amphetamines continue to be used for their anorectic properties in short-term starter diet regimes, other less euphorigenic anorectics are available. In chronic high doses, the stimulants produce psychotic states resembling normally occurring paranoid psychoses. Since these stimulants are potent dopamine agonists, they have reinforced the theory that psychoses such as schizophrenia may be related to an overactivity of dopamine. The fact that antipsychotic drugs also block dopamine effects and antagonize amphetamine and cocaine is consistent with the dopamine theory of psychosis. Dr. Ellinwood discusses some of the animal studies with these agents and the possible animal models of human psychosis. Acute and chronic toxicity of stimulant drugs is described. "Speed kills" by inducing hyperthermia, hypertension, and convulsions. Appropriate treatments are indicated.

amphetamine
and
cocaine

Everett H. Ellinwood, Jr., M.D.

Illegal or excessive use (abuse) of stimulant drugs, such as amphetamine or cocaine, is important because of the societal problems produced and also as a source of data for major theoretical positions in psychopharmacology. Acute and chronic stimulant intoxication in animals and humans provides a model for naturally occurring psychosis. Also, amphetamine self-administration permits the study of dependence upon and behavioral reinforcement by drugs without a major physiologic-dependence effect.

Patterns of Abuse of Amphetamine and Cocaine

There are at least two patterns of chronic abuse of amphetamine, the oral and the intravenous. With oral administration, as tolerance develops the individual gradually increases his dose of amphetamine, often over a period of weeks or months. Sedatives and alcohol are frequently used for sleep at night. The intravenous pattern is characterized by injection of large doses (up to 1500 mg daily) fairly frequently, over a period of 4 to 6 days, during which there is little or no sleep. Finally, the user stops from exhaustion, sleeps for 24 to 48 hours, awakens and starts the cycle again, often reaching successively higher doses with each cycle (Kramer 1969).

Oral amphetamine abusers are recruited mainly from the ranks of women who stay at home and are prescribed amphetamines for weight reduction, businessmen and professionals using them for antifatigue, activity sustaining, and weight reduction effects, students attempting to cram for exams, and truck drivers wanting to remain alert for a 1- to 2-day period of long-distance hauling. A considerable number of individuals are initially attracted to the recreational use of amphetamine for their euphoric properties.

The intravenous abusers of stimulant drugs are usually recruited from within the drug-using subculture. Whereas the oral use of amphetamine produces a sustained sense of euphoria associated with an energizing effect, the intravenous use of amphetamine or cocaine additionally produces the much desired "flash," an immediate ecstasy, at times compared to an orgasmic experience. This intensely euphoric feeling is sometimes described as an electrical shock running from the head, to the abdomen, to the groin; at other times, it is described as an expanding, flashing, buzzing, vibrating feeling.

Nasal insufflation (snorting, sniffing) is used with both cocaine and amphetamine, providing a less intense acute onset. This is the most widely practiced mode of cocaine administration, since cocaine is rapidly destroyed in the stomach. Rapid liver metabolism is also responsible for the relatively short duration of cocaine action. Currently cocaine enjoys a widespread reputation in both the drug subcultures and the general population as the cadillac or champagne of recreational drugs and as a potent aphrodisiac.

Stimulant Psychosis

The chronic use of several stimulants, eg, D- and L-amphetamine, methylphenidate, phenmetrazine, and cocaine, often appears to result in psychosis. However, more extensive descriptions have been made for amphetamine psychosis than for other stimulant psychoses. Thus, this section will focus on amphetamine psychoses; differences between various stimulant psychoses, if they exist, have not been documented. Clinical details of the cocaine psychosis have not been reported since the early 1900s (Maier 1926). Although one could expect differences between the syndromes secondary to the strong local anesthetic effect of cocaine, the similarities are more evident.

Amphetamine psychosis mimics paranoid schizophrenia so closely that many times it has been diagnosed as such by knowledgeable clinicians. Usually the amphetamine psychosis develops after the user increases his intake to more than 150 mg; at times up to 600 to 3000 mg per day.

Although there appear to be individual thresholds of sensitivity to the development of amphetamine psychosis, when it develops it is a fairly distinct syndrome, with delusions of persecution; ideas of reference; visual, auditory, and olfactory hallucinations; changes in body image; hyperactivity; and excitation (Ellinwood 1972). However, like syphilis, the amphetamine syndrome presents many forms, including hypomaniclike reactions. The absence of disorientation, the more developed and not infrequently fixed delusions, and the appearance of repetitious, compulsive behaviors are usually sufficient to distinguish the amphetamine psychosis from toxic psychosis. However, toxic hallucinatory psychosis also occurs with acute high-dose amphetamine intoxication.

Prominent primary delusional experiences are characteristic of amphetamine psychosis and, in part, are responsible for the great similarity between it and paranoid schizophrenia. In their purest form primary delusions appear suddenly as a "eurekalike solution or conviction," quite developed, and have an intense feeling of reality attached to them. These primary delusional experiences with further cognitive elaboration can lead to systematization of delusions. In the later stages one notes marked lability of affect, which is often oriented around these paranoid delusions; the amphetamine abuser is frequently seen by the physician in a hyperactive paranoid panic.

Behaviors Antecedent to the Psychosis

Prior to the primary delusion stage, amphetamine abusers describe and display behavior associated with an intense feeling of curiosity and meaningfulness, often manifested by repetitious, stereotyped cleaning, examining, searching, and sorting behaviors which often involve minute objects. A pleasurable stage of "suspiciousness" often occurs.

Experimental animals, chronically intoxicated with amphetamine, manifest evolving clusters of behavior comparable to those noted in humans, even though the important thinking and feeling components are more difficult to measure. Stereotyped movements are the hallmark of both acute and chronic amphetamine intoxication in animals. For example, in primates (monkeys, apes, and man) dermatologic excoriations may result from these repetitious grooming patterns (picking, probing). In man such behavior may evolve into delusions of parasitosis (eg, cocaine bugs). Over the latter period of chronic intoxication, one notes the investigatory attitude being replaced by an increasing hyperreactive attitude, most often consisting of sudden orienting or startle responses toward both real as well as "hallucinated" stimuli.

Neural Substrates of Amphetamine-Induced Behavior

There are considerable data (Randrup and Munkvad 1968, Wallach 1974) indicating that neural transmitters sustaining the amphetamine-induced behavioral response, at least in the acute stages of intoxication, are primarily dopamine and secondarily norepinephrine.

Amphetamine and cocaine not only block reuptake of but also release catecholamines from central dopamine and norepinephrine neurons (see Fig. 2, p 232). According to Scheel-Kruger (1972), both actions theoretically lead to an increase in the availability of neurotransmitters at the receptor. Blockade of reuptake has been overemphasized as a sole mechanism of action of cocaine and amphetamine. Since tricyclic antidepressants block noradrenergic neuron reuptake of norepinephrine (Carlsson et al 1969, Schildkraut et al 1967), anticholinergic compounds, ie, benztropine, block dopamine neuron reuptake (Farnebo et al 1970), and neither group of drugs is subject to chronic abuse liability nor produces the stimulant behavioral syndrome in laboratory animals, then the reuptake mechanism does not appear to be importantly involved in the stimulant abuse syndrome.

Increased motor activity and stereotyped behaviors induced in experimental animals are not dependent on stored catecholamines, since reserpine, which depletes stored norepinephrine and dopamine, does not block the effect of amphetamine on these behaviors. The action of amphetamine depends primarily on the release of newly synthesized catecholamines. Amphetamine does not have a major direct receptor stimulating action, since alpha-methylparatyrosine, which blocks the synthesis of both norepinephrine and dopamine, blocks amphetamine-induced behaviors (Randrup and Munkvad 1968, Weissman et al 1965). In contrast, cocaine as well as methylphenidate is antagonized by high doses of reserpine and is relatively uninfluenced by alpha-methylparatyrosine (Scheel-Kruger et al 1976).

Amphetamine-induced hypermotility in rats probably depends on norepinephrine (perhaps also with a permissive role for dopamine), since decreasing newly synthesized norepinephrine by blocking dopamine beta-hydroxylase (the enzyme converting dopamine to norepinephrine) blocks the amphetamine-induced hypermotility but not the stereotyped behavior; in fact, this behavior is often found to be prolonged (Scheel-Kruger and Randrup 1967). This evidence, in addition to the observation that dopamine receptor blocking agents, such as the phenothiazines, also inhibit stereotypy (Wallach 1974) indicates that dopamine plays a major role in the induction of

stereotypy. The most potent antipsychotic neuroleptics are also potent dopamine receptor blockers—a point that has strengthened the
analogy of amphetamine-induced stereotyped behavior in animals
to amphetamine psychotic symptoms, as well as to functional
psychoses in humans.

End-Stage Behaviors

Stereotypy is the main feature of the initial and intermediate stages
of chronic amphetamine intoxication in experimental animals (rats,
cats, and monkeys), but at the end-stage this component is part of a
much more complex behavioral expression (Ellinwood 1973). Possible analogies of these animal postural motor disorders are the dystonic and cataleptic reactions sometimes recorded with chronic amphetamine intoxication in humans (Tetetsu 1963, Kramer 1967). The
hyperstartle reactivity in animals may be analogous to the reactive
paranoid panic in human amphetamine psychosis.

Behavioral Fixations

The stimulant psychosis in humans cannot be explained entirely in
pharmacologic terms. The thought disorders sometimes persist during abstinence. There is also an increased potential for psychotic
reactions in abstinent individuals, not only by subsequent exposure
to amphetamine (often even smaller doses) (Kramer 1969), but also
by psychologic and physical arousal from stress (Utena 1974). Animal studies demonstrate analogous phenomena. Intravenous amphetamine abusers report that the injection process itself becomes
secondarily reinforcing, since they can obtain a moderate rein-
troduction of the "high" by injecting water or reinjecting blood. The
phenomenon is called "booting" and the individual a "needle freak"
in the speed subculture. Thus learning or conditioning mechanisms
must be invoked in explaining these phenomena (Ellinwood 1973).

Tolerance /Withdrawal Effects

Most of the original research indicated that chronic moderate doses
of amphetamine did not produce tolerance for the behavioral (central) effects in either man or animal (Rosenberg et al 1963, Kosman
and Unna 1968). Some recent evidence demonstrates that it is important to consider the animal species as well as the type of behavior
recorded. When a rat is administered amphetamine over days, the
gross body movements and exploratory behaviors decrease over
days with a concomitant increase in stereotyped behaviors (Segal

and Mandell 1974). Furthermore, cocaine apparently increases the
behavioral responsivity towards stereotyped behavior even more so
than amphetamines, and indeed this increased sensitivity has been
reported to persist for at least 10 days by the early studies of Tatum
and Seevers (1929) and more recently documented to persist for
weeks or more (Kilbey and Ellinwood 1976). There is also an associated drug-induced enhancement of electrical activity in the
mesolimbic forebrain which also persists for several weeks (Stripling and Ellinwood 1976).

Two effects of amphetamine, to which users develop marked tolerance, are the anorectic and the hyperthermic response. Tolerance
to the anoretic effect is clinically important when one considers the
number of extended amphetamine prescriptions for appetite suppression that were written in previous times. Most amphetamine
overdose-induced hyperthermic deaths are reported in nontolerant
individuals. There is a marked tolerance to the lethal effects of
high-dose amphetamine and probably to high-dose cocaine. The
LD$_{50}$ for daily injections of amphetamine over a period of weeks has
been noted to increase at least threefold in monkeys (Ellinwood
1971). Since propranolol significantly reduces the lethality from
amphetamine, there is good reason to suspect that at least one aspect
of the toxicity and secondary tolerance may result from beta-
adrenergic mechanisms operating peripherally.

Cocaine lethality tolerance is more complicated since cocaine is
both a local anesthetic and a stimulant. The local anesthetic seizure-
inducing effect develops little or no tolerance. In fact, Downs and
Eddy (1932) found a reverse tolerance (sensitization) for seizures
from cocaine administered on a daily basis, this effect persists weeks
after the termination of cocaine administration (Stripling and Ellinwood 1976).

The withdrawal response following chronic use of stimulants has
a more protracted, less well-defined pattern without the overwhelming dysphoria, autonomic, and somatic response noted with narcotics. The initial withdrawal is often characterized by exhaustion and
sleep. The ensuing withdrawal shows a rather prolonged period of
lassitude, fatigue, and depression. The increased sleep noted in
withdrawal has an increased percentage of rapid eye movement
(REM) sleep.

Abuse Potential of Stimulants

Clinical case reports and animal laboratory studies indicate that
there is a marked abuse potential with amphetaminelike stimulants.

Rats (Pickens 1968), monkeys (Balster and Schuster 1973, Deneau et al 1964), and cats (Balster et al 1975) will initiate and maintain intravenous self-administration of amphetamine and cocaine just as they do with opioids. In the self-administering animal the response patterns, pharmacologic response, and toxicity of stimulants are similar to those seen in humans who abuse stimulants. In humans the latency from the first stimulant experience to an overwhelming abuse cycle can be a very short period, frequently only 2 to 8 months following intravenous use. The original European example of cocaine abuse, Freud's friend Fleischl, occurred the same year that Freud obtained his first supply of cocaine. During the next year, cases of cocaine intoxication were being extensively reported. Several epidemics of stimulant abuse have arisen within a period of 2 to 3 years.

Amphetamine abusers report that intravenous high-dose use is the most addicting and that it produces an intense orgasmic experience unlike oral administration or "snorting." Rapid escalation of dosage often occurs. Regular administration of oral therapeutic doses of amphetamine over a period of 6 weeks or less probably does not have an overwhelming abuse potential, since literally millions of prescriptions have been written for this regime in weight reduction programs. Many amphetamine abusers indicate that they either were prescribed amphetamines for longer periods of time or subsequently sought out additional prescriptions of the drug and used higher doses.

As with opioids, stimulants demonstrate some capacity for a resolute grip on the individual after prolonged periods of abstinence. Occasionally amphetamine abuse may continue for 10 to 15 years or more; however there is a tendency for the amphetamine abuser, unlike the heroin addict, to "burn out" within 2 to 3 years or, alternately, to experience a psychosis or other difficulties and stop the drug habit.

Management of Acute Medical Complications

There are no case reports in the English literature of acute fatal cocaine overdoses in drug abusers who survive long enough to require treatment. Presumably this reflects the rapid, more lethal, local anesthetic effects of cocaine. Death due to overdose of local anesthetics, including cocaine, is usually a relatively acute effect after injection or after absorption from local application and is due most often to a respiratory arrest and, possibly at times, a cardiac arrest. Although it is rare that the clinician will see this type of acute toxicity from drug-abuse patients, occasionally acute toxic effects are noted with cocaine used as a local anesthetic in large doses when it is absorbed rapidly from the local site. Under these circumstances artificial respiration and cardiac massage can be lifesaving (Orr and Jones 1968, Ritchie et al 1970).

Work with experimental animals demonstrates that cocaine-induced seizures can be effectively treated with benzodiazepines, such as diazepam. After seizures are under control, the toxic effect secondary to adrenergic mechanisms should be easily managed by propanolol, since cocaine is rapidly metabolized.

The toxic fatal or subfatal syndromes with amphetamine overdose are occasionally seen in chronic, high-dose (300 to 1500 mg) intravenous users but infrequently because of the rapid tolerance developed to peripheral adrenergic mechanisms. Most of the reported fatal cases of amphetamine intoxication have been in relatively recent or neophyte users of amphetamine or with accidental intoxication. Death from overdose of amphetamines is usually associated with hyperthermia and indeed death often ends with hyperpyrexia, cardiovascular shock, and convulsions. Thus the environmental temperature and physical exertion may greatly potentiate the adverse amphetamine reaction. Stimulants not only affect the temperature-regulating mechanism in the hypothalamus but also by the nature of the stimulated motor activity and vessel constriction tend to conserve heat; heat strokes are often the initial symptom complex. Thus it is not rare for adverse effects among bicycle riders or other athletes, who have taken amphetamines in only moderately large doses, to occur on a hot day.

The signs and symptoms of the sublethal dose include dizziness, tremor, irritability, confusion, perhaps hostility and assaultiveness, auditory and visual hallucinations, panic states, skin flushing, chest pain, palpitation, cardiac arrythmias, hypertension, vomiting, abdominal cramps, and excessive sweating. With life-threatening toxic doses the above symptoms are noted as well as hyperpyrexia, hypertension, convulsions, systemic acidosis, and finally cardiovascular collapse and death. Other complications are encountered, including cerebral vascular occlusions and infarctions. By far the most life-threatening aspect is the hyperthermia and convulsions that precede cardiovascular collapse. The patient should be carefully monitored for these two complications, as soon as amphetamine intoxication is suspected, and removed to a hospital, if possible. A temperature rise above 102F (especially if there has been a rapid rise) should be treated vigorously and before the accelerated rise to the fatal level. If the temperature is not controlled by submersion in cool water, then it should be aggressively treated with full-body ice pack or hypothermic blanket, and judicious use of chlorpromazine to control shivering. Convulsions are most often associated with the hyperthermic condition. (In this case we are not discussing the convulsions secondary to the local anesthetic effect of cocaine.) Convulsions may culminate in status epilepticus. Intravenous administration of diazepam at a rate of 5 to 20 mg per minute can be given for the initial dose, repeated at intervals of 15 to 20 minutes, depending upon respiratory depression and hypotension. Certainly at this point one should have the capacity for intubation to control respiratory obstruction.

Treatment of sublethal doses of amphetamine can begin with general measures. If the patient has ingested a large oral dose of amphetamine, then gastric lavage or induction of vomiting is indicated, because there is often a delayed gastric emptying time. Excretion of amphetamines can also be enhanced by acidifying the urine with ammonium chloride. Judicious use of chlorpromazine (25 to 50 mg, intramuscularly) can have a remarkable calming effect on these individuals. Of course one needs to be aware of the possible anticholinergic contaminants in street stimulants and thus the possibility that an anticholinergic crisis induced by chlorpromazine is treatable with physostigmine. Chlorpromazine is recommended because of its blocking effect on norepinephrine as well as on dopamine, and indeed one wants to reduce cautiously the overwhelming peripheral adrenergic effects of amphetamine. In treating only the psychotic manifestations of amphetamine intoxication, haloperidol is probably the drug of choice, since it has a much more specific effect (dopamine) and does not retard the degradation of amphetamine as does chlorpromazine (Davis 1970). Alternatively, propranolol can be used to treat the peripheral adrenergic effects.

Other complications of amphetamine intoxication include effects secondary to hypertension, including subdural and subarachnoid hemorrhage (Gericke 1945). In some cases subarachnoid hemorrhage is from predisposing aneurysms and arteriovenous malformations (Goodman and Becker 1970, Kalant 1966, Kane et al 1969). Intracerebral hematoma formation (Weiss et al 1970) as well as cerebral vascular thrombosis have also been reported (Kane et al 1969). Multiple microhemorrhages have also been reported in cases coming to autopsy.

Amphetamine abusers also suffer from all medical complications of nonsterile, intravenous use of drugs in an unknown quantity similar to intravenous narcotic users. These conditions include hepatitis, pneumonia, embolic pneumonia, lung abscess, endocarditis, tetanus, syphilis, and generalized septicemia. Necrotizing angitis (Citron et al 1970) as well as beading and constriction of central nervous system arterioles (Rumbaugh et al 1971) has been reported in amphetamine users. Experimental animals chronically intoxicated with high doses of amphetamine have microhemorrhages; also, brain stem neuronal chromatalysis is noted, which would be expected in severe chronic exhaustive states.

Management of the Amphetamine Psychosis

The amphetamine psychosis frequently presents as an agitated or panic state, in the hospital emergency room. Cocaine psychosis is a rare occurrence at present, due to the overwhelming cost of maintaining a habit sufficient to develop psychosis; therefore this section will deal primarily with amphetamine psychosis. The diagnosis can usually be made from clinical examination and by history and confirmed by urinanalysis for drugs. Within 24 to 48 hours, most of the visual hallucinations have abated, and one notes that the delusional content decreases remarkably over the next week to 10 days. Delusions do continue, however, and occasionally more fixed delusions may still persist over a year after the last dose. Usually within 24 hours after the last dose the patient begins to spend increasing amounts of time sleeping and may sleep as much as 18 to 20 hours a day over the next 72 hours. The condition frequently resembles narcolepsy, with the patient half awake and half dreaming. In this state he can become confused and sometimes needs reassurance; frequently these dreaming stages are interpreted by clinicians as psychoses. Prior to the sleep stage the patient may be irritable and depressed. Depression can continue and indeed gather intensity up to 2 weeks after the intoxication, and without treatment can last over a more extended period. Suicidal ideation occasionally occurs. The depressive affect usually has a much greater component of neurasthenia than is usually noted in depression; the patients complain of fatigue and they appear emotionally flat and apathetic.

In the acute psychotic phase it is important to keep the patient relatively quiet and reassured. Most often the patient does not require antipsychotic drugs after the first 24 hours of admission. Patients are frequently aggressive and assaultive during this stage, especially if they reach the state of panic, and thus it is best to hospitalize amphetamine abusers even in the withdrawal stage. As the agitated state is replaced by depression, this can be treated with tricyclic antidepressants; in fact, antidepressant medication often aids in avoiding the period of 3 to 4 weeks of chronic apathy and fatigue combined with depression. During the first 2 weeks of withdrawal, it is important to set the stage for subsequent treatment of underlying personality problems and disabilities. Establishment of strong therapeutic relationship during this phase can often carry over the rough spots during the ensuing months. It is wise to explain to the patient that the expected depression, apathy, and lack of initiative will tend to wax and wane over the next 2 or 3 months and that these symptoms have a direct relationship to the previous extensive drug use and not just to situational or intrapsychic processes.

References

Balster RL, Kilbey MM, Ellinwood EH: Methamphetamine self-administration in the cat. Psychopharmacologia (Berl.) 46:229, 1976

———, Schuster CR: A comparison of D-amphetamine, L-amphetamine, and methamphetamine self-administration in rhesus monkeys. Pharmacol Biochem Behav 1:67, 1973

Carlsson A, Corrodi H, Fuxe I, Hofkelt T: Effects of some antidepressant drugs on the depletion of intraneural brain catecholamine stores caused by 4, α-dimethyl-meta-tryamine. Eur J Pharm 5:367, 1969

Citron BP, Halpern M, McCarron M, et al: Necrotizing angitis associated with drug abuse. N Engl J Med 283:1003, 1970

Davis J: The effects of haloperidol, chlorpromazine, amphetamine metabolism and amphetamine stereotyped behavior in the rat. J Pharmacol Exp Ther 175:428, 1970

Deneau GA, Yanagita T, Seevers MH: Psychogenic dependence to a variety of drugs in the monkey. Pharmacologia 6:183, 1964

Downs AW, Eddy NB: The effect of repeated doses of cocaine on the rat. J Pharmacol Exp Ther 46:199,1932

Ellinwood EH: Effect of chronic methamphetamine intoxication in rhesus monkeys. Biol Psychiatry 3:25, 1971

———: Amphetamine and stimulant drugs. In Drug Use in America (Second Report of the Natural Commission on Marihuana and Drug Abuse). Washington DC, US Govt Printing Office, 1973, pp 140–157

———, Sudilovsky A: Chronic amphetamine intoxication: behavioral model of psychoses. In Cole JO, Freedman AM, Friedhoff AJ (eds): Psychopathology and Psychopharmacology. Baltimore, Johns Hopkins, 1973, p 51

Farnebo LO, Fuxe K, Hamberger B, Ljungdahl H: Effect of some antiparkinsonian drugs on catecholamine neurons. J Pharm Pharmacol 22:737, 1970

Gericke OL: Suicide by ingestion of amphetamine sulfate. JAMA 128:1098, 1945

Goodman SJ, Becker DP: Intracranial hemmorrhage associated with amphetamine abuse. JAMA 212:480, 1970

Kalant OJ: The Amphetamines, Toxicity and Addiction. Springfield, Ill, Thomas, 1966

Kane EFJ, Keeler MF, Reifler CB: Neurological crises following metamphetamine. JAMA 210:556, 1969

Kilbey MM, Ellinwood EH Jr.: Chronic administration of stimulant drugs: Tolerance and response potentiation. In Ellinwood EH, Kilbey MM (eds): Cocaine and Other Stimulants. New York, Plenum Press, 1976

Kosman ME, Unna KR: Effects of chronic administration of the amphetamines and other stimulants on behavior. Clin Pharmacol Ther 9:240, 1968

Kramer JC: Introduction to amphetamine abuse. J Psyched Drugs 2:1, 1969

————, Fischman US, Littlefield DC: Amphetamine abuse—patterns and effects of high doses taken intravenously. JAMA 201:305, 1967

Maier HW: Der Kokainismus. Liepzig, Verlag, 1926, p 108

Orr D, Jones I: Cardiovascular effects of cocaine and lignocaine. Anesthesia 23:194, 1968

Pickens R: Self-administration of stimulants by rats. Int J Addic 3:215, 1968

Randrup A, Munkvad I: Behavioral stereotypies induced by pharmacological agents. Pharmakopsychiatrie and Neuropsychopharmacologia 1:18, 1968

Ritchie JM, Cohen PJ, Dripps RD: Cocaine, procaine and other synthetic local anesthetics. In Goodman LS, Gillman A (eds): The Pharmacological Basis of Therapeutics. New York, Macmillan, 1970, p 371

Rosenberg DE, Wolbach AB, Miner EJ, Isbell H: Observations of direct and cross tolerance with LSD and D-amphetamine in man. Psychopharmacologia 5:1, 1963

Rumbaugh CL, Bergeron T, Fang F, McCormick R: Cerebral angiographic changes in the drug abuse patient. Radiology 101:335, 1971

Scheel-Kruger J, Randrup A: Stereotype hyperactive behavior produced in the absence of noradrenaline. Life Sci 6:1389, 1967

————: Behavioural and biochemical comparison of amphetamine derivatives, cocaine, benzotropine and tricyclic anti-depressant drugs. Eur J Pharmacol 18:63, 1972

————, Braestrup C, Nielson M, Golembiowska K, Mogilnicka E: Cocaine: Discussion on the role of dopamine in the biochemical mechanism of action. In Ellinwood EH, Kilby MM (eds): Cocaine and Other Stimulants. New York, Plenum Press, 1976.

Schildkraut JJ, Schanberg SM, Breese GR, Kopin IJ: Norepinephrine metabolism and drugs used in the affective disorders: a possible mechanism of action. Am J Psychiatry 124:600, 1967

Segal DS, Mandell AJ: Long-term administration of D-amphetamine: Progressive augmentation of motor activity and stereotypy. Pharmacol Biochem Behav 2:249, 1974

Stripling JS, Ellinwood EH Jr.: Sensitization to cocaine following chronic administration in the rat. In Ellinwood EH, Kilbey MM (eds.): Cocaine and Other Stimulants. New York, Plenum Press, 1976

Tatum AL, Seevers MH: Experimental cocaine addiction. J Pharmacol Exp Ther 36:401, 1929

Tetetsu S: Methamphetamine psychosis. Folia Psychiat Neurol Jap 7:(Suppl)377, 1963

Utena H: On relapse-liability; schizophrenia, amphetamine psychoses and animal model. In Mitsuda H, Fukuda I (eds): Biological Mechanisms of Schizophernia and Schizophrenia-Like Psychosis. Tokyo, Igaku Shorn, 1974, p 285

Wallach MB: Drug-induced stereotyped behavior: similarities and differences. In Usdin E (ed): Neuropsychopharmacology of Monoamines and Their Regulatory Enzymes. New York, Raven, 1974, p 241

Weiss SR, Raskind R, Morganstern N, Pytlyk P, Paiz T: Intercerebral subarachnoid hemorrhage following use of metamphetamine. Int Surg 53:123, 1970

Weissman A, Koe BK, Tenen SS: Antiamphetamine effects following inhibition of tyrosine hydroxylase. J Pharmacol Exp Ther 151:339, 1965

nicotine
and
tobacco

commentary

Tobacco has been used in Western civilization for nearly 500 years. Although it is not officially recognized as a drug, it functions like one in every way. Hundreds of millions of people have become addicted to tobacco, or at the very least, have developed very strong smoking habits. The health hazards of smoking have been investigated and widely publicized only during the last decade and more information is being gathered daily. We know much less about the desirable effects of smoking or indeed why people smoke at all. Circumstantial evidence for the central role of nicotine is strong, but much more research is needed. Curing the smoking habit is as difficult as treating alcoholism or heroin addiction. The fact that 25 percent of physicians continue to smoke, in the face of evidence of danger, shows how difficult it will be to convince their patients to stop. The following chapter examines possible reasons why people smoke, what smoking does, and why and how some people stop smoking.

nicotine
and
tobacco

Murray E. Jarvik, M.D., Ph.D.
Ellen R. Gritz, Ph.D.

Columbus introduced the American Indian habit of tobacco use to Europeans in 1492. Since then it has played a prominent role in Western civilization (Wagner 1971). In 1604 shortly after assuming the British throne from his aunt Queen Elizabeth, James I published his *Counterblaste to Tobacco*, a treatise attacking the custom of tobacco smoking and warning of its health hazards. Ironically if one takes a trip down the James River to Jamestown, Virginia today, one sees immense plantations of tobacco along its banks. The credit for establishing the tobacco industry, America's oldest, belongs to John Rolfe, who developed the first successful tobacco plantation in Virginia around 1612. By 1652 tobacco production in England was prohibited in order to help agriculture in the infant American colony. Sporadic and often Draconian attempts to suppress tobacco use in various countries always failed, illustrating the tenacity of the habit. Tobacco is one of the major industries in the United States and one of the more important exports that maintain the balance of payments.

In most developed countries almost half of the men and one-quarter of the women smoke cigarettes, but the proportion of women smoking is rising everywhere. This is clearly illustrated in studies of the prevalence of teen-age smoking, where the percentage of teen-age boys who smoke has remained essentially constant over the years 1968 through 1974, while the percentage of teen-age girls smoking has risen progressively and approaches the prevalence in males (DHEW publication NIH 76-931). Despite vigorous attempts by various public and private health agencies to discourage smoking, there is actually an increase in smoking in the younger portion of the population.

It is clear that the initiation of smoking is dependent upon social factors, such as peer pressure, parental example, advertising, and the growth of the women's liberation movement. In fact, in certain primitive societies smoking is eagerly adopted by almost all adults, except where it is forbidden by religion (Damon 1973). The prevalence of smoking in every country in the world strongly suggests that there is a physiologic substrate for reinforcement of tobacco use. Genetic factors apparently play a role in the tendency to smoke (Kety 1972) just as they have in alcoholism and possibly other drug addictions (Goodwin et al 1976). Since such a large proportion of mankind smokes, it would be important to identify the determinants of smoking.

Why Do People Smoke?

There are many purely psychologic theories of smoking (surveyed in Jarvik 1970). Freud, who fought a lifelong losing battle with cigar smoking, compared it to thumb sucking. He considered smoking an autoerotic manifestation of deprivation of breast sucking, to be equated with masturbation (Menninger 1975). This is an example of a psychologic theory that does not even consider pharmacologic factors; it is assumed that people smoke because of some interaction between personality and experience. Others have stressed the role of social reinforcement (Larson and Silvette 1971). The personality of smokers appears to differ from that of nonsmokers. There is evidence that smokers on the average are more extroverted, antisocial, externally oriented, impulsive, oral, and mentally deviant than nonsmokers, although more information is needed on these hypotheses (Smith 1970).

Even though these personality traits have been associated with smokers, they do not provide a satisfactory explanation of why people smoke. Our hypothesis and that of a number of other investigators is that nicotine is the primary reinforcing agent in tobacco, and that smoking is a form of drug-seeking behagior most likely controlled by nicotine. Tobacco is used only in ways that result in a significant level of nicotine in the blood. Since nicotine is so efficiently detoxified by the liver, tobacco is never swallowed as are barbiturates, alcohol, amphetamines and even opium. However, studies of the levels of nicotine in blood after oral administration in humans have not yet been conducted. Animal studies indicate that although a large proportion of nicotine is detoxified in the liver, some of it does reach the systemic circulation. Of course smoking, chewing, and nasal insufflation are commonly used methods of bypassing the hepatic circulation and provide circumstantial evidence that nicotine-seeking underlies tobacco use.

The evidence that smoking is drug-seeking behavior is not as firm as that found with other drug dependencies. If a subject (or animal) is dependent upon a drug, he will work to keep the blood level fairly constant. Attempts with animals or man to demonstrate this kind of titration behavior with nicotine have been only partially successful. Experimenters have varied the amount of nicotine the subject can obtain in a cigarette, or in some less natural form such as nicotine chewing gum, nicotine aerosols, nicotine tablets, or parenterally. Objective measures studied have included the number of cigarettes smoked, heart rate, catecholamines, nicotine and its metabolites excreted in the urine, and plasma nicotine levels. Ratings of satisfaction and strength of cigarettes, or well-being and desire to smoke when nicotine is otherwise administered, have been used as subjective measurements.

Until recently, inability to measure actual nicotine intake in humans has posed a methodologic problem. In addition to estimates of intake from nicotine-in-smoke figures provided by the FTC (1975) or chemical butt analysis, nicotine levels in humans can now be measured directly in blood plasma (Russell et al 1975, Langone et al 1973) and from the nicotine excreted in urine (Beckett et al 1971).

There appears to be quite a bit of evidence supporting the titration hypothesis from studies in which plasma nicotine levels were measured when subjects smoked cigarettes varying in nicotine content (Russell et al 1975); in which mecamylamine, a centrally acting nicotine antagonist, produced an increase in smoking (Stolerman et al 1973); and in which nicotine readministered either in gum or by cigarette reduced smoking by quantity and latency measures (Kozlowski et al 1975).

Some of the earlier studies usually cited in support of titration (Ashton and Watson 1970, Frith 1971) are flawed by methodologic problems in the manner of assessing nicotine intake, in confounding task difficulty variables with ease of puffing using different filters (so being unable to account for differences in inhalation or puffing style), and by inadequate statistical analysis.

Sometimes experimental cigarettes were so aversive as to mask any natural titration. Thus, lettuce cigarettes injected with nicotine were intensely disliked by subjects who did not vary the number smoked according to the amount of injected nicotine (Goldfarb et al 1970). Yet these subjects continued to smoke one-half to one pack of the lettuce cigarettes per day. Such persistence may be seen as a

demonstration of nicotine-seeking behavior, the "secondary reinforcement" or indirect pleasure derived from smoking per se, or else
an example of how long it takes to give up smoking when even a
little nicotine is supplied. Similarly, when cigarettes were cut in half
(Goldfarb and Jarvik 1972), subjects did not double the number
smoked but may have compensated for the shorter length by inhal-
ing more deeply or taking more than the normal number of puffs.

It is clear that it would be difficult to show that people regulate
their nicotine intake precisely. The large number of variables involved in smoking, the highly overlearned motor aspects of the
habit, plus all the social factors make the area very complex. But the
physiologic and carefully performed behavioral studies of smoking
titration do strongly suggest that people make some attempt, albeit
not a very precise one, to keep themselves "dosed" with nicotine.

Is Smoking an Addiction?

Even though Samuel Johnson used smoking as an example when he
defined addiction in his dictionary, there is considerable controversy as to whether it truly qualifies as an addiction. One would
have to demonstrate a pharmacologic agent sought by the smoker as
well as some type of abstinence syndrome on acute withdrawal of
the drug.

A wide variety of dysphoric changes occur in smoking abstinence,
many suggesting that the arousal level drops from that chronically
induced by nicotine. Anecdotal reports of withdrawal syndromes
appear frequently in the scientific and popular literature (USPHS
Report 1103, 1964, Brecher 1972, Larson and Silvette 1971). The
desire to smoke (craving) and abstinence symptomatology vary according to the time of day, and decrease with length of abstinence
(Gritz and Jarvik 1973, Shiffman and Jarvik, personal communication). It has been difficult to measure a definable, physiologic abstinence syndrome under controlled experimental conditions, but decreases in heart rate and blood pressure have been found (Knapp et
al 1963, Weybrew and Stark 1967). In addition, significant decreases
in adrenalin and noradrenalin levels, increased skin temperature,
and improved hand steadiness were observed over 5 days of nonsmoking (Myrsten et al 1974).

All of the above changes could be the result of a gradual readjust-
ment in arousal level rather than a classic abstinence syndrome
characterized by central nervou system hyperexcitability. Although
the American Psychiatric Association is probably going to include
compulsive tobacco use as a new diagnosis in the next edition of the

DSM III, it is not yet clear how it will be defined. Very likely any individual who feels his smoking is a problem and wants to be cured is a candidate for the diagnosis. Whether smokers who don't want to stop will be considered suffering from this disorder is still a debatable question.

The argument has been made, particularly by antismoking forces, that smoking is an insidious illness, while 50 years ago smoking was considered a sophisticated habit attacked only by puritans or religious fundamentalists. In the early stages the smoker is trapped by a habit he can break only with great difficulty. Today it is recognized that a variety of disabling and fatal illnesses (emphysema; Buerger's disease; coronary atherosclerosis; cancer of the lung, mouth, pharynx, larynx, esophagus, bladder or prostate; peptic ulcer; or cirrhosis of the liver) are associated with heavy smoking over a 30- to 40-year period.

Psychologic and Physiologic Effects of Smoking

Cigarette smoking produces a panoply of physiologic responses, most of which can be reproduced by the administration of nicotine. These include electroencephalographic effects characteristic of arousal though other complex actions may supervene (Ulett and Itil 1969).

Nicotine releases a variety of biogenic amines, both peripherally and centrally. Possibly the central release of catecholamines is responsible for the reinforcing effect (Hall and Turner 1972). The release of epinephrine from the adrenal medulla must be responsible in part for the noticeable sympathetic effects of smoking, including tachycardia, vasoconstriction and rise in blood pressure, rise in free fatty acids, and tremor. Excitation of respiration is a prominent effect and may be a direct action of nicotine on the medulla and peripheral chemoreceptors. Nausea and vomiting, so prominent in novice smokers, is due to stimulation of the chemoreceptor trigger zone in the medulla. Nicotine also causes an increase in gastrointestinal activity. The morning cigarette is used as a laxative by some heavy smokers.

Does Nicotine/Smoking Produce Stimulation or Sedation?

There have been a variety of psychoactive effects of nicotine, ranging from stimulant to tranquilizer, reported in the animal as well as human (Dunn 1973). This is not surprising since nicotine is a complex drug acting on central and peripheral nervous systems as well as directly on various organs, such as the heart. Most of the psychoactive effects relate to the arousal level of the organism. In examining various studies it is important to differentiate acute from chronic effects, and to consider the nature of the task that is being either facilitated or disrupted by nicotine. It thus becomes easier to relate experimental results to ordinary human smoking, which is a chronic behavior occurring in a variety of circumstances.

Some recent animal work sheds an interesting light on the brain mechanisms affected by nicotine. In a provocative study in rats, Nelson (1976) found that nicotine could antagonize the disrupting effect upon behavior of stimulating the reticular formation. Furthermore when rats first learning a task were injected with nicotine, their learning was impaired, but their postacquisition behavior was facilitated. The overall impression to be derived from these studies is that chronic nicotine administration facilitates motivated well-learned task performance, especially in an arousal-oriented vigilance task such as the one described above.

Researchers in smoking behavior (Tomkins 1966, Russell 1971, Myrsten et al 1975) have attempted to characterize the situations in which people choose to smoke, for example, those low on the arousal continuum (lying in bed) or high on the continuum (meeting a deadline on a project). Trying to distinguish smokers in such a manner is part of the previously mentioned extensive literature on the "smoking personality." We will concentrate here upon studies relevant to the question of raised or lowered arousal level and the need to smoke.

When subjects were selected by questionnaire for smoking exclusively in high arousal or exclusively in low arousal situations, it was possible to show impaired or facilitated performance on difficult-to-easy vigilance tasks. Performance on a sensorimotor task was facilitated in the situation in which the subject would choose to smoke, and impaired in the situation in which he would ordinarily not have smoked (Myrsten et al 1975). This study used only light smokers (fewer than 15 cigarettes per day), and was highly selective in choosing the two subject samples; most people smoke in a range of situations in a fairly automatic fashion, especially as the number of cigarettes smoked per day increases.

The same group of researchers (Myrsten et al 1972) established that smoking facilitated performance over nonsmoking levels in a boring, simple reaction-time task, and also improved performance over time in a difficult, stressful reaction-time task in which performance usually deteriorated. In all of these studies smoking increased physical indices of arousal, such as heart rate and catecholamine excretion, over baseline nonsmoking levels. Subjective reports of arousal and mental efficiency did not differ much among conditions, probably because people are not aware of changes in mood or performance while smoking regularly, only when deprived for "substantial" periods of time (even a few hours for some smokers). In fact, showing a "gruesome" medical film to both heavy and light smokers reduced smoking in both groups; lying on a couch produced an increase in smoking for all subjects (Fuller and Forrest 1973).

In sum, it would appear that the predominant central actions of nicotine and smoking are toward arousal. On the other hand, depression of the patellar reflex in man accounts for some of the relaxation experienced by smokers (Domino 1973). The most likely possibility is that it may have either effect, depending on the state of the smoker and on the dose of nicotine taken (Tomkins 1966, Myrsten et al 1975).

Does Nicotine/Smoking Have an Effect on Learning and Memory?

Stimulant drugs, such as amphetamine, improve cognitive and psychomotor performance by raising arousal levels and reversing fatigue effects, but under certain circumstances may directly facilitate learning (Weiss and Laties 1962, Hunter et al 1976). Nicotine has stimulant effects as well, which may facilitate performance and learning.

Enhancement of attention and arousal by nicotine have been obtained in animals (Nelsen 1976, Bovet-Nitti 1969, Garg 1969). Although claims were made for facilitation of learning processes in some of these studies, it was not possible to rule out arousal as the basic mechanism, especially when nicotine was administered before the learning trials on a daily basis. Prompted by suggestive animal findings, studies were conducted on humans. Facilitated learning of the pursuit rotor, a psychomotor tracking task, was reported by Frith (1968). However, on nonsense syllable learning, a cognitive task, smoking impaired immediate performance but had a facilitating effect on recall scores 45 minutes later, after the effects of the single cigarette had worn off (Andersson 1975). Smokers claim they concentrate better, work more efficiently, and think more clearly while smoking, claims that should be carefully investigated.

Toxicity of Tobacco

The acute debilitating effects of smoking are rarely noted by smokers who are tolerant to the actions of nicotine. Nonsmokers, however, can become acutely ill from smoking only a single cigarette, with evidence of nausea, vomiting, diarrhea, salivation, abdominal cramps, sweating, headache, dizziness, disturbed hearing and vision, and marked weakness. Pallor may be seen and faintness may occur, with circulatory shock in severe cases of nicotine poisoning. Nicotine is much more toxic when smoked than when swallowed because of the protective activity of the liver.

Very sensitive nonsmokers may react adversely to cigarette smoke in a closed room. It is unlikely that pharmacologic levels of nicotine can be inhaled from smoke in such a dilute form, but carbon monoxide may reach significant levels in a small, close space, and some individuals are allergic to smoke components.

The major health hazards from smoking result from the chronic use of cigarettes; they have been extensively described in the medical literature since the influential Surgeon General's Report (1964). Smoking still has its advocates who feel that the health hazards have been exaggerated. A drug that produces illness in an animal, even after several hours, is subsequently frequently avoided (Garcia et al 1974). The delay between onset of smoking and appearance of illness (negative reinforcement) may be 40 years, whereas positive reinforcement takes only a few seconds. This discrepancy in latency of positive (immediate) and negative (delayed) reinforcement accounts for the difficulty in extinguishing the habit.

Treatment of the Smoking Habit

Should the physician try to stop his patients from smoking? If they want to stop, then it is clear that he has the obligation to try. This will be much more difficult if the physician himself smokes, as 25 percent of physicians do. If the patient does not want to stop, then there is the difficult issue of intrusion by the physician. Advising the patient about the health risks involved in smoking and establishing whether there is any personal risk to the patient are of crucial importance. However, heavy smokers are rarely disturbed by some nebulous future risk to themselves or even demonstrable damage by smoking to a friend or relative.

While the pharmacologic basis of the smoking habit may be self-administration of nicotine, the act of smoking involves many complex behaviors. Extinguishing the smoking habit involves reducing to very low levels, or completely eliminating the longing for nicotine as well as the motor and social aspects of the habit, which are so routine and comforting by themselves (secondary reinforcement). Behavior therapy (operant conditioning), overt or covert aversion training (smoking-induced sickness, shock, disease data), psychotherapy, and hypnotherapy have all been tried on smokers seeking to quit. Many smoking clinics, both profit-making and nonprofit, use variants of behavior therapy. Some of the factors involved in successful treatment include the amount of personal attention, the length of the treatment, and the desire of the smoker to quit. But the relapse rate is high for all types of treatment, about 80 percent after only 3 months to 1 year of abstinence (Hunt and Bespalec 1974). Although purely behavioral therapies are most commonly employed to cure the smoking habit, pharmacotherapy has occasionally been used with the aim of easing dysphoria and facilitating the learning of substitute behaviors.

If nicotine seeking is the basis of the cigarette smoking habit, then substitution of nicotine ought to relieve the craving for cigarettes. There are a few studies in which nicotine was administered intravenously (Lucchesi et al 1967) or orally (Jarvik et al 1970) and in which nicotine antagonists were administered orally (Stolerman et al 1973). Significant, although small alterations in the number of cigarettes subjects chose to smoke occurred in each study; nicotine decreased smoking, and the nicotine antagonist mecamylamine increased it. Judging from these experimental results, the selection of a cigarette was only partially determined by blood level of nicotine. Subjects in these studies were not trying to give up smoking, thus altering their smoking behavior was quite impressive. A chewing gum containing nicotine bound to an ion exchange resin has recently been developed (Brantmark et al 1973). There has been evidence of short-term beneficial effects, but long-term benefit has not yet been demonstrated.

Lobeline, a drug that resembles nicotine in some repects, has been tried as a substitute, but most well-controlled studies show no advantage of lobeline over a placebo (Davison and Rosen 1972). Only Ejrup (1963) had marked success with lobeline in Sweden, using large parenteral doses over a 6-month period.

The impression from a recent survey of the literature on drug therapy for smoking was that none of the following agents has been particularly useful in helping smokers to quit: amphetamine, methylphenidate (Ritalin), fenfluramine (Pondimin), diazepam (Valium), phenobarbital, or meprobamate. Placebo or drug therapy seems to be equally effective in the short run in helping smokers to cease smoking or to cut down sizably on the daily number of cigarettes. Combined with some form of psychotherapy, initial success rates are even higher (Schwartz and Dubitsky 1967, 1968; Hunt and Bespalec 1974). However, what really counts is the long-term effects of any form of therapy. To be effective a smoking cure should be permanent, which means that 1- and 5-year follow-ups are essential.

It is entirely conceivable that either a nicotine substitute or some new method of adminstering nicotine, which will satisfy a smoker's need, will be found. At the moment no one has succeeded in substituting nicotine for smoking on a long-term convincing basis. Either there is some other component to the cigarette habit besides the nicotine, which makes it very reinforcing, or for some as yet unknown reason the cigarette smoking route of administering nicotine is more reinforcing than any other. Only further research will throw light on this important question.

A compromise between ignoring the patient's smoking habit and trying to make him stop if he cannot, is to convert him to a less hazardous form of tobacco—none without attendant risk. He might try cigarettes with tighter filters or lower tar and nicotine content. In the absence of any illness feedback from cigarettes, chances are that smoking patients will revert to their accustomed smoking levels. It may be useful to send the patient to a smoking clinic, such as those sponsored by the American Cancer Society, where a certain percentage of patients are actually permanently cured of smoking.

The only reason why a person will give up a pleasurable habit is because he realizes that the cost to him will be greater than the benefits he experiences. Attempts should be made to increase the immediacy and the personal relevance of the dangers of cigarette smoking to be sure that smokers feel personally threatened. How to accomplish such indoctrination most successfully must be the subject of future research. Epidemiologic evidence shows us that highly educated individuals (such as physicians) are much more apt to be influenced by evidence about the harm of smoking than the poorly educated, but intellectual factors alone are clearly not enough to inhibit smoking. One can see the utilization of defense mechanisms, such as denial, rationalization, and projection, to counter the threat of cigarette-caused disease and death. More intensive study of the factors responsible for success in ex-smokers should result in the development of more effective and rational therapies.

References

Andersson K: Effects of cigarette smoking on learning and retention. Psychopharmacologia 41:1–5, 1975

Ashton H, Watson DW: Puffing frequency and nicotine intake in cigarette smokers. Br Med J 2:679–681, 1970

Beckett, AH, Gorrod JW, Jenner P: The analysis of nicotine-1′-noxide in urine in the presence of nicotine and cotinine, and its application to the study of in vivo nicotine metabolism in man. J Pharm Pharmacol 23:55S–61S, 1971

Bovet-Nitti F: Facilitation of simultaneous visual discrimination by nicotine in four "inbred" strains of mice. Psychopharmacologia 14:193–199, 1969

Brantmark B, Ohlin P, Westling H: Nicotine-containing chewing gum as an anti-smoking aid. Psychopharmacologia 31:191–200, 1973

Brecher EM: Licit and Illicit Drugs. Boston, Little Brown, 1972

Damon A: Smoking attitudes and practices in seven preliterate societies. In Dunn WL Jr (ed): Smoking Behavior: Motives and Incentives. Washington DC, Winston, 1973, pp 219–230

Davison GC, Rosen RC: Lobeline and reduction of cigarette smoking. Psychol Rep 31:443–456, 1971

Domino EF: Neuropsychopharmacology of nicotine and tobacco smoking. In Dunn WL Jr (ed): Smoking Behavior: Motives and Incentives. Washington DC, Winston, 1973, pp 5–31

Dunn WL Jr (ed): Smoking Behavior: Motives and Incentives. Washington DC, Winston, 1973

Ejrup B: Experience in smoking withdrawal clinics. New York American Cancer Society News Service, 1963, pp 1–7

Federal Trade Commission: Tar and Nicotine Content of Cigarettes. DHEW Publication No. (CDC) 74–8703, 1975

Frith CD: The effects of varying the nicotine content of cigarettes on human smoking behavior. Psychopharmacologia 19:188–192, 1971

————: The effects of nicotine on the consolidation of pursuit rotor learning. Life Sci 7:77–84, 1968

Fuller RGC, Forrest DW: Behavioral aspects of cigarette smoking in relation to arousal level. Psychol Rep 33:115–121, 1973

Garcia J, Hankins WG, Rusiniak KW: Behavioral regulation of the milieu interne in man and rats. Science 185:824–831, 1974

Garg M: The effects of nicotine on two different types of learning. Psychopharmacologia 15:408–414, 1969

Goldfarb TL, Jarvik ME, Glick SD: Cigarette nicotine content as a determinent of human smoking behavior. Psychopharmacologia 17:89–93, 1970

————, Jarvik ME: Accommodation to restricted tobacco smoke intake in cigarette smokers. Int J Addict 7:559–565, 1972

Goodwin DW, Schulsinger F, Moller N, et al: Adoption and psychiatric illness in a nonpatient population. Arch Gen Psychiatr 1976

Gritz ER, Jarvik ME: A preliminary study: forty-eight hours of abstinence from smoking. Proceedings of the 81st Annual Convention of the American Psychological Association 1:1039–1040, 1973

Hall GH, Turner DM: Effects of nicotine on the release of ^{3}H-Nordrenaline from the hypothalamus. Biochem Pharmacol 21:1829–1831, 1972

Hunt WA, Bespalec DA: An evaluation of current methods of modifying smoking behavior. J Clin Psychol 30:431–438, 1974

Hunter B, Zornetzer SF, Jarvik ME, McGaugh JL: Modulation of learning and memory: effects of drugs influencing neurotransmitters. In Dversen LL, Dversen SD, Snyder SH (eds): Handbook of Psychopharmacology. New York, Plenum, 1976

Jarvik ME: The role of nicotine in the smoking habit. In Hunt WA (ed): Learning Mechanisms in Smoking. Chicago, Aldine, 1970, pp 155–190

————, Glick SD, Nakamura RK: Inhibition of cigarette smoking by orally administered nicotine. Clin Pharmacol Ther 11:574–576, 1970

Kety SS: The motivational factors in cigarette smoking: a summary. In Dunn WL, Jr (ed): Smoking Behavior: Motives and Incentives. New York, Wiley, 1973, pp 287–295

Knapp RP, Bliss CM, Wells H: Addictive aspects in heavy cigarette smoking. Am J Psychiatry 119:966–972, 1963

Kozlowski LT, Jarvik ME, Gritz ER: Nicotine regulation and cigarette smoking. Clin Pharmacol Ther 17:93–97, 1975

Langone JJ, Gjika HB, Van Vunakis H: Nicotine and its metabolities, radioimmunoassays for nicotine and cotinine. Biochemistry 12:5025–5030, 1973

Larson PS, Silvette H: Tobacco: Experimental and Clinical Studies, Supplement 2. Baltimore, Williams & Wilkins, 1971

Lucchesi BR, Schuster CR, Emley GS: The role of nicotine as a determinant of cigarette smoking frequency in man with observations of certain cardiovascular effects associated with the tobacco alkaloid. Clin Pharmacol Ther 8:789–796, 1967

Menninger K: Whatever Became of Sin? New York, Hawthorn, 1973

Myrsten A-L, Andersson K, Frankenhaeuser M, Elgerot A: Immediate effects of cigarette smoking as related to different smoking habits. Percept Mot Skills 40:515–523, 1975

————, Elgerot A: Effects of Abstinence from Tobacco Smoking on Physiological Arousal Level in Habitual Smokers. Reports from the Psychological Laboratories, University of Stockholm, No 428, 1974

————, Post B, Frankenhaeuser M, Johansson G. Changes in behavioral and physiological activation induced by cigarette smoking in habitual smokers. Psychopharmacologia 27:305–312, 1972

Nelson JM: Psychobiological consequences of chronic nicotine administration. In Lal H, Singh J (eds): Neurobiology of Drug Dependence, Vol 1: A Behavioral Analysis of Drug Dependence. Mt. Kisco, NY, Futura, 1976

Russell MAH: Cigarette smoking: natural history of a dependence disorder. Br J Med Psychol 44:1–16, 1971

————, Wilson C, Patel UA, Feyerabend C, Cole PV: Plasma nicotine levels after smoking cigarettes with high, medium and low nicotine yields. Br Med J 6:414–416, 1975

Schwartz JL, Dubitzky M: The smoking control research project: purpose design and initial results. Psychol Rep 20:367–376, 1967

————: One-year follow-up results of a smoking cessation program. Can J Pub Health 59:161–165, 1968

Smith GM: Personality and smoking: a review of the empirical literature. In Hunt WA (ed): Learning Mechanisms in Smoking. Chicago, Aldine, 1970, pp 42–61

Stolerman IP, Goldfarb T, Fink R, Jarvik ME: Influencing cigarette smoking with nicotine antagonists. Psychopharmacologia 28:247–259, 1973

Teenage Smoking: National Patterns of Cigarette Smoking, Ages 12 Through 18, in 1972 and 1974. DHEW Publication No. (NIH) 76–931, Department of Health, Education and Welfare, Public Health Service.

Tomkins SS: Psychological model for smoking behavior. Am J Pub Health 56:17–20, 1966

Ulett JA, Itil RM: Quantitative electroencephalogram in smoking and smoking deprivation. Science 164:969–970, 1969

United States Public Health Service: Smoking and Health. Report of the Advisory Committee to the Surgeon General of the Public Health Service, Publication 1103, 1964

Wagner S: Cigarette Country. New York, Praeger, 1971

Weybrew BB, Stark JE: Psychological and Physiological Changes Associated with Deprivation from Smoking. U.S. Naval Submarine and Medical Center Report 490, 1967

Weiss B, Laties VG: Enhancement of human performance by caffeine and the amphetamines. Pharmacol Rev 14:1–36, 1962

the hallucinogens

commentary

Hallucinogenic drugs are of interest to the practitioner because they are so popular in the community. Today there are strong advocates and opponents of the nonmedical use of these agents, and Dr. Jones adopts a balanced view. Even though a great deal of research has been done with the hallucinogens, it is not yet clear exactly how dangerous they are. Dr. Jones considers the evidence and concludes that more research is needed. From time to time, medical uses for hallucinogenic drugs have been proposed, but attempts to evaluate these uses have been sabotaged by the popular illegal traffic and counterattempts to prohibit their use. These drugs have been proposed and tried in the treatment of terminal cancer, as an aid in psychotherapy, and in the treatment of other drug addictions, such as alcoholism. Hallucinogenic drugs are still useful tools for studying physiologic and chemical mechanisms underlying behavior. Dr. Jones summarizes some of the vast literature in this area. He discusses LSD and its congeners, cannabis, the anticholinergic hallucinogens, and phencyclidine. The early hope that these drugs might produce a model psychosis that would explain the etiology of naturally occurring psychoses has not been fully realized, but much important chemical and physiologic knowledge has been revealed through their use.

the hallucinogens

Reese T. Jones, M.D.

Hallucinogens refer to a large number of drugs that induce marked changes in perception, thought, and mood. At certain doses and under certain conditions many drugs commonly used in medicine can produce delusions, illusions, hallucinations, and the mood and cognitive changes seen in naturally occurring psychoses. Just a few examples include anticholinergics, antimalarials, antidepressants, bromides, opiate antagonists, stimulants, and corticosteroids. However, lysergic acid diethylamide (LSD) and related hallucinogens differ in that they induce profound changes in sensation and mood coexisting with a relatively clear and unclouded sensorium and consciousness and at doses which result in comparatively slight physiologic activity.

The classification of hallucinogens is somewhat arbitrary. Even the term *hallucinogen* is not completely satisfactory. By a precise definition, a hallucination is a sensory experience, not resulting from a stimulus in the external environment. Most drugs thought of as hallucinogens only rarely, if ever, produce true hallucinations (Hollister 1968, Hoffer and Osmond 1967). *Illusionogenic* is probably a more appropriate term. Another label is *psychotomimetic*, but such drugs do not always produce or mimic a psychosis. *Psychedelic* was a term coined in 1957 (Hoffer and Osmond 1967), but the drugs may not always be "mind manifesting," and many observers would argue the agents only distort rather than expand consciousness. *Phantasticum*, a term used by Lewin (1931) in the early part of this century, may come the closest to describing the actual reaction of the subject given such agents. Whatever the label, the class of drugs does share the property of enhancing awareness of self and environment—both internal and external—even though they may differ in other aspects of their pharmacology.

LSD and Related Hallucinogens

Lysergic acid diethylamide and its psychedelic relatives have been the most popular and notorious recreational hallucinogens in recent years (Hollister 1968). Lysergic acid diethylamide, psilocybin, psilocin, dimethyltryptamine (DMT), and diethyltryptamine (DET) are all indolalkylamines. The structurally more simple phenethylamine types include mescaline and a series of drugs that are a cross between amphetamine and mescaline, such as 2, 5-dimethyoxy-4-methyamphetamine (DOM or STP), 2, 5-dimethoxy-4-ethylamphetamine (DOE), methylene dioxyamphetamine (MDA), and others (MMDA, TMA, and so on). Despite marked differences in chemical structure and potency, these drugs produce very similar subjective effects. Thus, LSD, the most extensively studied drug of the group, can be used as a prototype of the effects of the others (Hollister 1968).

Hallucinogenic Drugs Inducing Delirium

Anticholinergic Hallucinogens

The prototypes of the anticholinergic substances are atropine and scopolamine. However, any drug with atropinelike effects has a potential for producing a delirium. This includes commonly used drugs like the tricyclic antidepressants and the phenothiazines. Even the instillation of mydriatic anticholinergics into the conjunctival sac can produce central effects in sensitive individuals. Because many of the symptoms are unpleasant, it seems that only sporadic recreational use occurs. However, a sampler of plants may inadvertently ingest something with fairly high concentrations of belladonna alkaloids, for example, Jimson weed. On occasion, various anticholinergics appear in the illicit drug market, usually because of misrepresentation or ignorance of their true nature. This usually leads to a brief flurry of bad trips at a particular rock festival, rather than a pattern of sustained merchandising and use.

In contrast to the hallucinogens of the indole group, the confusional picture following anticholinergic drugs is usually accompanied by decreased alertness, apprehension, and diminished contact with the environment. At low doses the expected peripheral autonomic effects predominate. As the dose is increased, euphoria, drowsiness, restlessness, and motor incoordination progress rapidly to a state marked by impaired memory, confusion, hallucinations, hyperreflexia, convulsions, hyperthermia, and finally coma. Although the symptoms may be dramatic, death is rare and, only with supportive treatment does the patient recover from the coma. The syndrome can last 48 hours or longer (Ketchum et al 1973).

Supportive and symptomatic treatment is usually adequate. However, an uncommonly used rational treatment is physostigmine, given as a slow intravenous injection of 1 to 3 mg (Ketchum et al 1973). If salivation, sweating, and intestinal hyperactivity do not occur soon after the beginning of the injection of physostigmine, this confirms the diagnosis of belladonna intoxication. Delirium and coma should rapidly diminish. Because of physostigmine's brief duration of action, repeat doses in 1 to 2 hours may be needed. Diazepam is suitable to provide sedation, if needed, or to control convulsions. Phenothiazines may worsen the symptoms and should not be used.

Anesthetic Drugs

Phencyclidine is one of a series of 1-arylcyclohexylamine compounds developed in the late 1950s as possible anesthetic agents (Domino 1964). Phencyclidine was evaluated in clinical trials under the name Sernyl for use as a general anesthetic. After considerable clinical testing, its use in humans was discontinued because of anesthetic emergent reactions characterized by hallucinations and agitation. It is still marketed for veterinary purposes, hence one of its names on the illicit market is *animal tranquilizer*. A structurally related compound, ketamine was subsequently developed and is now marketed as an anesthetic.

Although available on the illicit market since 1967, phencyclidine has received little attention until recently. In some areas it is now said to be the most readily available illicit drug. Phencyclidine goes by a wide variety of street names, including PCP, Angel Dust, Mist, Hog, Rocket Fuel, Crystal, and Peace Pill. It is sold alone or in combination with LSD. It is commonly misrepresented as tetrahydrocannabinol, mescaline, or psilocybin. Phencyclidine has been rarely identified as such on the illicit market (Commission of Inquiry Report 1973). However, recent unpublished reports suggest that it is becoming a popular drug in its own right, with even groups of chronic users now appearing. Phencyclidine is readily synthesized in illicit laboratories; hence if there is a market for the drug, its manufacture and distribution will be difficult to control.

This class of compounds may represent an entirely new type of psychoactive agent with some properties of gaseous anesthetics, stimulants, analgesics, barbiturates, and hallucinogens (Domino et al 1974). Oral use, nasal insufflation, or smoking (by adding it to parsley or marihuana) is currently popular. At low doses (under 5 mg) effects resembling alcohol intoxication are produced. However, at moderate-to-high doses, depersonalization, hallucinations, delusions, and loss of time sense develops, progressing with increasing dose to coma. Catalepsy with marked difficulty in speaking is common. Some investigators think that the symptoms of phencyclidine more closely resemble those of schizophrenia than those induced by LSD (Cohen et al 1962).

Central nervous system depression, hypotension, bradycardia, and convulsions develop at the highest doses. At more moderate dose levels, dystonic reactions, vertical and horizontal nystagmus, miosis, and elevated blood pressure are common. Recovery from coma takes at least 24 hours, with return of normal mental status taking up to a week. Unlike the situation with other hallucinogens, death from overdose may occur and is usually related to recurrent seizures and respiratory depression (Kessler 1974).

Phencyclidine intoxication should be suspected when the mental state resembles that induced by other hallucinogens, but with ataxia, horizontal and vertical nystagmus, dystonic symptoms, or status epilepticus. The drug is so readily available and so commonly misrepresented in the illicit drug market that a high index of suspicion of its presence is appropriate.

The treatment of reactions at low doses is similar to that for other hallucinogens—supportive care and reduction of sensory stimulation. Diazepam, carefully given intravenously in 2- to 3-mg doses, appears useful in the case of severe agitation or seizure activity. The interaction of high doses of phencyclidine and other drugs is not well studied, hence caution is indicated. For example, there is a marked potentiation of the effects of pentobarbital in animals pretreated with phencyclidine. It is not clear whether significant tolerance and dependence develop after regular use of phencyclidine.

Other Anesthetic Hallucinogens

Almost any anesthetic drug whose action is characterized by a prolonged Stage II anesthesia can produce delirium with psychotomimetic features, for example, nitrous oxide, ether, or chloroform. In many areas, nitrous oxide is a popular deliriant when available. The main hazard is inadvertent overdosage, with resultant respiratory and cardiovascular problems.

Naturally Occurring Hallucinogens

A number of the hallucinogens are naturally occurring substances that have been used for centuries (Schultes 1969). Mescaline from the peyote cactus and psilocybin from the "sacred mushrooms" (teonanctl) are perhaps the best known. A full description of mescaline's actions and discussion of its use in therapy and diagnosis were published in the 1920s and relatively ignored (Kluver 1928). Peyote is used in ceremonies by the Native American Church, with relatively few problems.

Other plant materials often considered for recreational hallucinogenic use include the Mexican Morning Glory, DMT (dimethyl tryptamine), in South American Indian snuffs, the fly agaric mushroom, nutmeg, and a variety of belladonna alkaloids. Of course, cannabis sativa is the most popular natural hallucinogen in current use. A review of Kluver (1928) or Lewin's writings (1931) is useful whenever one thinks something new has been discovered in the recent hallucinogen era. One cannot help but be impressed with how facts about drug effects are continually rediscovered by investigators who are loath to go to the library.

LSD and Related Hallucinogens—Historical Perspective

Lysergic acid diethylamide was synthesized in 1938 but appeared to be relatively uninteresting in animal physiologic studies. While working in his laboratory, Hofmann accidentally ingested a small amount of LSD and recognized an unusual mental state (Hofmann 1959). A few days later, he swallowed what he considered a small dose (0.250 mg) to confirm his hypothesis that LSD produced the intoxication. Within a few minutes the onset of usual somatic effects, largely sympathomimetic, were perceived along with giddiness, restlessness, nausea, difficulty in concentration, visual distortions, and paresthesias. In the second and third hour, the wavelike visual illusions with micropsia, macropsia, auditory distortions, synesthesias, and time sense changes followed. All this occurred in the presence of intact and even hypervigilant consciousness. This relative preservation of a clear sonсorium is in marked contrast to that produced by anticholinergic hallucinogens and other deliriants. The nature of the experience is fairly similar for LSD, mescaline, psilocybin, DMT, and DOM, the main differences involving duration of effect and intensity of somatic symptoms. Details of the various forms and types of LSD "trips" have been well described elsewhere

(Brecher 1972, Freedman 1968, Hoffer and Osmond 1967, Hollister 1968).

Hofmann's original descriptions of the LSD experience (Hofmann 1959) are of particular interest, since they are among the few not influenced by prior expectations on the part of the recipient or the experimenter. In an historical overview, Brecher (1972) describes how LSD was popularized and how the wide publicity given to various "adverse" effects to some extent determined them (Freedman 1968). Lysergic acid diethylamide represents a classic example of a drug where sociocultural factors possibly changed its psychopharmacology.

In reading the post Timothy Leary (about 1963 onward) hallucinogen literature, it is easy to develop a distorted impression of not only the effects but also the relative dangers of the hallucinogens. Both the psychedelic apologists of the 1960s and those who believe LSD use leads to permanent madness tended to ignore the vast amount of research done with LSD between 1943 and 1963 (about 2000 reports) (Hoffer and Osmond 1967). This older literature suggests that LSD given under proper circumstances was not only an interesting drug, but a relatively safe one (Cohen 1960). The more recent hallucinogen literature also tends to ignore Lewin's (1931) and Kluver's (1928) early twentieth-century studies of mescaline and other hallucinogens.

Prolonged psychoses, panic reactions, or related adverse mental effects are rare, even in experimental or clinical settings using psychiatric patients as subjects. Cohen's survey in 1959 (Cohen and Ditman 1963) found that psychotic reactions lasted over 48 hours in 0.18 percent of psychiatric patients and 0.08 percent of experimental subjects. Only a few flashbacks were noted. The four suicides in the 5000-person sample is a lower figure than one would expect without any treatment in the population of drug addicts, psychopaths, depressions, and personality problems treated with LSD. The most common prolonged reaction in the experimental studies was a mild depression. The few cases of prolonged psychosis tended to occur in prepsychotic individuals.

Psychologic Effects

A noticeable psychologic effect develops after 20 to 30 µg of LSD. The onset of effects on oral doses is about 1 hour, with a peak at 2 or 3 hours and a gradual return to normal over 6 to 10 hours. Peak psychologic and behavioral effects follow blood levels nicely. Psilocybin produced effects lasting only a few hours, and DMT effects may wear off in less than an hour. Mescaline is said to produce more somatic, vegetative symptoms than LSD (Hollister 1968). The effects are all related to dose to some extent. Confusion, disorientation, and prolonged trips are more likely at high doses.

Performance on tests involving attention, concentration, and motivation is impaired. Tests of learning, memory, and other cognitive functions are usually impaired or unchanged. Effects on other perceptual motor functions would suggest impaired driving ability. Although enhancement of subjective qualities of most sensory modalities is commonly reported, evidence of objectively measured change is lacking. Studies of hallucinogenic effects on creativity produced inconsistent results. Specific aphrodisiac or other alterations in sexual functioning are not evident, though decreased inhibitions, and altered time and tactile sense may enhance enjoyment. The validity of hallucinogen-induced religious experience is probably scientifically untestable and will probably remain an area of controversy.

Tolerance, Dependence, Toxicity

A marked degree of tolerance to the psychologic and many of the physiologic effects of LSD develops after only three or four daily doses and is lost equally rapidly. Cross-tolerance between LSD, mescaline, and psilocybin develops, but no cross-tolerance with amphetamine or other classes of hallucinogens is seen. The cross-tolerance between compounds with very different chemical structures, but not between mescaline and amphetamine which have similar configurations, suggests common sites of action exist. There is no evidence of significant dependence; withdrawal phenomena are not seen, nor is sustained drug-seeking behavior evident.

The lethal dose of LSD in man must be exceedingly high. No deaths due to direct drug effects have been reported, although fatal accidents during LSD intoxication do occur. In terms of lethal physical toxicity, LSD must be considered one of the safest drugs. In contrast, MDA appears to be the only one of the hallucinogens in this class that involves a significant risk of fatal overdose. A number of fatalities after oral use have been reported (Cimbura 1972).

Adverse Psychologic Reactions

What is a desirable or pleasurable effect in one individual in a certain situation may well be an adverse effect in another individual or situation. For example, phencyclidine was withdrawn from use as a human anesthetic because of adverse psychologic reactions during the postanesthetic recovery period, yet it is used as a recreational drug *because* it produces these very same psychologic reactions.

The most commonly accepted adverse psychologic reaction to

hallucinogens is the "bad trip"—a relatively brief (less than 24 hours, often an hour or less) episode of panic, anxiety, and fear of death, insanity, and so forth. These can best be treated by reassurance and a supportive, quiet, consistent, and nonstimulating environment. Antianxiety drugs or mild sedation with barbiturates may occasionally be useful. Phenothiazines are rarely needed and can produce troublesome side effects of their own, particularly when given in large parenteral doses.

The unpleasant psychologic reactions can occur even in users who have had many previous satisfactory experiences. They only rarely appear to be due to adulterants or contaminants in the drug, though misrepresented drugs (for example, phencyclidine sold as mescaline) or drugs of greater than advertised potency can contribute to such reactions.

More puzzling, and fortunately rarer, adverse psychologic reactions include prolonged depressions, paranoid behavior, and psychotic episodes. These may last far beyond the 8 to 10-hour period of acute drug effects and may, in some instances, persist for years. It is unclear whether such episodes would have occurred without the drug (Cohen and Ditman 1963, Freedman 1969). In most cases prior psychopathology existed, although in a few cases prolonged adverse psychologic effects persisted in individuals without obvious preexisting psychopathology.

Persistent recurrences of drug effects known as "flashbacks" are another puzzling phenomena related to the use of hallucinogens. Many reports may simply represent increased awareness of the "psychopathology of everyday life" on the part of an experienced hallucinogen user and may not represent a direct drug effect. It is worth noting that no "flashback" phenomena were reported in the first 20 years of LSD research. It was only after the phenomena received widespread publicity in the media that investigators began to give estimates like 5 percent of all users experience them.

The use of hallucinogens does not seem to enhance criminal activity nor violence, except in rare instances of drug-induced panic reactions (Tinklenberg 1973). In fact, hallucinogen use may reduce the inclination for assaultive behavior.

Repeated use of hallucinogens has been said to be associated with subtle changes in the ability to engage in abstract thinking, personality changes, and something termed the *amotivational syndrome* (McGlothlin and West 1968). However, these clinical impressions are not always supported by the results of objective testing (McGlothlin and Arnold 1971). Without proper prospective studies, the complexity of determining a direct causal relationship between drug use and such changes will continue to remain an area of controversy (McWilliams and Tuttle 1973).

Physical Toxicity

Although they have a close structural similarity with amphetamine, MDA and STP (DOM) have little amphetaminelike peripheral physiologic effects. Despite much speculation, there is, as yet, no firm evidence of brain damage due to repeated hallucinogen use. A concern over chromosomal aberrations and teratogenic effects led to a number of studies reporting contradictory evidence of uncertain biologic significance (Jarvik et al 1974). Optimal cytogenetic techniques have not usually been used in the studies. Even if chromosomal breakage is related to hallucinogen use, its biomedical significance is unknown. Temporary or permanent breakage results from a variety of factors—x-rays, pollutants, fever, viral infections, and commonly used drugs like caffeine and aspirin. Drug users may differ from nonusers on a number of these factors. The effects of hallucinogens (and most other drugs) on the fetus during pregnancy are uncertain (Jacobson and Berlin 1972). Most investigators would agree that the use of hallucinogens for either medical or nonmedical purposes by pregnant women is unwise.

Therapeutic Uses

Some of the first studies of hallucinogens investigated their use as adjuncts in psychotherapy for the treatment of alcohol or opiate dependence or to reduce the need for analgesics in terminal cancer patients. The initial impressive reports of success have not been substantiated in subsequent controlled studies (Hoffer and Osmond 1967, Hollister 1968, Ludwig et al 1970). Currently there is no widely accepted medical use of hallucinogens.

Hallucinogens and Interactions With Other Drugs

Users of hallucinogens often use a variety of other psychoactive drugs. Interactions of various combinations have not been systematically studied. For example, mixtures of LSD and phencyclidine often appear in illicit samples. Animal studies indicate that such a combination might be antagonistic, but human confirmatory studies are lacking. Amphetamine is said to prolong and intensify the effects of hallucinogens. Yet the combination rarely appears in illicit samples. Many of the psychologic effects of the hallucinogens are reduced by phenothiazines and, to a lesser extent, by sedatives and minor tranquilizers.

The problems of assessing the possible interactions of recreational drugs is illustrated by the sequence of events following the appearance of STP on the illicit market. The toxic effects of STP were reportedly potentiated by the chlorpromazine used in the treatment of adverse effects (Smith 1969). Notice of this apparent potentiation was widely circulated. However, in subsequent laboratory studies chlorpromazine clearly lessened the effects of DOM (STP). The explanation is that the assumed DOM (STP) responsible for the alleged STP-chlorpromazine interaction was really an anticholinergic drug instead of or in addition to the DOM.

Cannabis

Cannabis was probably one of the first deliberately used to produce psychotic or psychoticlike states in normal people in an experimental situation (Jones 1973, Moreau 1973). Most users of marihuana in the United States would argue that the sense of well-being or euphoria, relaxation, drowsiness, mild perceptual changes, and altered time sense that follows the smoking of a marihuana cigarette are not what they would expect from an hallucinogen. Cannabis can appear to be an hallucinogen or not, depending on the dose under consideration, along with personality of the user, setting, expectations, and all other determinants of the effect of any hallucinogen. For the past few years, cannabis research has been a high-priority area in terms of funding and other support. A number of excellent reviews cover the outpouring of recent research findings (Cannabis 1972, Hollister 1971, Marihuana 1972, Marihuana and Health 1974, Mechoulam 1973, Miller 1974).

Botany and Chemistry of Cannabis

Cannabis comes from hemp plants. Marihuana refers to the leaves and other parts of the plant chopped up and usually smoked in a pipe or cigarette. Hashish is the dried resinous exudate of the flowering tops of the plant and tends to contain the highest concentration of chemicals thought to be psychoactive. The group of chemicals called cannabinoids, particularly delta-9-tetrahydrocannabinol (THC) seems to be the substance responsible for the major part of the plant's potency.

Tetrahydrocannabinol can be synthesized but the process is expensive and the yields are low. What is claimed to be THC on the illicit market usually is phencyclidine or various combinations of other drugs (Cannabis 1972). Concentrated extracts of cannabis (hashish oil) containing very high concentrations of THC are easily prepared and increasingly available (Marihuana and Health 1974).

After smoking, absorption is rapid, with effects appearing within minutes. Up to 95 percent of an oral dose is absorbed, but the rate is variable and erratic, taking as long as 2 or 3 hours for peak effects and lasting up to 4 to 6 hours. Tetrahydrocannabinol is about three times more potent when smoked as compared to oral ingestion. Because of poor solubility, preparations of cannabinoids suitable for parenteral use are complicated to prepare and not commonly available for recreational use. Drug kinetics are similar after smoking or after intravenous injection. A rapid phase of disappearance of THC, with a half-life of about 30 minutes, is followed by a slow phase with a half-life of 36 to 48 hours. Metabolites appear in the urine for several days following single doses, but repeated doses show no evidence of build-up of metabolites in urine. The 11-hydroxy metabolite may prove to be the principal source of THC activity. However, it remains to be seen whether other metabolites are active as well.

Psychologic Effects of Cannabis

The dose is an important determinant (Domino et al 1974). A mild and brief "high" follows a low dose smoke and can be altered by many nonpharmacologic variables. A prolonged hallucinogenic experience will reliably follow a large oral dose. An initial, relatively short period of stimulation (euphoria, often anxiety, and enhanced perceptions) is usually followed by a more prolonged period of sedation marked by a drowsy, relaxed, dreamlike state. The effects are similar to those produced by other hallucinogens and include altered time sense, paresthesias, difficulty concentrating, speaking, and remembering, visual illusions, and occasional hallucinations. The syndrome is similar whether produced in the laboratory or in the outside world.

Physiologic Effects of Cannabis

Dose-related tachycardia is a sensitive and reliable change. Blood pressure can be slightly elevated at lower doses, with often marked orthostatic hypotension following large doses. Conjunctival reddening tends to follow subjective symptom changes. A slight decrease in intraocular pressure may be related to cardiovascular changes. Muoolo woakness, decreased coordination, tremor, nystagmus, and ataxia tend to be dose related. The sleep electroencephalogram is more reliably altered than the waking electroencephalogram (Feinberg et al 1975). The former is marked by eye movement and rapid eye movement sleep (REM) decrements with relatively little effect on slow-wave sleep and increments in total sleep time when the drug is begun. REM rebound occurs on discontinuation of the drug. The effects of cannabis on the waking electroencephalogram include minimal increases in alpha activity, minimal slowing of rhythms, and a tendency toward greater synchronization.

Plasma testosterone levels were decreased in a group of marihuana smokers (Kolodny et al 1974). Other endocrine system changes have been reported following marihuana use. None of the reported alterations are outside the limits of normality, so their biomedical significance is open to question. Reported effects of marihuana smoking on cell-mediated immunity and chromosome alterations are also of uncertain biologic significance (Marihuana and Health 1975). No clear-cut evidence of teratogenesis in humans has appeared. Many of the findings in this area are not uniformly reproduced in other laboratories (Mendelson et al 1974).

Cognitive and Psychomotor Function Effects of Cannabis

Most cognitive functions can be altered by cannabis (Cannabis 1972, Marihuana 1972, Marihuana and Health 1974). Dose is all important, but complexity of the task, prior practice, past drug history, and other variables also determine outcome of any experiment. Tests of recent memory functions are sensitive to impairment. Altered time sense is the most consistent measurable perceptual alteration.

Tolerance and Dependence

Tolerance to many of the behavioral, physiologic effects and the lethal effects of cannabis develops rapidly in animals (Cannabis 1972, Marihuana and Health 1974). Functional and pharmacodynamic adaptation to the drug seem more important than changes in metabolism, although the mechanisms of tolerance are still unclear. Tolerance must develop in man at certain dosage levels since regular users in countries where potent material is readily available consume enormous amounts. Volunteers in chronic experiments tend to increase the number of marihuana cigarettes smoked or show decreased effects from a constant dose (Szara and Braude 1975). There is some evidence for cross-tolerance between alcohol and cannabis, but not between THC and LSD. After high doses of cannabis, taken for a period of time, irritability, restlessness, sleep disturbance, perspiration, tremor, weight loss, salivation, and nausea rapidly follow sudden cessation of the drug. These symptoms of physical dependence are not usually evident in more infrequent users (Szara and Braude 1975). The importance of such symptoms as a partial determinant of drug-seeking behavior is unclear.

Adverse Psychologic Effects

The patterns of adverse psychologic reactions attributed to cannabis are very similar to those associated with other hallucinogens (Jones 1973). The acute onset of panic, confusion, disorientation, delusions, and depersonalization seems to be determined by the same multiplicity of factors associated with LSD-induced "bad trips." The rarer but long-lasting psychosis or toxic confusional states are equally puzzling and raise the same unanswered questions concerning the interaction between preexisting psychopathology and drug-induced mental illness. The transient bad trips are apparently very common if one is to believe surveys of marihuana users. For example, in Tart's 150-person sample of enthusiastic and experienced marihuana smokers, 21 percent reported "freaking out" one or more times (Tart 1970). Twenty percent reported losing control and being taken over by a hostile outside force after smoking. Tart believes this population probably underreported negative effects. The fact that such adverse reactions rarely come to the attention of medical treatment facilities suggests that most are self-limited and need no specific intervention other than support and the passage of time.

The *amotivation syndrome* (Cannabis 1972, Marihuana 1972, Marihuana and Health 1975) manifested by loss of interest, ambition, lack of self-esteem, apathy, introversion, and other subtle personality changes has been a topic of much discussion. Whether it represents a consequence or cause of marihuana use is uncertain. During the period of chronic intoxication, it appears that motivation is impaired. If and how long this persists after a period of use has not been determined.

The same sort of "flashbacks" reported after LSD use has been reputed to occur with cannabis use (Marihuana 1972). The etiology and significance is as poorly understood.

Adverse Physiologic Effects

The lethal dose of a cannabis must be exceedingly high. Respiratory system changes may be common with frequent use (Tennant et al 1971). Allergic reactions to the plant material should be fairly common, though seldom reported. Cerebral atrophy as measured by brain ventricular dilatation was reported in a small group of patients who had used cannabis frequently (Campbell et al 1972). These findings are controversial. Studies of chronic users in other countries can be misleading and falsely reassuring or may cause undue alarm if sample size, cultural differences, etc., are not carefully considered. For example, the popular press has written much about the

so-called *Jamaica Study* in which a small sample of chronic cannabis users and nonusers were compared on a battery of psychologic
and biomedical measures (Rubin and Comitas 1975). If cannabis-
induced brain damage is as rare and hard to measure an event as
alcohol-induced brain damage, it would be very easy to miss its
occurrence in a sample size of 30. One might also worry that tobacco
and alcohol appeared to be relatively nontoxic substances based on
the results of such a study. Many adverse effects, if they exist, may
be exceedingly uncommon and not apparent on small sample surveys.

References

Brecher EM: Licit and Illicit Drugs. Boston, Little, Brown, 1972

Campbell AM, Thomson JL, Evans M, Williams MJ: Cerebral atrophy in
young cannabis smokers. Lancet 1:202, 1972

Cannabis: A Report of the Commission of Inquiry into the Non-Medical Use
of Drugs. Ottawa, Information Canada, 1972

Cimbura G: 3,4-Methylenedioxyamphetamine (MDA): Analytical and forensic aspects of fatal poisoning. J Forensic Sci 17:329, 1972

Cohen BD, Rosenbaum G, Luby ED, Gottlieb JS: Comparison of phencyclidine (Sernyl) with other drugs. Arch Gen Psychiatry 6:79, 1962

Cohen S: Lysergic acid diethylamide: side effects and complications. J Nerv
Ment Dis 130:30, 1960

———, Ditman KS: Prolonged adverse reactions to lysergic acid diethylamide. Arch Gen Psychiatry 8:475, 1963

Commission of Inquiry into the Non-Medical Use of Drugs: Final report.
Ottawa, Information Canada, 1973, p 363

Domino EF: Neurobiology of phencyclidine (Sernyl), a drug with an unusual spectrum of pharmacological activity. Int Rev Neurobiol 6:303, 1964

———, Rennick P, Pearl JH: Dose-effect relations of marihuana smoking on
various physiologic parameters in experienced male users—observations on
limits of self-titration of smoke. Clin Pharmacol Ther 15:514, 1974

Feinberg I, Jones R, Walker JM, Cavness C, March J: Effects of high dosage
delta-9-tetrahydrocannabinol on sleep patterns in man. Clin Pharmacol Ther
17:458, 1975

Freedman DX: On the use and abuse of LSD. Arch Gen Psychiatry 18:330,
1968

———: The psychopharmacology of hallucinogenic agents. Annu Rev Med
20:409, 1969

Hoffer A, Osmond H: The Hallucinogens. New York, Academic, 1967

Hofmann A: Psychotomimetic drugs: chemical and pharmacological aspects. Acta Physiol Pharmacol Neerlandica 8:240, 1959

Hollister LE: Chemical Psychoses. Springfield, Ill., Thomas, 1968

————: Marihuana in man: three years later. Science 172:21, 1971

Jacobson CB, Berlin CN: Possible reproductive detriment in LSD users. JAMA 222:1367, 1972

Jarvik LF, Yen FS, Dahlberg CC, et al: Chromosome examinations after medically administered lysergic acid diethylamide and dextroamphetamine. Dis Nerv Syst 35:399, 1974

Jones RT: Drug models of schizophrenia. In Cole JD, Freedman AM, Friedhoff A (eds): Psychopathology and Psychopharmacology. Baltimore, Johns Hopkins, 1973

Kessler GF Jr.: Phencyclidine and fatal status epilepticus (letter). N Engl J Med 291:979, 1974

Ketchum JS, Sidell FR, Crowell EB Jr., Aghajanian GK, Hayes AH Jr.: Atropine, scopolamine and ditran: comparative pharmacology and antagonists in man. Psychopharmacologia 28:121, 1973

Kluver H: Mescal—The Devine Plant and Its Psychological Effects. London, Kegan Paul, 1928

Kolodny RC, Masters WH, Kolodner RM, Toro G: Depression of plasma testosterone levels after chronic intensive marihuana use. N Engl J Med 290:872, 1974

Lewin L: Phantastica, Narcotic and Stimulating Drugs. London, Routledge and Kagan Paul, 1931

Ludwig AM, Levine J, Stark LH: LSD and Alcoholism, Clinical Study of Treatment Efficacy. Springfield, Ill., Thomas, 1970

Marihuana: A Signal of Misunderstanding. First Report of the National Commission on Marihuana and Drug Abuse. Washington, DC, US Government Printing Office, 5266–0001, 1972

Marihuana and Health: Fourth Annual Report to Congress. Washington, DC, US Government Printing Office, 1974, p 75

McGlothlin WH, Arnold DO: LSD revisited: a ten year follow-up of medical LSD use. Arch Gen Psychiatry 24:35, 1971

————, West LJ: The marihuana problem: an overview. Am J Psychiatry 125:126, 1968

McWilliams SA, Tuttle RI: Long term psychological effects of LSD. Psychol Bull 79:341, 1973

Mechoulam R (ed): Marihuana, Chemistry, Pharmacology, Metabolism and Clinical Effects. New York, Academic, 1973

Mendelson JH, Kuehnle J, Ellingboe J, Babor TF: Plasma testosterone levels before, during and after chronic marihuana smoking. N Engl J Med 291:1051, 1974

Miller LL (ed): Marihuana. Effects on Human Behavior. New York, Academic, 1974

Moreau JJ: Du Hachisch et de l'Alienation Mentale. Paris, Masson, 1845. Translated by Barrett GJ: Hashish and Mental Illness. New York, Raven, 1973

Rubin V, Comitas L: Ganja in Jamaica. A Medical Anthropological Study of Chronic Marihuana Use. The Hague, Mouton, 1975

Schultes RE: Hallucinogens of plant origin. Science 163:245, 1969

Smith DE: The psychotomimetic amphetamines with special reference to STP (DOM) toxicity. J Psyched Drugs 2:73, 1969

Szara S, Braude M: The Pharmacology of Cannabis. New York, Raven, 1976

Tart CT: Marihuana intoxication: common experiences. Nature 226:701, 1970

Tennant FS, Preble M, Prendergast TJ, Ventry P: Medical manifestations associated with hashish. JAMA 216:1965, 1971

Tinklenberg J: Drugs and crime. In Drug Use in America: Problem in Perspective, Patterns and Consequences of Drug Use. Washington, DC, US Government Printing Office 1:242, 1973

part V
concluding
remarks

Murray E. Jarvik, M.D., Ph.D.

One of the problems with psychopharmacology, especially in its early days, is that drugs with unknown mechanisms of action are being used to treat diseases of unknown etiology. Today, we know more about the biologic basis of psychiatric disorders, though admittedly not enough. We also have reasonable hypotheses about how these drugs work. The connecting link seems to be the neurotransmitter systems in the brain. Presently, we think that schizophrenia implies an overactivity of dopamine in the limbic system, depression an imbalance between norepinephrine and serotonin, with too much of the former and too little of the latter; and mania just the opposite. Anxiety also seems to involve hyperactivity of norepinephrine and perhaps insufficient activity of gamma aminobutyric acid. Effective drugs, such as the phenothiazines, tricyclic antidepressants, or benzodiazepines, are presumed to normalize the neurotransmitter activity. Direct evidence for the neurotransmitter link between drug and diagnosis is still relatively weak, but should be established in the foreseeable future.

Clearly, in all conditions, it is desirable that an accurate diagnosis be made before treatment is started. Most psychiatric drugs are fairly safe, so even a mistake may not be too serious. However, valuable time can be lost if the diagnosis is delayed, and the patient may be forced to suffer longer than he has to. Titration of the dose of drug to an effective level would be desirable but may be difficult in an individual case. Side effects should be guarded against, looked for, treated, and, if necessary, the drug may have to be stopped.

The two most important properties of a drug that a clinician wants

515

to know are its efficacy and its toxicity. Its general efficacy has to be determined by controlled studies. The clinician's judgment comes in approximating his diagnosis and treatment regimen with those used in controlled studies. General rules of treatment have been indicated in the preceding chapters, but the clinician will have to rely on his own intuition to match individual idiosyncratic needs of the patient to the general rules. Similarly, though we have provided guidelines for guarding against side effects, because every patient reacts differently, vigilance is necessary to spot the onset of toxic effects of drugs. There may be a tendency among more dynamically oriented psychiatrists to avoid medication because of the risk of toxic effects. But an error of omission may be far worse than one of commission. Drugs have a proven value in the treatment of psychiatric disorders, and no patient who can benefit should be denied such assistance.

author index

subject index

Subject Index 541

Subject Index 541

Imipramine (cont.)
  EEG, effect on, 181
  for enuresis, 300, 375, 379,
    380–381
  historical aspects, 16
  hormones and, 195
  indications for, 262
  maintenance on, 278
  for minimal brain dysfunction, 300
  for narcolepsy, associated
    symptoms of, 111
  neurotransmitters and, 195, 275
  for panic anxiety, 316
  partial conversion to
    desmethylimipramine,
    283–284
  partition coefficient, 172
  for pavor nocturnis and
    somnambulism, 385–386
  in pediatric therapy, 297, 300, 375,
    379, 380–381, 382–383,
    385–386
  pituitary hormone release and, 196
  predicting response by
    amphetamines, 255, 270
  for school phobia, 375, 382–383
  side effects, 263, 380–381, 383
  structure of, 261
  triiodothyronine and, 285
Inderal. See Propranolol
5-Indo-2-deoxyuridine, 172
Indolalkylamines, 500
Indoleamines, 191, 231
Indoles, 206, 207. See also specific
  drug
Insomnia, 105, 110–111, 329–330
  drug-withdrawal, 329–330, 340
  forms of, 110–111
  5-HT depletion and, 109
  illness and, 5
  mania and, 329, 331
  produced by PCPA in animals, 109
  treatment of, 110–111, 330–331
    bromides, 325
    pseudotherapy, 49
    proprietary drugs, 343, 345
    sedative-hypnotics, 331–340
  as symptom of psychiatric

Insomnia (cont.)
  disorders, 329
Instrumental conditioning, 59, 61.
    See also Conditioning
Insulin, 187
  alcohol elimination and, 410
  coma therapy, 16, 64, 210
  conditioning and, 63, 64, 65
Interactions, drug, 184. See also
    specific drug
Involutional syndromes, 223, 226,
    262, 269
Iproniazid, 265
  mood elevation and, 233
  structure of, 266
Isocarboxazid
  dose range, 265
  structure of, 266
Isoniazid
  hepatotoxicity of, 264
  structure of, 266
Isopropanol, 172
Isoxsuprine, 368

Jamaica Study, 512
Janimine. See Imipramine
Jimson weed. See Datura

Kava, 12
Kemadrin. See Procyclidine
Katamine, 77, 501
Kidney disease, 415
Kola nut, 451, 453

Lactic acid, 409
Laennec's cirrhosis, 409
Lamina 5 cells, 148, 149
Learning, 4, 5, 59, 61–68, 489. See
    also Conditioning;
    Memory; State-dependent
    learning
Levo-Dromoran. See Levorphanol
Levodopa
  accentuation of choreiform and
    athetoid movements in